AF334018

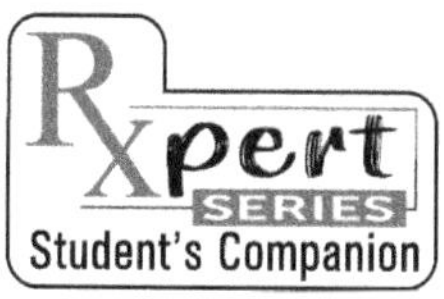

Human Anatomy and Physiology-II

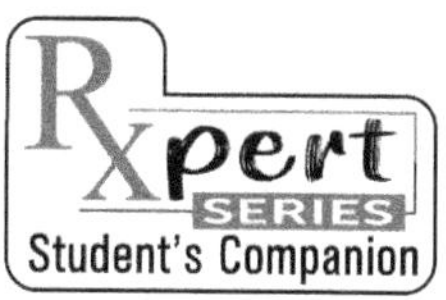

Human Anatomy and Physiology-II

Amteshwar Singh Jaggi
M. Pharm., Ph.D.
Punjabi University,
Patiala, Punjab.

N. Anitha
M. Pharm., Ph.D.
Sultan-ul-Uloom College of Pharmacy
Hyderabad, Telangana.

Anjana Bali
M. Pharm., Ph.D.
Central University of Punjab,
Bathinda, Punjab.

Manish Kumar
M. Pharm.
Punjabi University,
Patiala.

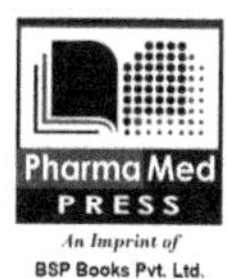

PharmaMed Press

An imprint of BSP Books Pvt. Ltd.

4-4-309/316, Giriraj Lane,
Sultan Bazar, Hyderabad - 500 095.

Human Anatomy and Physiology-II
by **Amteshwar Singh Jaggi, Anjana Bali, N. Anitha and Manish Kumar**

Published by

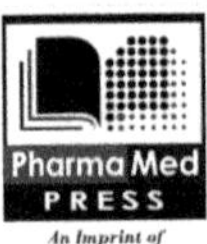

PharmaMed Press

An imprint of BSP Books Pvt. Ltd.
4-4-309/316, Giriraj Lane, Sultan Bazar, Hyderabad - 500 095.
Phone: 040-23445688; Fax: 91+40-23445611
E-mail: info@pharmamedpress.net
www.bspbooks.net/www.pharmamedpress.net

ISBN: 978-93-95039-32-1 (Hardback)

Preface

Human Anatomy and Physiology is an integral subject in Pharmaceutical Sciences and the strong knowledge about the structure and functions of human body organs in essential to understand the pathophysiology, basic and clinical pharmacology. The present book attempts to clarify the basic aspects of human anatomy and physiology in a simple and lucid manner. The book is written for B Pharmacy IInd Semester students as per new syllabus drafted by Pharmacy Council of India (PCI). The book has been divided into nine chapters i.e. nervous tissue, central nervous system, digestive system, energetics, respiratory system, urinary system, endocrine system, reproductive system and introduction to genetics. At the start of each chapter, the important points related to that chapter have been added in the form of 'chapter at glance". In each chapter, the special emphasis has been made to explain the structures of organs with appropriate figures. A good number of tables have also been incorporated to summarize the key features of each chapter. At the end of each chapter, review questions of two marks, five marks, ten marks and multiple choice have been added, which will be very helpful to students as well as teachers. We hope that the book shall cater the need of graduate as well as young faculty in understanding the basic aspects related to human anatomy and physiology. The authors wish to acknowledge their family members, friends, colleagues and students for their support, love and encouragement that helped in completing this book.

-Authors

Contents

Nervous Tissue

After completing this lesson, the Reader should be able to understand:

- *Introduction*
- *Overview of nervous system*
- *Organization of nervous system*
- *Coverings of the Central Nervous System (CNS)*
- *Neurons*
- *Neuroglia*
- *Membrane potential*
- *Synapse*
- *Neurotransmitters*
- *Receptors*
- *Ligands*

1.1   Introduction

The nervous system is mainly composed of nerve cells neurons (electrically, excitable cells) and neuroglia (also called glia or glial cells). In other words, neurons and neuroglia are the main two nerve cells of the nervous system. The neurons and neuralgia are also of different types and these perform specialized functions to control the body functions. These cells are interconnected through synapses (specialized connections to communicate with cells). The nervous system has three main functions including sensory, integrative and motor functions **(Table 1-1).**

1. **Sensory function:** The information is conveyed from the periphery to the brain through sensory neurons.
2. **Integrative function:** The information obtained from the periphery is perceived, analyzed (mainly in the cerebral cortex) and decisions are taken.
3. **Motor function:** The information is conveyed from the brain to the periphery through motor neurons.

Table 1-1 Functions of the nervous system

Sr. No.	Type of Functions	Comments
1	Sensory	Sensory or afferent neurons convey information from periphery to brain
2	Integrative	Inter-neurons interpret the information received from sensory neurons, decisions are taken
3	Motor	Motor or efferent neurons receive the information from inter-neurons and produce a response at the organ

Organization of the Nervous System

Based on structure, the nervous system is divided into two main subdivisions i.e. the central nervous system (CNS) and peripheral nervous system (PNS). The CNS consists of the brain and spinal cord. Further, the CNS has different centers, which carry out the various functions including sensory, motor and integration of data. These centers can be further divided into lower centers, including the spinal cord and brain stem, and higher centers, communicating with the brain via effectors (peripheral organs). The peripheral nervous system is composed of cranial nerves from the brain, spinal nerves from the spinal cord, ganglion, and plexuses **(Figure 1-1).** The peripheral nervous system is further subdivided into the somatic

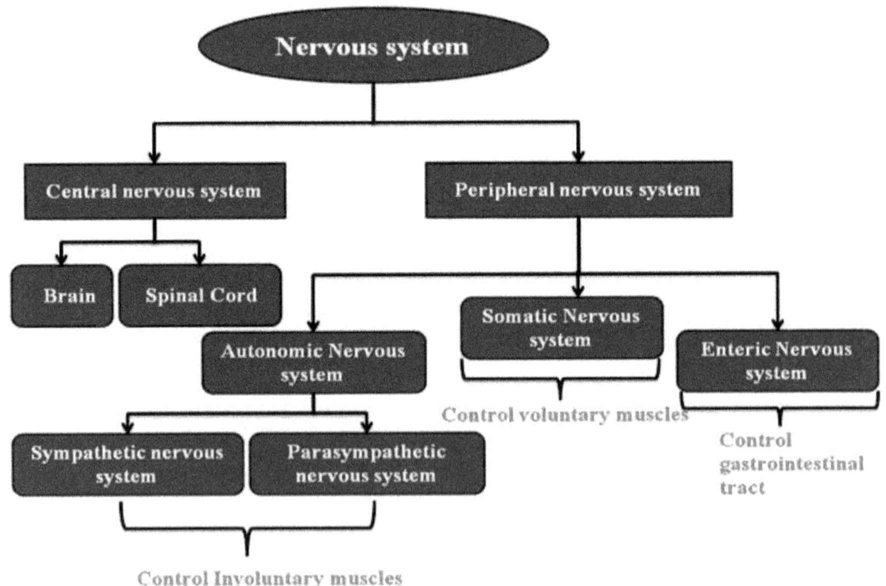

Figure 1-1. Classification of nervous system

nervous system (SNS), autonomic nervous system (ANS), and enteric nervous system (ENS). The function of the peripheral nervous system is to convey impulse to and from the CNS **(Table 1-2)**. The afferent nerves bring the information to the sensory neurons of CNS from the sensory receptors. On the other hand, the efferent nerves carry the information from the motor neurons of the CNS towards different peripheral tissues or organs. The somatic nervous system controls the voluntary (skeletal muscles) i.e. muscles which are under the control of the will of the person such as limbs. The autonomic nervous system is further divided into the sympathetic nervous system and the parasympathetic nervous system. The autonomic system controls the organs, which are not under the control of the will of the persons i.e. involuntary (smooth muscles and heart) such as the uterus, bronchi, blood vessels, etc. Another key difference between the autonomic and somatic nervous systems is that the autonomic nervous system uses two neurons between the CNS and target organ, while the somatic nervous system uses one neuron. Another system called the enteric nervous system innervates the visceral organs i.e. gastrointestinal tract, pancreas and gall bladder.

In the CNS, the collection of the neuron is called nuclei and the collection of the axon is called tracts. Whereas in the peripheral nervous system, the collection of the neuron is called ganglia and the collection of the axon is called nerves.

Table 1-2 Different types of the peripheral nervous system and their functions

Sr. No.	Types of Peripheral nervous system (PNS)	Functions
1	SNS (Somatic nervous system)	The nervous system controls the voluntary muscles (skeletal muscles). In other words, it controls the muscles that are under the control of the will of a person e.g. limbs
2	ANS (Autonomic nervous system)	The nervous system controls the involuntary muscles (smooth muscles and heart). In other words, it controls the muscles that are not under the control of the will of a person e.g. heart, uterus, bronchi, etc.
3	ENS (Enteric nervous system)	This is the local nervous system in the gastrointestinal tract. These monitor chemical changes within the GI tract, control stretching of its walls and control secretions from glands.

Coverings of the Central Nervous System (CNS)

The brain and spinal cord are protected by bones termed as cranium (cover brain) and vertebral column (surround spinal cord), respectively. The human cranium contains eight bones i.e. 1 frontal bone; 1 occipital bone; 2 parietal bones; 1 sphenoid bone; 2 temporal bones. Inner to the cranium and vertebral column, there are membranous coverings called meninges. The three protective membranes are **(Figure 1-2)**:

1. **Dura mater (Outer membrane):** It is the outermost layer of the meninges, which protects the brain and spinal cord. It is almost attached to the cranium.
2. **Arachnoid mater (Middle layer):** The arachnoid mater is the middle layer of the meninges, lying directly underneath the dura mater. There is a space between arachnoid and pia mater, which is termed as subarachnoid space and is filled with 'subarachnoid fluid'.
3. **Pia mater (Inner layer):** It is the innermost layer, which directly covers the brain and spinal cord.

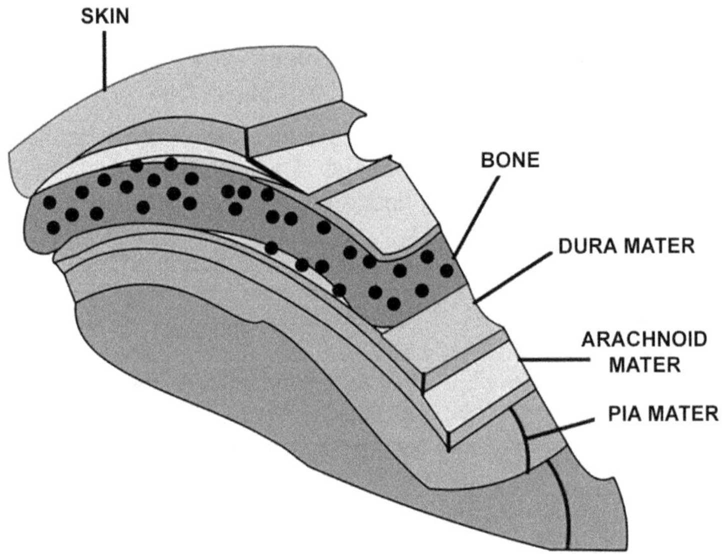

Figure 1-2 Protective coverings of the brain, including skin, a bony portion (cranium) and membranous coverings (meninges)

Neurons

Neurons are the basic functional units of the nervous system and are estimated to be as 100 billion in our nervous system. They generate electrical signals called action potentials, which assist them to rapidly transmit information over long distances. Neuron communicates with other cells in a unique way via specialized connections called synapses. Structurally, neuron consists of three parts a cell body, an axon and dendrites **(Figure 1-3)**.

1. **Cell Body:** The cell body contains the nucleus, which serves as the control center of the cell. It is surrounded by the cytoplasm and it has typical cell organelles such as mitochondria, Golgi bodies, lysosomes, and extensive rough endoplasmic reticulum (ER). The rough ER has granular structures and these are referred to as Nissl bodies in neurons. These serve as a site of protein synthesis. Another important structure in the cytoplasm is the presence of neurofibril, which forms the cytoskeleton and provides support and shape to the cell. The cell body connects to the dendrites, which bring information to the neuron, and the axon, which sends information to other neurons.

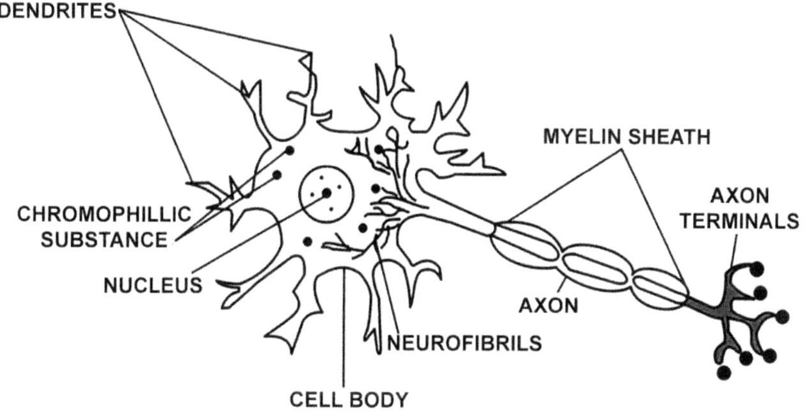

Figure 1-3 Structure of a Neuron

2. **Axon:** Usually, there is a single large branch of a neuron, which is termed as the axon and it is attached to the cell body at the axon hillock. The axon extends from the cell body and divided into many smaller branches (axon terminals) before ending at nerve terminals. The tips of the axon terminal swell into a bulb-like structure called synaptic end bulbs, which are filled with neurotransmitters. The cytoplasm of the axon is called axoplasm and is surrounded by the plasma membrane known as axolemma. The axoplasma also contain neurofibrils. Mostly, there is a single branch of axon; however, some branches may arise from the axon called axon collaterals (Figure 1-4). The main function of the axon is to transmit an electrochemical signal to other neurons.

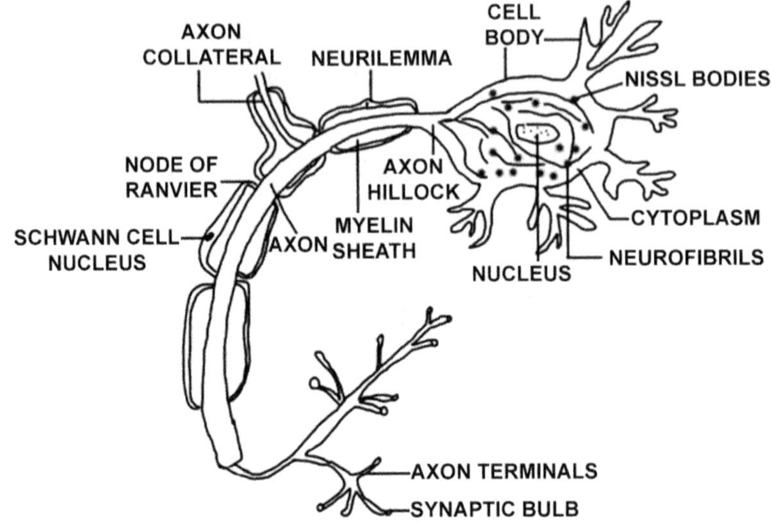

Figure 1-4 A detailed structure of a neuron

The longer axons are usually covered with a myelin sheath, which performs similar functions as insulation around an electrical wire. Moreover, due to the presence of myelin sheath, the speed of nerve conduction is increased. On the other hand, the nerve conduction velocity is significantly less in non-myelinated fibers (absence of myelin sheath). Myelin is a lipid-rich substance formed in the CNS by glial cells (oligodendrocytes) and in the peripheral nervous system by the Schwann cells **(Figure 1-5)**.

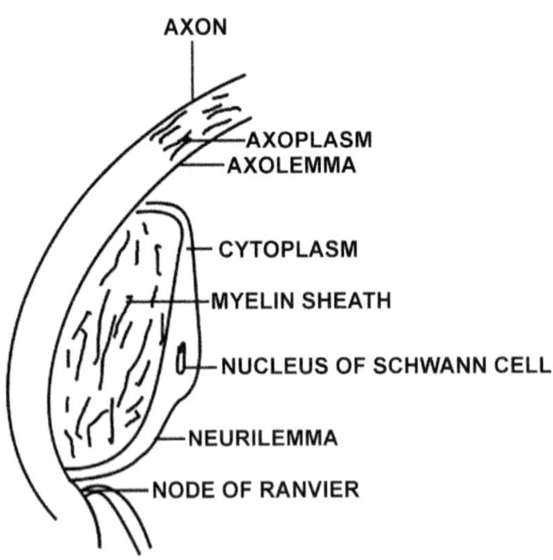

Figure 1-5 Magnified view of Schwann cells

The action potential propagation in myelinated neurons is much faster than in unmyelinated neurons due to saltatory conduction. In other words, there is the propagation of action potentials (by jumping) along the myelinated axons from one node of Ranvier to the next node of Ranvier. In unmyelinated neurons, action potential has to travel all along the axon; therefore, the conduction velocity of action potentials is relatively slow.

3. **Dendrites:** The neuron has a number of extensions called dendrites, which receive messages from other neurons. In other words, dendrites obtain information from surrounding neurons and convey to the cell body of its neurons. These are usually much smaller in length, not covered with myelin. In contrast to a single axon for a neuron, there are a number of dendrites connected to the cell body.

Table 1-3 Structural components of Neuron and its functions

Sr. No.	Structure	Function
1	Dendrites	These are branched, and provide a large surface area for receiving stimuli and passing impulses to the cell body
2	Chromatophillic substances (Nissil Body)	Layers of rough endoplasmic reticulum, whose function is protein synthesis
3	Neurofibrils	The filamentous strands of protein that support the cell body
4	Collateral branches (Axon Collaterals)	In some cases, there are extensions of the axon that may also transmit impulses
5	Axons	Conduct the impulse away from the cell body to another neuron or organ
6	Axon terminals	These enlargements at the ends of the branched axon; also contain synaptic vesicles that produce or secrete neurotransmitters into synapses
7	Microtubules	Minute channels that transport material within the cell

Table 1-4 Key differences between Axon and Dendrites

Sr. No.	Axons	Dendrites
1	Only one axon is present in a neuron	Usually multiple in number in a neuron
2	It carries nerve impulses away from the cell body	It carries nerve impulses to the cell body
3	Axon contains neurofibrils and no Nissl's granules.	Dendrites contain both neurofibrils and Nissl's granules

Table 1-4 Contd...

Sr. No.	Axons	Dendrites
4	Axon forms the efferent component of the impulse	Dendrites from the afferent component of the impulse
5	It is a thin, long process of uniform thickness and smooth surface	These are short, multiple processes, thickness diminishes as these divides repeatedly
6	The branches of the axon are fewer (axon collaterals) and at right angles to the axon.	The dendrites branch profusely and are present at different angles

Classification of Neurons

The neurons can be classified into two categories according to structure and function **(Table 1-5** and **Table 1-6)**.

Structural Classification

The neurons can be classified into three categories based on structure i.e. multipolar neurons, bipolar neurons, and unipolar neurons.

I. **Multipolar neurons:** These types of neurons have several dendrites and only one axon. The neurons of the brain and spinal cord come under this category.

II. **Bipolar neurons:** These types of neurons have one dendrite and one axon. These are found at the retina of the eye and olfactory area of the brain.

III. **Unipolar neurons (Pseudounipolar neuron):** In this neuron, only one process is attached to the cell body. These are the sensory neurons. Originally, they are developed as a bipolar neuron. However, during development, axons and dendrites fuse to form a single process.

Table 1-5 Structural classification of neuron

Sr. No.	Type of Neuron	Structure
1	Multipolar neurons (several dendrites and one axon)	

Table 1-5 Contd...

Sr. No.	Type of Neuron	Structure
2	Bipolar neurons (one dendrite and one axon)	
3	Unipolar neurons (only one process is attached to the cell body)	

Functional Classification

The neurons can be classified into three categories based on the direction of nerve impulse conduction i.e. afferent neurons, efferent neurons and interneurons **(Table 1-6).**

I.   **Afferent neurons:** These neurons carry the signal from the periphery i.e. from the skin, muscles, joints, sense organs to the brain and spinal cord.

II. **Efferent neurons:** These neurons convey the motor nerve impulse from the CNS to peripheral organs. These can be subdivided into alpha or gamma motor neurons.

III. **Inter-neurons or association neurons:** These neurons carry nerve impulses from one neuron to another. Most neurons in the brain (90%) are association neurons.

Table 1-6 Structural classification of neuron

Sr. No.	Types of Neurons	
Based on structure		
1	Multipolar neurons	These have one axon, several dendrites
2	Bipolar neurons	These have one axon and one dendrite. Two cell processes are attached to the cell
3	Unipolar neurons	These have a single process attached to the cell body
Based on function		
1	Afferent neurons	Transmit nerve impulses from periphery to the spinal cord and brain
2	Efferent neurons	Conduct impulses away from the spinal cord or brain to peripheral organs
	Alpha motor neurons	Innervate and stimulates skeletal muscles
	Gamma motor neurons	Innervate specialized muscle tissue called muscle spindle
3	Association (Interneurons)	Conduct nerve impulses from one neuron to another neuron

Myelin sheath

Myelin sheath is a multilayered, lipid and protein covering that surrounds the axons. The nerve fibers that are surrounded by myelin sheath are called myelinated nerve fibers, while the nerve fibers that are not containing myelin sheath are called unmyelinated nerve fibers. Myelin sheath is produced by two types of neuroglia: neurolemmocytes and oligodendrocytes. In the peripheral nervous system, neurolemmocytes (Schwann cells) produce the myelin sheath. Structurally, the axon is surrounded by two layers: Inner layer which is made up of myelin sheath. It is a non-living deposition or covering; The Outer layer is a living layer that surrounds the inner layer. It contains the nucleus and cytoplasm of neurolemmocyte. This is also called neurolemma or sheath of Schwann (**Figure 1-6**). When an axon is injured, the neurolemma helps in the regeneration of axon and myelin sheath. In the CNS, oligodendrocytes produce myelin sheath around the axons. In contrast to the peripheral nervous system, only the myelin sheath is present and neurolemma (living layer) is absent. If any injury takes place to the axon, then there is no regrowth after injury due to the absence of neurolemma. The amount of myelin increases from birth to maturity. The presence of myelin increases the speed of nerve impulse conduction. In the PNS, there are small gaps called nodes of Ranvier between segments of the sheath which are less in CNS (**Table 1-7**).

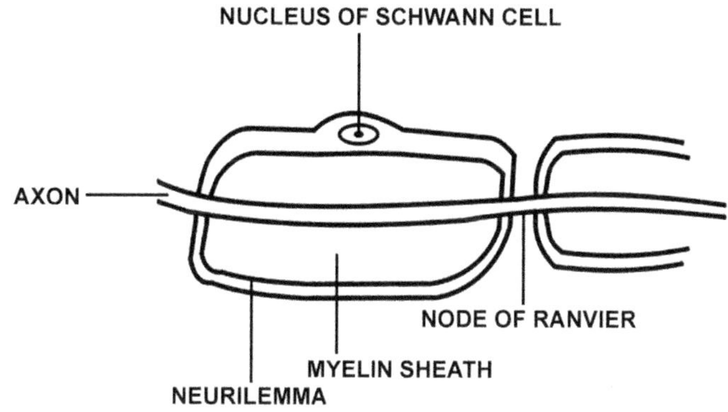

Figure 1-6 Typical structure of axon, myelin sheath, and nucleus of Schwann cell

Table 1-7 Key differences between myelin in CNS and PNS

Sr. No.	Myelin in CNS	Myelin in PNS
1	Formed by oligodendrocytes	Formed by Schwann cells
2	Neurolemma (living layer) is absent	Neurolemma is present
3	Fewer nodes of Ranvier	More nodes of Ranvier
4	Less regeneration after injury due to absence of neurolemma	More rapid regeneration after injury due to presence of neurolemma

Neuroglia

Neuroglia is also called glia or glial cells. These are the specialized cells of the nervous system. These physically and physiologically support, nourish, and protect the neurons and maintain homeostasis in the interstitial fluid. These are about half of the volume of CNS; smaller than neurons in size; but 5-50 times more in number. These cells can divide and multiply, but cannot propagate action potential. During an injury, these cells fill up space and help in healing. The neuroglial cells of the CNS include astrocytes, oligodendrocytes, microglial cells and ependymal cells **(Tables 1-8 and 1-9)**. In the PNS, two types of neuroglial cells are found i.e. neurolemmocytes (Schwann cells) and satellite cells.

1. **Astrocytes (Astro-star; cytes-cell):** These are the cells, which are having a star-like structure and have many processes. These cells help in the metabolism of neurotransmitters, maintain the proper concentration of K+ ions, help in brain development, help in the formation of the blood-brain barrier, provides a link between neurons and blood vessels and regulates the entry of substances into the brain.

Table 1-8 The different types of neuroglia and its functions

Sr. No.	Types	Function
Neuroglia in the central nervous system		
1	Astrocytes	Star-shaped structure, largest, most numerous, many processes, forms structural support between capillaries and neurons within the CNS. These contribute to the blood-brain barrier (BBB) formation
	Protoplasmic astrocytes	Present in the gray matter; have short branches
	Fibrous astrocytes	Present in white matter; have long branches
2	Oligodendrocytes	Smaller, similar to astrocytes, fewer processes; form myelin sheath (multilayered protein and lipid layer) in CNS; guide development of neurons within the CNS
3	Microglia	Small, numerous spine-like projections, phagocytize pathogens and cellular debris within CNS
4	Ependymal cells	Cuboidal-columnar cells, line ventricles of the brain and central canal of the spinal cord; form CSF; form blood-CSF
Neuroglia in the peripheral nervous system		
5	Schwann cells	Forms myelin sheath, participate in axonal regeneration (more easily in PNS than CNS). Support ganglia within PNS
6	Satellite cells	Forms myelin within PNS; surround cells of PNS ganglia; regulate the exchange of material between neurons and interstitial fluid

2. **Oligodendrocytes: (Oligo-few; dendro-processes):** They are smaller in size as compared to astrocytes and also have few processes. They provide supports to neurons and produce myelin sheath.

3. **Microglial cells: (Micro-small; glia-adhere):** These are small phagocytic cells that are present in central nervous system. They protect by engulfing microorganism that enters the central nervous system.

4. **Ependymal cells:** They line the brain ventricles and they help in the formation of cerebrospinal fluid. The shape of ependymal cells varies. It can be ciliated squamous or columnar epithelial cells.

5. **Neurolemmocytes or Schwann cells:** These produce cells the myelin sheath and regulate the exchange of material between neurons and interstitial fluid.

6. **Satellite cells**: These cells provide supports to neurons present in ganglia.

Table 1-9 Structures of astrocytes, dendrites, and ependymal cells

Sr. No.	Neuroglia	Shape
1	**Astrocytes** (Star-shaped, many processes)	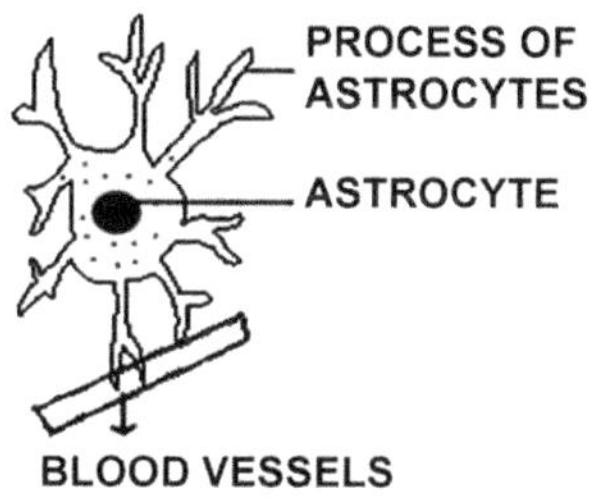
2	Oligodendrocytes (Few processes attached to cell)	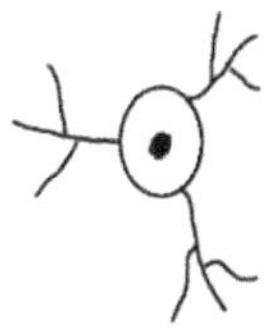
3	Ependymal Cells	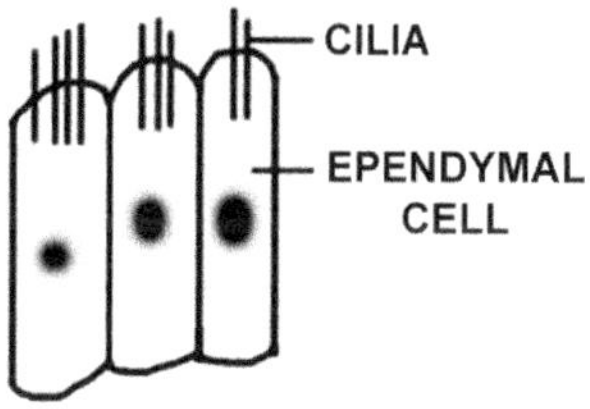

Membrane Potential

There are various terms concerning voltage changes across the plasma membrane that need to be understood. These include the following:

1. **Resting membrane potential:** In the resting neuron, a resting membrane potential (potential difference) exists across the cell membrane. In other words, there is a potential difference across the cell membrane even in the resting state. This potential difference is due to the imbalance of charged particles across the cell membrane i.e. between the extracellular and intracellular fluids. Therefore, a cell membrane is said to be polarized (separation of charges). In the resting state, there is a net negative charge inside the cell (intracellular space) in comparison to the outside (extracellular space) (Figure 1-7).

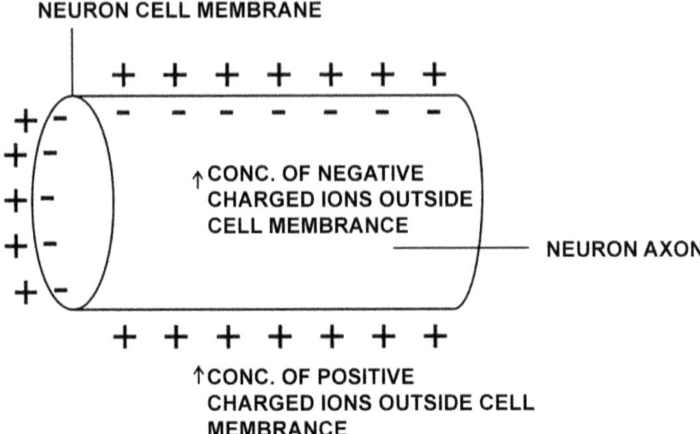

Figure 1-7 A segment of a neuron showing the separation of anions and cations across the cell membrane, leading to the development of net negative membrane potential (in the resting state) inside the cell.

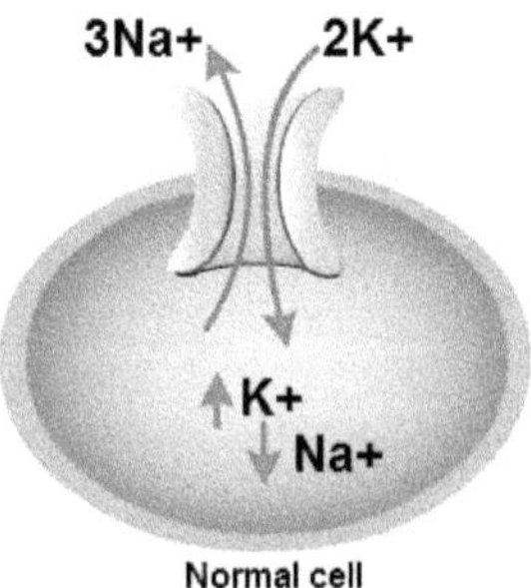

Figure 1-8 Normal functioning of Na+-K+ ATPase pump to pump three sodium outside the cell and pump two potassium ions inside the cells, leading to the development of resting membrane potential.

The resting membrane potential is around -70 to -80 MV (inside negative). The presence of a sodium-potassium pump (Na+-K+ ATPase pump) helps in maintaining the resting membrane potential. Indeed, this pump uses ATP (energy) to actively transport three sodium ions (Na+) ions from inside the cell to the outside. In return, two potassium ions (K+) are transported inside the cell from the outside **(Figure 1-8).** The net result is the movement of one extra positive ion outside the cell in each cycle and the continuation of this process leads to an accumulation of negative charge inside the cells.

2. **Action potential:** A rapid change in the membrane potential is termed as an action potential. In the resting state, the membrane potential is negative and in response to a stimulus, there is a rapid change in the membrane potential from negative to positive. Action potential comprises of depolarization

followed by repolarization (discussed below). An important point is that the events of depolarization and repolarization occur very rapidly **(Figure 1-9)**.

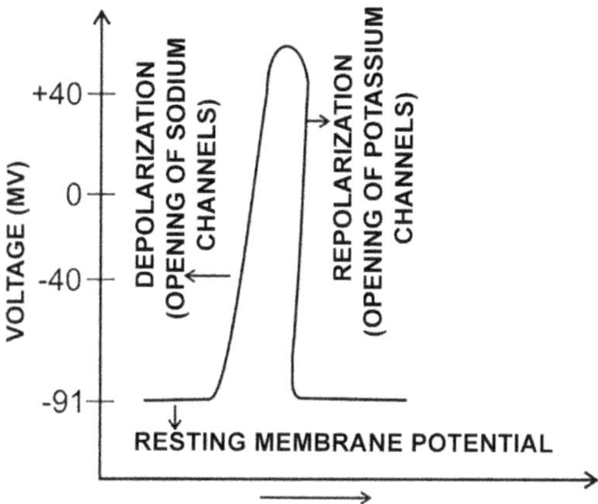

Figure 1-9 A Representation of action potential comprising of depolarization and repolarization

The action potential is a way of passing nerve impulses from one point to another point. In other words, the traveling disturbance in membrane potential is called the action potential. The following sequences are associated with action potential:

1. **Depolarization:** During depolarization, the membrane potential tends to increase and becomes less negative/zero or even positive. Depolarization means loss of the state of polarization, which occurs in a resting state. Actually, in response to a stimulus, there is the opening of fast operating, voltage-gated sodium channels, which allows the rapid movement of sodium ions from outside (present in excessive amount) to inside the cell (present in lesser amount). The net movement of positive sodium ions is responsible for the increase in membrane potential. This state ends with the closure of sodium channels, which are closed due to the development of positive membrane potential inside the cell (Figure 1-10).

2. **Repolarization:** Depolarization is rapidly followed by repolarization in which the membrane potential again becomes decreases from positive to negative. When the membrane potential becomes positive, there is a closure of sodium channels (discussed above) and the opening of voltage-gated potassium channels. This opening leads to the rapid movement of potassium ions from inside the cells (present in excessive amounts) to the outside (present in lower amount). The outward movement of positive ions decreases the membrane potential and inside membrane potential again becomes negative **(Figure 1-10)**.

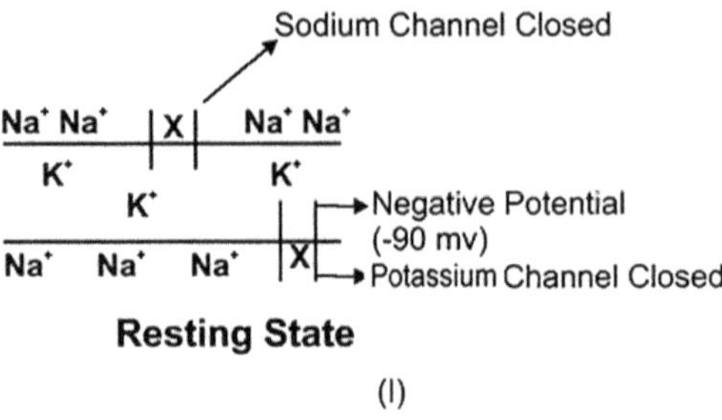

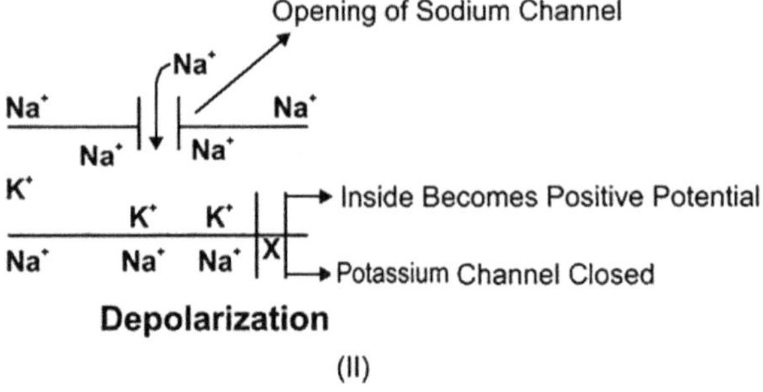

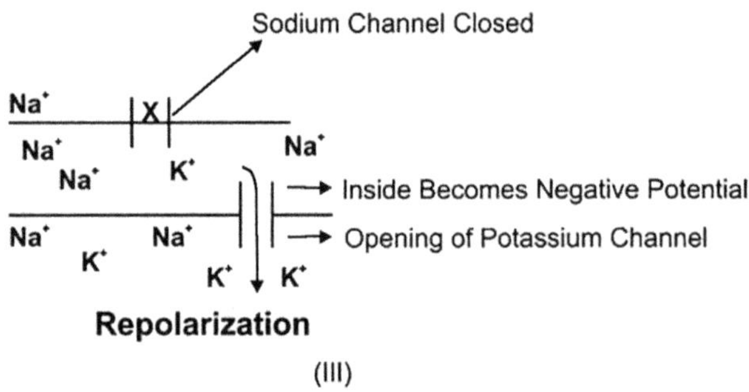

Figure 1-10 Schematic representation of events taking place in resting state (I), during depolarization (II) and repolarization (III)

A synapse is a specialized junction through which impulse passes from one neuron to another and the process of passage of impulses is termed as synaptic neurotransmission. In the nervous system, a synapse is formed between axon terminals of one neuron and dendrites of another neuron. Therefore, the impulse is passed from axon terminals (one neuron) to dendrites (another neuron) as synaptic neurotransmission **(Figure 1-11).** A typical synapse comprises of presynaptic membrane of axon terminal, synaptic/neural cleft (space) and postsynaptic membrane of the dendrite. An important point of the presynaptic and postsynaptic membrane is that these are expanded in the synaptic region to increase the surface area. Inside the presynaptic membrane, there are several synaptic vesicles, which store chemical messengers termed as neurotransmitters. On the other hand, there are specific receptors (depending on the type of neurotransmitter released) present on the postsynaptic membrane. The different steps involved in synaptic neurotransmission are as follows:

1. An action potential spreads over the axon terminal and depolarizes the presynaptic membrane
2. Depolarization of the presynaptic membrane is associated with an influx of calcium ions. The increase in calcium ions causes the movement of synaptic vesicles towards the presynaptic membrane. It is followed by the fusion of vesicles with the presynaptic membrane
3. It leads to release of neurotransmitters from the synaptic vesicles by exocytosis into the synaptic (neural) cleft
4. The neurotransmitter diffuses across the synaptic cleft to the postsynaptic membrane and binds to the specific receptor present on the postsynaptic membrane
5. The binding of the neurotransmitter to receptors leads to initiation of nerve impulse on the second neuron
6. The neurotransmitter is removed from the synapse by different methods including its enzymatic degradation or reuptake by a pump present on the presynaptic terminals

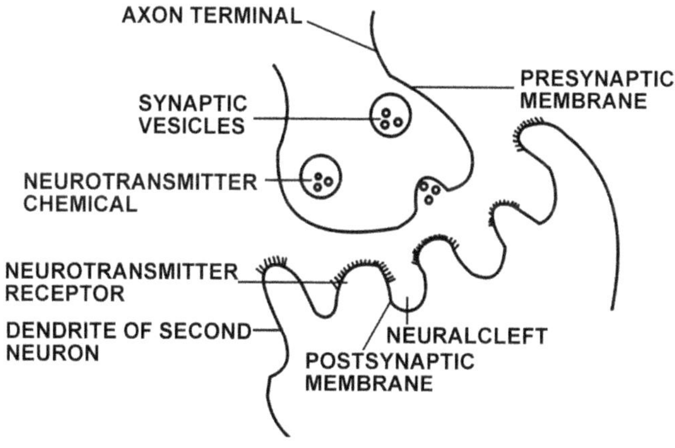

Figure 1-11 Schematic of synapse and synaptic transmission

Neurotransmitters

These are the chemicals that are normally stored inside the synaptic vesicles and released in the synaptic cleft to bind with receptors on the postsynaptic membrane to trigger the action potential. These are of various types depending on their chemical nature and functions performed. The common examples of neurotransmitters include acetylcholine, adrenaline, noradrenaline, dopamine, glutamate, histamine, serotonin (5-HT), GABA (gamma-aminobutyric acid) and bradykinin, etc. All these neurotransmitters perform different functions by activating on their specific receptors **(Table 1-10).** Based on their functions, neurotransmitters may be excitatory or inhibitory.

1. Excitatory neurotransmitters are those that produce excitation on the postsynaptic membrane. These act on the postsynaptic membrane and initiate the generation of excitatory postsynaptic potential (EPSP). Generally, there is the opening of sodium channels on the postsynaptic membrane after the binding of receptors with neurotransmitters. Examples of this type include glutamate.

2. Inhibitory neurotransmitters are those that produce inhibition on the postsynaptic membrane. These act on the postsynaptic membrane and initiate the generation of inhibitory postsynaptic potential (IPSP). Generally, there is an opening of chloride ion channels on the postsynaptic membrane after the binding of receptors with neurotransmitters. Examples of this type include GABA.

Table 1-10 Name of common neurotransmitters and their receptors

Sr. No.	Name of Neurotransmitters	Receptors
1	Acetylcholine	Muscarinic (M) and nicotinic (N) receptors
2	Adrenaline, noradrenaline	Alpha and beta receptors
3	Glutamate	NMDA and AMPA receptors
4	Dopamine	Dopamine (D) receptors
5	Histamine	Histamine (H) receptors

Receptors

Receptors are the molecules, mostly protein in nature, which receive the signals from the neurotransmitters or drugs and convert the signals into a biological response. In other words, neurotransmitters or drugs produce their effects on different tissues/organs by binding to their specific receptors. The agents that bind specifically to a receptor are termed as ligands. Receptors are located either on the plasma membrane or these are present inside the cells i.e. in the cytoplasm or nucleus **(Table 1-11).**

1. **Receptors Present on Plasma Membrane:** Most of the receptors are located on the cell surface i.e. on the plasma membrane. The ligands for these receptors are generally hydrophilic (water-soluble). Examples: muscarinic receptors, nicotinic receptors, alpha receptors, beta receptors, dopamine receptors, etc.

2. **Intracellular Located Receptors located intracellularly:** Sometimes, receptors are located inside the cells i.e. in the cytoplasm. The ligands for these receptors are generally lipophilic. These ligands cross the plasma membrane and bind with cytoplasmic receptors. The ligand and receptor

complex moves to the nucleus and binds to specific DNA elements, termed as 'Response Elements'. Examples of such receptors include glucocorticoid receptors, mineralocorticoid receptors, thyroid receptors, estrogen receptors, testosterone receptors, and progesterone receptors.

Table 1-11 Name of common neurotransmitters and their receptors

Sr. No.	Cell Surface Receptors	Intracellular Receptors
1	Receptors are present on the cell surface	Receptors are located inside the cytoplasm
2	The ligands are hydrophilic	The ligands are lipophilic and cross the cell membrane to bind with cytoplasmic receptors
3	The response produced due to binding of the ligand with these receptors is generally quick	The response produced due to binding of the ligand with these receptors is generally slow
4	There is no alteration in transcription and protein synthesis	The binding of ligands with these receptors alters transcription and protein synthesis.
5	The examples of these receptors include: muscarinic receptors, nicotinic receptors, alpha receptors, beta receptors, dopamine receptors	The examples of these receptors include: glucocorticoid receptors, mineralocorticoid receptors, thyroid receptors, estrogen receptors, testosterone receptors, and progesterone receptors

Ligands

Receptors are very specific i.e. specific ligands can bind to specific receptors. The ligands can further be of different types, depending on whether they activate the receptors or they inhibit the receptors **(Table 1-12)**.

1. **Agonist:** It is a ligand that binds to the receptors and produces a biological response by inducing its activation. For example, acetylcholine is an agonist of muscarinic and nicotinic receptors; adrenaline and noradrenaline are agonists are alpha and beta receptors.

2. **Antagonist:** It is a ligand that binds to the receptor and prevents the actions of an agonist by inhibiting the binding of agonist to the receptor. In other words, antagonist inhibits the receptors and prevents agonist-induced activation of receptors. For example; atropine is an antagonist of muscarinic receptors and inhibits the actions of acetylcholine; beta receptor blockers inhibit beta receptors and inhibit the actions of adrenaline and noradrenaline.

Table 1-12 Types of ligands, depending on their ability to activate or inhibit the receptors

Sr. No.	Agonist	Antagonist
1	It binds to receptors and induces its activation	It binds to receptors but does not induce activation
2	It produces a biological response	It prevents the biological response of an agonist
3	Examples include acetylcholine as an agonist of muscarinic and nicotinic receptors; adrenaline and noradrenaline as agonists of alpha and beta receptors	Example include atropine as an antagonist of muscarinic receptors

1.2 Chapter at a Glance

Term	Description
Synapses	Specialized connections for communication
Sensory function	Information is conveyed from periphery to brain
Motor function	Information is conveyed from brain to periphery
ANS	Autonomic nervous system
ENS	Enteric nervous system
SNS	Somatic nervous system
Multipolar neurons	Neurons with several dendrites and only one axon.
Bipolar neurons:	Neurons with one dendrite and one axon
Ependymal cells	Line brain ventricles and forms the cerebrospinal fluid
Microglial cells	Small phagocytic cells
Action potential	A rapid change in the membrane potential
Neurotransmitters	Chemicals released in the synaptic cleft to trigger the action potential
EPSP	Excitatory postsynaptic potential
IPSP	Inhibitory postsynaptic potential
GABA	Gamma-aminobutyric acid
Agonist	The ligand binds to the receptors and produces a biological response
Antagonist	The ligand binds to a receptor and prevents actions of agonist

Exercises

Multiple Choice Questions

1. Nervous system manly consists of
   (a) Spinal cord
   (b) Nerves
   (c) Brain
   (d) All of the above

2. A unit of Nervous system is
   (a) Spinal cord
   (b) Neuron
   (c) Brain
   (d) Nerves

3. Multipolar neurons have
   (a) Several dendrites and one axon
   (b) One dendrites and one axon
   (c) Only one process is attached to the cell body
   (d) None

4. Bipolar neurons have
   (a) Several dendrites and one axon
   (b) One dendrites and one axon
   (c) Only one process is attached to the cell body
   (d) None

5. Afferent neurons transmit nerve impulses from
   (a) From periphery to the spinal cord and brain
   (b) From spinal cord to periphery
   (c) Both a and b
   (d) None of the above

6. Which of the following neuroglial cell is not found in the CNS?
   (a) Astrocytes
   (b) Oligodendrocytes
   (c) Microglial cells
   (d) Neurolemmocytes

7. Which of the following neuroglial cells are found in the PNS?
   (a) Schwann cells
   (b) Satellite cells
   (c) Both a and b
   (d) None

8. Which of the following is not a feature of Myelin in CNS?
   (a) Formed by oligodendrocytes
   (b) Neurolemma is present
   (c) Fewer nodes of Ranvier
   (d) Less regeneration after injury

9. Efferent neurons
   (a) Conduct impulses away from the spinal cord or brain to peripheral organs
   (b) Conduct impulses to spinal cord or brain from peripheral organs
   (c) Both a and b
   (d) None of the above

10. Neuron communicates with other cells uniquely via specialized connections called
    - (a) Neurofibril
    - (b) Neurolemma
    - (c) Synapses
    - (d) None of the above

Short Answer Questions

1. Classify the nervous system..
2. What are the functions of the nervous system?
3. What are the coverings of the central nervous system?
4. Write about different types of the peripheral nervous system and their functions.
5. What are the different types of nerve cells?
6. What is an action potential?
7. Define the cell body, axon, and dendrites.
8. Define synapse.
9. What is the myelin sheath?
10. What are astrocytes?
11. What are Schwann cells?
12. What are oligodendrocytes?
13. What do you mean by depolarization and repolarization?
14. What is the resting membrane potential?
15. What are neurotransmitters?

Long Answer Questions

1. Explain the structural component of the neuron and its functions.
2. Explain the different types of neuroglial cell and their functions.
3. Write a note on action potential with all events taking placing during an action potential.
4. Write a note on synapse and synaptic transmission.
5. Write a note on the myelin sheath
6. Explain the differences between axons and dendrites.
7. Write the differences between myelin in CNS and PNS.
8. Write about common neurotransmitters and their receptors.
9. Write about depolarization and repolarization.
10. What are unipolar, multipolar and bipolar neurons?

Bibliography

Costanzo LS. Physiology. 4th Edition. Lippincott Williams & Wilkins.

Guyton AC, Hall JE. Textbook of Medical Physiology. 11th Edition. Elsevier Saunders. 2006.

Jaggi AS, Bali A, Singh N. Pathophysiology. 1st Edition. Vallabh Prakashan. 2019.

Jain AK. Human Anatomy and Physiology for Pharmacy. 3rd Edition. Arya publications. 2017.

Lodish H, Berk A, Kaiser CA. Molecular Cell Biology. 6th Edition. W. H. Freeman & Co Ltd. 2007.

Tortora GJ, Derrickson B. Principles of Anatomy and Physiology. 15th Edition. John Wiley and Sons, Inc. 2017.

Waugh A, Grant A. Ross and Wilson Anatomy and Physiology in Health and Illness. 12th Edition. Churchill Livingstone. 2014.

Answer Key MCQs

1. (d)	2. (b)	3. (a)	4. (b)	5. (a)
6. (d)	7. (c)	8. (b)	9. (a)	10. (c)

Central Nervous System

After completing this lesson, the Reader should be able to understand:

- *Introduction*
- *Overview of the Central Nervous System*
- *The Brain*
  - *Covering Membranes (Meninges)*
  - *Cerebrospinal fluid (CSF)*
- *Ventricles of brain*
- *Structural Features of Brain*
  - *Olfactory Lobes*
  - *Cerebrum*
  - *Basal Ganglia (Extrapyramidal Pathway)*
  - *The Diencephalon*
  - *Mid Brain*
  - *Cerebellum*
  - *Pons varolii (Pons-bridge)*
  - *Modulla oblongata*
- *Reticular formation*
- *Limbic System*
- *Blood Brain Barrier (BBB)*
- *Electroencephalogram (EEG)*
- *Human spinal cord*
- *Reflex actions*
- *Functions of afferent and efferent nerve tracts*

2.1   Introduction

The central nervous system (CNS) consists of the brain and spinal cord. Both are derived from the embryonic neural tube and are surrounded by protective membranes called the meninges. The adult human brain is comprised of four major regions including the cerebrum, the diencephalon, the cerebellum, and the brain stem, whereas the spinal cord is a single structure (Figure 2-1).

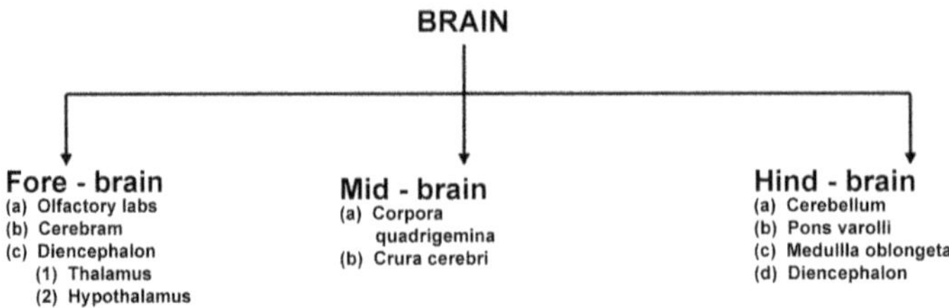

Figure 2-1 Different regions of the brain

The Brain

The brain is an anterior part of the central nervous system. It is located in the cranial cavity or cranium. The human brain weighs about 1.2 kg -1.4 kg and constitutes about 2 percent of total body weight. The brain is composed of about 100 billion neurons. Although these neurons contain genetic material DNA, yet there is no DNA replication or mitosis in the brain. In other words, the cells of brain do not under cell division. The different parts of the brain are explained below:

Covering Membranes (Meninges)

The brain is covered with three membranes dura mater, arachnoid mater and pia mater also called as meninges (explained earlier) (Figure 2-2). There is a subarachnoid space between the pia mater and the arachnoid membrane. It is filled with a fluid called cerebrospinal fluid (CSF). There is another space called as subdural space, which as a space between the dura mater and arachnoid membrane. It is also filled with some fluid (Table 2-2).

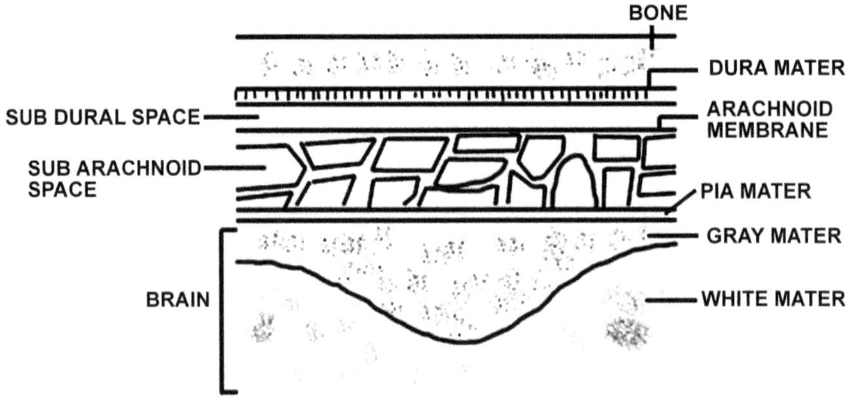

Figure 2-2 Three different meninges covering the brain and spinal cord

Table 2-1 Different types of spaces, fluid, and their functions

Sr. No.	Spaces	Fluid	Function of Fluid
1	Subarachnoid space (between the pia mater and arachnoid membrane)	CSF	Nourish the cells of CNS, acts as a shock absorber, provide buoyancy and protect brain against damage from its own weight
2	Subdural space (between the dura mater and arachnoid membrane)	Serous fluid	Acts as a lubricant; as a consequence, the dura mater can freely move over the arachnoid.

Cerebrospinal fluid (CSF)

It is a clear lymph-like fluid formed by the transport of active substances from blood plasma in the choroid plexus. The CSF runs through the brain as well as the spinal cord through the central canal. The total volume of CSF is approximately 150 ml and is produced at a rate of 800 ml per day.

Composition of CSF

CSF is a clear, colorless and transparent fluid, alkaline in nature. It has a specific gravity of 1.005 and 0.3 ml of CSF is produced/min (Table 2-2).

Table 2-2 Composition of CSF

Sr. No.	Content	Amount
1	Water	99.13%;
2	Solids-	0.87
3	K^+	3.00 mEq
4	Cl^-	114.0 mEq
5	Glucose	60 mg%
6	Protein	20 mg%

Functions of CSF

(i) CSF acts as a shock absorber as it forms a protective cushion around and within the CNS to protect the brain from any kind of injury.

(ii) CSF maintains the homeostasis surrounding nervous tissue cells and nourishes the cells of the CNS. It also partially provides the supply of nutrients, exchange of gases and disposal of the metabolic waste products and forms a medium through which diffusion of various signal molecules (like neurotransmitters) takes place.

(iii) The components of the immune system present in the CSF fluid (leukocytes and immunoglobulins) provide protection against various pathogens.

(iv) CSF provides buoyancy i.e. 1500 gram brain suspended in CNS, has a buoyed weight of approximately 45 grams. It protects the brain against the damage caused by its own weight

Ventricles of brain

There are 4 hollow, fluid-filled spaces in brain that are called ventricles. Two lateral ventricles are present in cerebral hemisphere with one ventricle in each hemispheres. The third ventricle is located in the diencephalon and is connected to the lateral ventricles by the two interventricular foramina. The fourth ventricle is located in the brain stem. It is connected to the third ventricle by the cerebral aqueduct and meets the central canal inferiorly.

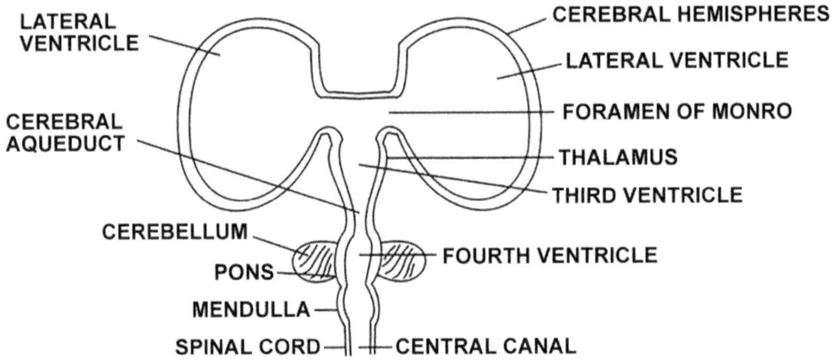

Figure 2-3 Representation of four ventricles of the brain, interconnected with one another   and continuing with the central canal of the spinal cord.

Structural Features of Brain

The brain is a very complex structure and it has been divided into different parts, both structurally as well as functionally (Figures 2-4 and 2-5). The different parts of the brain include the following:

1. **Olfactory Lobes:** These are pairs (two in number) of club-shaped structures present in the brain. These consist of two parts i.e. olfactory bulb and olfactory tract. These lobes are visible only in the ventral view of the brain.

   Functions of lobes: Olfactory nerve arises from the olfactory lobe and it is termed as 1st cranial nerve (described in next chapter). It is sensory in nature and is concerned with sense of smell. In other words, it brings the impulses related to smell from the nose to this region of the brain and helps in distinguishing/perceiving the smell.

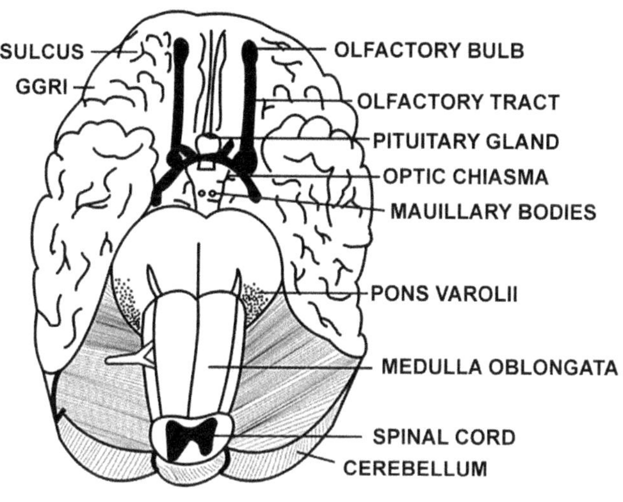

Figure 2-4 Ventral view of Human Brain

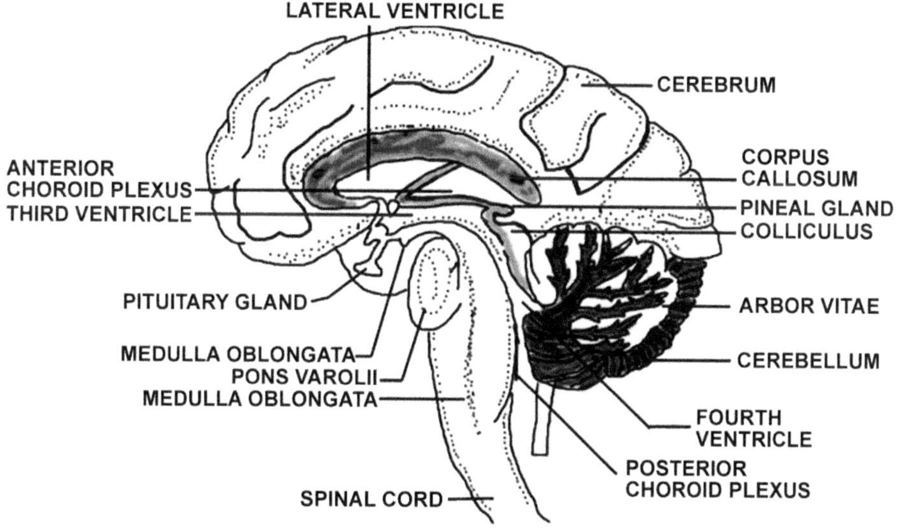

Figure 2-5 Median Section of Human Brain

2. **Cerebrum:** It constitutes a bulk of the brain portion and it includes cerebral cortex (outer region) and cerebral medulla (inner region). The cerebral cortex is made up of grey matter (unmyelinated neurons) and contains 75% of all neurons in the nervous system. On the other hand, the cerebral medulla is made up of white matter (myelinated neurons) and contains myelinated nerve fibers (Table 2-3). The cerebrum consists of two hemispheres i.e. left

hemisphere and right hemisphere, which are separated by the longitudinal fissure at the center of cerebrum. Both hemispheres are connected by the corpus callosum.

Table 2-3 Key differences between the gray and white matter

Sr. No.	Gray Matter	White Matter
1	It is grayish in appearance	It is whitish in appearance
2	It is the outer portion of cerebrum i.e. cerebral coretx	It is inner portion of cerebrum i.e. cerebral medulla
3	It is composed of millions of non-myelinated neurons that impart grey colour.	It is composed of myelinated nerve fibers that impart white colour.

Lobes of cerebral cortex

The surface of cerebral cortex is highly convulated (not smooth) and is greatly folded inwards. The upward folds are termed gyri (singular: gyrus) and the downward deeper grooves are called sulci (singular: sulcus). Sulci and gyri form a more or less constant pattern on the entire cerebral cortex. Each hemisphere of cerebrum is divided into four lobes: Frontal lobe, Parietal lobe, Temporal lobe and Occipital lobe (Figure 2-6; Table 2-4). The frontal lobe and parietal lobes are separated by central sulcus. The frontal lobe and temporal lobes are separated by lateral sulcus. The parietal lobe and occipital lobes are separated by parieto-occipital sulcus (Table 2-5).

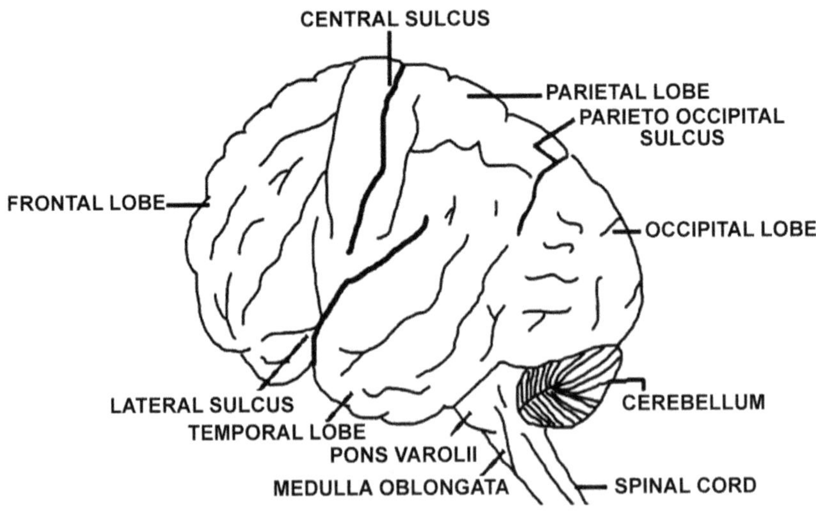

Figure 2-6 Lateral view of Human Brain showing different lobes along with Sulci

Table 2-4 Different types of lobes, their features and functions

Sr. No.	Lobes	Features	Functions
1	Frontal	Located at the front of the brain	Voluntary motor control of skeletal muscles; personality, intellectual process, verbal communication
2	Occipital	Located at the back portion of the brain	interprets visual information i.e. color, shape and structure
3	Temporal	Located on the bottom section of the brain	interprets auditory sensations i.e. smell, sound, hearing and memory
4	Parietal	Located in the middle section of the brain	It interprets taste, touch, pain, heat and cold

(i) **Frontal lobe:** This lobe controls skeletal muscle movement. It also control the intellectual processes including complex thought, creative ideas and their monitoring, translation of perceptions and memory into action, ability to abstract, reasoning, decision making, emotional behavior, willpower and personality

(ii) **Occipital lobe:** It interprets the visual information i.e. their colour, shape, structure etc.

(iii) **Temporal lobe:** It interprets auditory sensations i.e. smell, sound, hearing and memory.

(iv) **Parietal lobe:** It interprets taste, touch, pain, heat, cold. It is involved in taking information of environment and passing to rest of brain as well as knowing the position in the space.

Table 2-5 Different types of sulci and their significance

Sr. No.	Different types of sulci	Anatomical Significance
1	Lateral sulcus	Separates frontal lobe and temporal lobes
2	Central sulcus	Separates frontal lobe and parietal lobes; and the primary motor cortex from the primary somatosensory cortex.

Functional Areas of Cerebrum

Functionally, the cerebrum is divided into three portions. The three types of functional areas present in cerebrum include Sensory, Associate and Motor areas (Table 2-6). The sensory area receives the impulses from the peripheral areas i.e. receptors (Figure 7). The motor area transmits the impulses from the brain to the effector organs i.e. target organs. The associate areas store the input impulses, interpret the impulses and initiate the response according to impulse. These areas are involved in learning and memory etc.

On gross examination, the brain appears the same on two sides. However, the functional difference exists between two hemispheres of brain. The left hemisphere controls the right side of body, and right hemisphere controls the left side of body. Moreover, left hemisphere is more important for language, skill, reasoning, and intelligence. On the other hand, right hemisphere is more important for musical or artistic awareness and imagination etc. The presence of functional differences between two different hemispheres of brain is called as brain lateralisation.

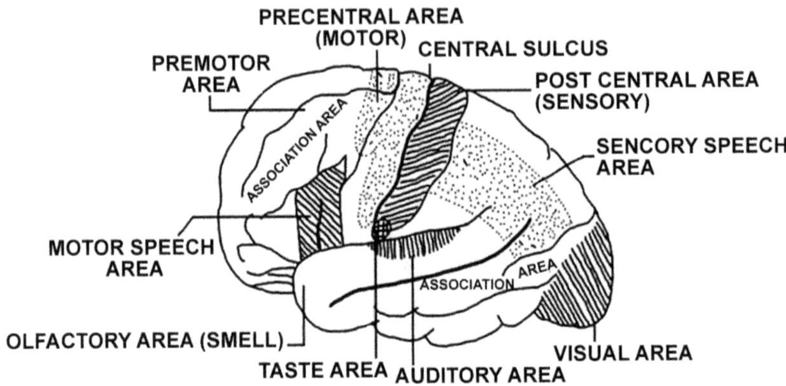

Figure 2-7 Cerebral hemisphere showing the different functional areas

The different motor and sensory functional areas include the followings (Table 2-6):

(i) Precentral area (Motor area): This area is present in the frontal lobe.

(ii) The neurons present in this area send impulses to initiate the contraction of voluntary muscles (skeletal muscles) e.g. limbs.

(iii) Postcentral area (sensory area): It is present in the parietal lobe.

(iv) It is present posterior to central sulcus. It receives impulses from periphery related to pain, touch, temperature etc.

(v) Sensory speech area: This area is present in lower part of the parietal lobe.

(vi) It also extends up to the temporal lobe. It perceives the spoken language and words.

(vii) Auditory area (Hearing area): It is present in the temporal lobe.

(viii) It is located immediately below the lateral sulcus. It is the centre of hearing.

(ix) Visual area: It is present in occipital lobe and is the centre for vision.

(x) Gaustatory area (taste area): It is present in parietal lobe.

(xi) It lies immediately above the lateral sulcus. It interprets the taste signals transmitted by tongue.

(xii) Olfactory area (smell area): It lies in temporal lobe. It interprets the signals transmitted by nose related to smell.

(xiii) Motor speech area (Broca's area): It lies in frontal lobe.

(xiv) It is connected with speech i.e. for speaking words.

Table 2-6 Different types of functional areas, their location, nature and functions

Sr. No.	Functional areas	Sensory/motor	Locations	
1	Precentral area	Motor	Frontal lobe	It initiates the contraction of voluntary muscles (skeletal muscles) e.g. limbs.
2	Post central area	Sensory	Parietal lobe	It receives impulses from periphery related to pain, touch, temperature etc
3	Sensory speech area	Sensory	Lower part of parietal lobe	It perceives the spoken language and words
4	Auditory area	Sensory	Temporal lobe	It is the centre of hearing
5	Visual Area	Sensory	Occipital lobe	It is the centre for vision
6	Gaustatory area	Sensory	Parietal lobe	It interprets the taste signals transmitted by tongue.
7	Olfactory area	Sensory	Temporal lobe	It interprets the signals transmitted by nose related to smell.
8	Motor speech area	Motor	Frontal lobe	It is connected with speech i.e. for speaking words.

3. **Basal Ganglia (Extrapyramidal Pathway):** It consists of a group of nuclei that are present at the base of cerebral cortex in the forebrain region. The various nuclei present in basal ganglia include the caudate nucleus, the putamen, and the globus pallidus. The globus pallidus is referred as the paleostriatum, and the caudate nucleus and putamen are together called as the neostriatum or striatum (Table 2-7).

Table 2-7 Different types of nuclei of basal ganglia and their group

Sr. No.	Individual Nuclei	Group of nuclei
1	• Caudate nucleus • Putamen	Neostriatum
2	• Putamen • Globus pallidus	lentiform nucleus
3	• Caudate nucleus • Putamen • Globus pallidus	Corpus striatum

Further, the putamen and the globus pallidus together are known as the lentiform nucleus, while the caudate nucleus, putamen, and globus pallidus form the corpus striatum (Table 2-8).

Table 2-8 Different types of nuclei in basal ganglia and their functions

Sr. No.	Individual Nuclei	Functions
1	Caudate nucleus	It is involved in storing and processing of memories, control communication skills and also works as a feedback processor i.e. uses information from past experiences to influence future actions as well as decisions
2	Putamen	It carries out complex functions related to movement and emotion. It is actively involved in a variety of cognitive functions such as episodic memory, cognitive control and category learning.
3	Globus pallidus	It is involved in regulation of voluntary movement

The pathway originating from basal ganglia is also termed as the extrapyramidal system and it is responsible for the fine control of motor activity and posture maintenance. Dopamine is the main neurotransmitter in this extrapyramidal system, particularly in the nigrostriatal tract. The nigrostriatal pathway originates from the substantia nigra and then innervates neostriatum. The substantia nigra consists of 2 parts, Substantia nigra pars compacta and Substantia nigra pars reticularis (Figure 2-8).

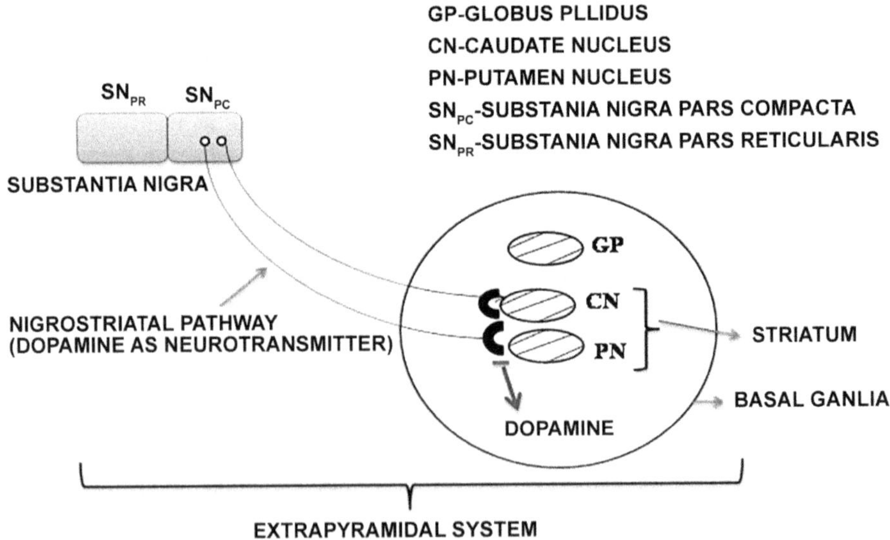

Figure 2-8 Representation of the extrapyramidal pathway

Functions of Basal Ganglia

(i) The main function of basal ganglia is control the movements of the body (motor functions). It controls the timing and intensity of movements. It determines how rapidly the movements are to be performed. Moreover, they also control how large the movements will be.

(ii) Indeed, these control the intensity and extent of muscle movement initiated by cerebrum. It means these do not initiate the movement; rather the extrapyramidal pathway helps in fine tuning the movements initiated by the pyramidal cells of the cerebrum.

(iii) The cognitive control of motor activity is also controlled by basal ganglia. It means those activities that arise from the thoughts generated in mind e.g. a movement of person on seeing the lion is controlled by basal ganglia and there is an important role of caudate nucleus in these types of movements.

(iv) The complex patterns of motor activities are also controlled by basal ganglia e.g. writing, performing which require some sort of skill.

(v) They also control (plan and execute) the stereotypic movements.

Parkinson Disease

It is the progressive neurodegenerative disorder in old age persons characterized by irreversible loss of dopaminergic neurons in the substantia nigra region of the brain i.e. in the nigrostriatal pathway. It is called as shaking palsy or paralysis agitans due to shaking hands and lack of motor coordination. The typical symptoms include rigidity, tremors, slow body movements (bradykinesia), postural difficulties appear. Non-treatment leads to progression to akinetic condition (no body movements) leading to immobility and death usually occurs due to pulmonary embolism or aspiration pneumonia. The drugs that increase the levels of dopamine such as levodopa or directly activate dopamine receptor are found to reduce the symptoms of disease (Table 2-9).

Table 2-9 Key features of Parkinson Disease

Sr. No.	Cells Affected	Pathway Affected	Neurotransmitter affected	Symptoms	Treatment
1	Substantia nigra	Nigrostriatal pathway	Dopamine	Rigidity, tremors, slow body movements, postural defects	Increase in dopamine by giving l-DOPA

4. **The Diencephalon:** The diencephalon is located deep below the cerebrum and constitutes the walls of the third ventricle. The two major regions of the diencephalon are the thalamus and the hypothalamus. There are other

structures, such as the epithalamus, which contains the pineal gland, and the subthalamus, which includes the subthalamic nucleus.

Epithalamus

It is very thin layer and is present above the thalamus. It does not function as nervous tissue. Its anterior part is folded and is highly vascular, is called as anterior choroid plexus that secretes CSF. Its posterior end has a pineal gland that secrets melatonin. In humans, melatonin helps in the regulation of circadian rhythm (sleep cycles). The melatonin production is influenced by the detection of light and dark by the retina of the eye. The melatonin production is inhibited when the retina detects light and is stimulated in the absence of light (Table 2-10).

Thalamus: It is located above the mid brain and is made up of gray matter. The major function of the thalamus is that it acts as a major relay centre. It means all the impulses passing to the cerebral cortex from the periphery or passing from cerebral cortex to periphery are first passed through thalamus. In other words, all impulses are relayed at thalamus before entering the cerebrum or passing from the cerebrum.

Indeed, it is involved in the relay and distribution of sensory and motor signals to specific regions of the cerebral cortex. Sensory signals generated in receptors are passed to the specific relay nuclei in the thalamus, where they are segregated and systematically organized. The relay nuclei in turn supply the information to the primary and secondary sensory areas of the cerebral cortex. Sensory input to thalamic nuclei is contralateral for the sensory and visual systems; bilateral and contralateral for the auditory system, and ipsilateral for the gustatory and olfactory systems. It is also regulates consciousness, sleep and alertness (Table 2-10).

Table 2-10 Parts of epithalamus and thalamus and their functions

Sr. No.	Parts	Subparts	Secretion	Functions
1	Epithalamus	Anterior choroid plexus	CSF	CSF acts as a shock absorber to protect the brain, provide buoyancy and protect brain from any kind of injury.
		Pineal gland	Melatonin	Melatonin helps in the regulation of circadian rhythm (sleep cycles).
2	Thalamus	-	-	The thalamus is involved in relaying sensory and motor signals to the cerebral cortex and regulating consciousness, sleep and alertness.

Hypothalamus: It lies below the thalamus. The optic nerves arise from eye and cross in front of hypothalamus to form optic chiasma. The hypothalamus is connected to the pituitory gland by stalk called infundibulum. The

Mammillary bodies are small rounded structures present behind the infundibulum (Table 2-11).

Table 2-11 Different centres of hypothalamus and their functions

Sr. No.	Centre	Functions
1	Endocrine gland	It releases a number of neurosecretory substances that stimulate the pituitary gland to release hormones that regulate growth and reproduction
2	Thermoregulatory centre	It regulates the body temperature and keep it at 37° C.
3	Hunger centre	It controls the body weight by controlling the amount of food consumed
4	Satiety centre	Activation of satiety centre induces the person to stop consuming the food and give feeling of satisfaction after taking food
5	Thirst centre	It controls the amount of water consumed
6	Limbic system	It helps in controlling the emotions of person like happiness, excitement, reward, punishment and fear etc.

Functions of hypothalamus

(i) It acts as an endocrine gland. It releases a number of neurosecretory substances that stimulate the pituitary gland to release hormones that regulate growth and reproduction. The details of hormones are described in endocrine chapter.

(ii) It is a thermoregulatory centre and it also called as the thermostat of body. It keeps the body temperature at 37° C. During fever, the thermoregulatory point is increased from 37° C and this is done in the presence of endogenous molecules called as prostaglandins. The antipyretics (that reduce fever e.g. paracetamol) reduce the formation of prostaglandins and bring the thermoregulatory point back to 37° C.

(iii) It also contains a hunger centre (appetite centre) and hence, it controls the body weight by controlling the amount of food consumed.

(iv) It also contains a satiety centre. Satiety refers to feeling of satisfaction after taking food. Activation of   hunger centre induces the person to consume the food, while activation of satiety centre induces the person to stop consuming the food.

(v) The posterior and lateral hypothalamus stimulation causes increased heart rate and blood pressure. However, pre-optic area causes decreased blood pressure and heart rate. Thus, it helps in regulating the cardiovascular functions.

(vi) It regulates the amount of water in the body. When the body fluids become too concentrated, then thirst centre is activated. It will result in drinking behaviour. Moreover,   when body fluid is concentrated, the supra-optic nuclei releases anti-diuretic hormone (ADH) hormone, which helps in reabsorbing the water from the renal system. Thus, this helps in increasing the water levels in the body.

(vii) It is part of limbic system, which helps in controlling the emotions of person like happiness, excitement, reward, punishment and fear etc.

5. **Mid Brain:** It is the small part of brain and consists of following regions:

Corpora quadrigemina: These are two pairs of rounded structures. One upper pair is called superior colliculi and lower pair is called inferior colliculi. One superior colliculi and one inferior colliculi of each side form corpora bigemina (tectum). The superior colliculi are concerned with the sense of sight. The inferior colliculi are concerned with hearing (Table 2-13; Figure 2-9).

Cerebral Peduncles (Crura cerebri)

These are two bundles of fibers that lie on interior (lower) surface of mid brain. These serve as a relay centre for the impulses passing between cerebrum, cerebellum, pons varolli and medulla oblongata (Figure 2- 9, Table 2-12).

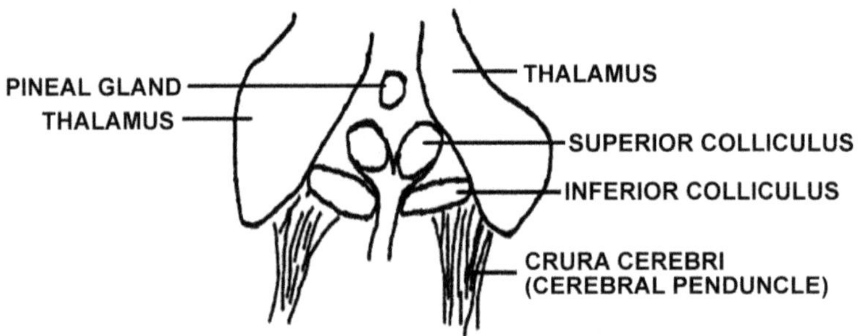

Figure 2-9 Mid Brain and Thalamus

Table 2-12 Parts and functions of mid brain

Sr. No.	Centre	Functions	
1	Corpora quadrigemina	Superior colliculi	Concerned with the sense of sight
		Inferior colliculi	Concerned with the sense of hearing
2	Cerebral Peduncles	—	Function as relay centre for impulses passing through different brain areas

6. **Cerebellum:** It is the second largest part of brain after cerebrum. It is a part of hind brain and it consists of three parts including two cerebellar hemispheres and vermis. Vermis is present between two cerebellar hemispheres. The shape of cerebellum is like butterfly. The gray matter is present on outer surface and white matter is located to inner surface. A very

large flask shaped cells called Purkinje cells are present in cerebellum. These are very complex cells of brain. Purkinje cells release a neurotransmitter called gamma-aminobutyric acid (GABA), which exerts inhibitory actions on other neurons of cerebellum i.e. deep cells and thereby, reduces the transmission of nerve impulses. These inhibitory functions enable Purkinje cells to regulate and coordinate motor movements (Table 2-13; Figure 2-10). It is very much different from other brain region described above i.e. cerebrum (Table 2-14).

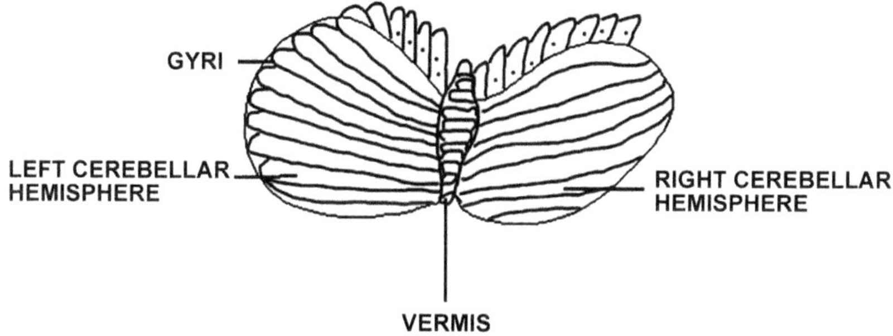

Figure 2-10 Different parts of cerebellum

Table 2-13 Different parts of cerebellum and their functions

Sr. No.	Parts of Cerebellum	Functions
1	Right cerebellar hemispheres	Right hemisphere control muscle movements on the left side of the body
2	Left cerebellar hemispheres	Left hemisphere control muscle movements on the right side of the body
3	Vermis	It is concerned with regulation of muscle tone for posture and locomotion.

Functions

(i) It controls the fast muscular movements (ballistic movements) of the body such as typewriting, running and talking etc.

(ii) It controls the motor movements initiated by the cerebrum (motor functions). In other words, it helps the cerebral cortex to coordinate patterns of movements e.g. hands, fingers, feet.

(iii) It helps the cerebral cortex to plan the timing and sequencing of the next successive movements that will be performed after the completion of present movement.

(iv) It helps to maintain the posture and equilibrium of the body. It functions in association with vestibular apparatus (present in the brain stem) to control postural and equilibrium movements. It is especially important for controlling equilibrium during rapid changes in body position.

(v) Cerebellum receives information from the motor cortex, which keep the cerebellum informed about the intended plan of movement. Moreover, it also receives input from the periphery, which keeps the cerebellum informed about the actual movement that has taken place. If these are not same (means intended movement and actual movement), then cerebellum brings necessary changes to bring them same.

(vi) Cerebellum helps to prevent the overshoot of movements and helps in dampening the excessive movement.

Table 2-14 Differences between cerebrum and cerebellum

Sr. No.	Cerebrum	Cerebellum
1	It is the largest part of brain	It is second largest part of brain
2	It is the part of fore-brain	It is the part of hind brain
3	It controls many functions of body like intelligence, memory etc	It is mainly concerned with maintaining posture and equilibrium
4	Arbor vitae is absent	Arbor vitae is present

7. Pons varolii (Pons-bridge): It is another part of hind brain and it lies below the mid brain and above the medulla oblongata. It consists of nerve fibers that form bridge between two cerebellar hemispheres.

Functions

(i) It contains respiratory centre and controls the respiration (explained in respiratory system)

(ii) Two cranial nerves arise from pons and these include trigeminal nerve (5th cranial nerve) and facial nerve (7th cranial nerve).

(iii) It acts as relay centre for impulses passing between medulla and higher brain parts; between hemispheres of cerebellum and between cerebrum and cerebellum.

8. Medulla oblongata: It has a pyramidal shape and is another part of the hind brain. It is present below the Pons varolii and is continuous with the spinal cord below. The lower side of medulla has a thin, vascular layer called Posterior choroid plexuses (Table 2-15).

Functions

(i) It contains the centers that regulate heart rate, blood pressure, respiratory, vomiting, coughing, sneezing, swallowing and salivation

(ii) It receives signals from the spinal cord and passes to the thalamus and cerebrum. It also passes signals (acts as relay centre) to the spinal cord that comes from the cerebrum, thalamus, etc.

(iii) Four cranial nerves originate from the medulla oblongata: glossopharyngeal nerve (9th), vagus nerve (10th), accessory nerve (11th) and hypoglossal nerve (12th)

Table 2-15 Functions of Pons and Medulla oblongata

Sr. No.	Functions of Pons	Functions of Medulla Oblongata
1	It contains the respiratory centre and controls the respiration	It contains the centers that regulate heart rate, blood pressure, respiratory, vomiting, coughing, sneezing, swallowing and salivation
2	It acts as a relay centre for impulses passing between the medulla and higher brain parts; between hemispheres of the cerebellum and between cerebrum and cerebellum	It receives signals from the spinal cord and passes to the thalamus and cerebrum. It also passes signals (acts as relay centre) to the spinal cord that come from the cerebrum, thalamus etc.
	Two cranial nerves arise from pons and these include trigeminal nerve (5th cranial nerve) and facial nerve (7th cranial nerve)	Four cranial nerves originate from the medulla oblongata: glossopharyngeal nerve (9th), vagus nerve (10th), accessory nerve (11th) and hypoglossal nerve (12th)

Transmission of signals from the motor cortex to muscles

The cerebral cortex is divided into the motor cortex and somatic sensory cortex. Further, the motor cortex is divided into three areas i.e. primary motor cortex, pre-motor area and supplemental motor area.

(i) Primary motor cortex: This area is responsible for controlling the muscles of the hand and   muscles of speech.

(ii) Pre-motor area: This area helps in controlling the muscles which control specific functions e.g.   positioning   of shoulders and arms. This area sends a signal to the primary motor cortex either directly   or   indirectly through the basal ganglia and thalamus.

(iii) Supplemental motor area: This area helps in fine control of muscles that are regulated by the primary motor area.

Most of the signals are transmitted from the motor cortex to the spinal cord directly through the corticospinal tract (pyramidal tract). However, some of the signals are also transmitted from the cortex to the spinal cord indirectly involving basal ganglia, cerebellum and brain stem. These tracts are called as the extra-pyramidal pathway.

(i) Corticospinal tract (pyramidal tract): About 30% of the corticospinal tract originates from the primary motor cortex and about 30% from the pre-motor and supplementary areas. The corticospinal (pyramidal) tract originates from the giant pyramidal cells (Betz cells), located inside the primary motor cortex region. These cells are very large in size and are of pyramidal shape.

The velocity of nerve transmission through these fibres is about 70 m/sec. After leaving the cortex, these fibers passes through the internal capsule (of basal ganglia) and then to the medulla (of the brain stem). The majority of pyramidal fibres cross to the opposite side and form the lateral corticospinal tract.

(ii) **Extrapyramidal system:** It is that part of the motor system that is not the part of direct corticospinal system. It includes tract passing through the motor cortex to the spinal cord indirectly through basal ganglia, reticular formation, vestibular nuclei and red nuclei. Some of the common extrapyramidal tracts include the followings:

(a) **Reticulospinal tract:** Some of the fibres originating from the motor cortex pass to the reticular substance, before entering the spinal cord and this pathway is termed as a reticulospinal tract.

(b) **Corticorubrospinal pathway (corticorubral and rubrospinal tract):** Some of the fibres originating from the motor cortex pass to the red nuclei of the mid brain via corticorubral tract. Thereafter, the neurons of the mid brain give rise to the rubrospinal tract that innervates the spinal cord. The corticorubrospinal pathway serves as an accessory route for transmission of relatively discrete signals from the motor cortex.

Reticular Formation

Reticular The reticular formation is a diffused, ill defined mass of nerve cells and fibres forming a meshwork of reticulum in the central portion of the brain stem. This portion is not well defined anatomically because it includes neurons located in different regions of the brain. The reticular formation is situated in the brain stem, and extends downwards into the spinal cord and upwards up to the thalamus and sub thalamus. Indeed, the reticular formation has been primarily designated on the basis of functional properties, not anatomically. On the basis of functions, two systems exist namely, ascending reticular activating system and descending reticular activating system.

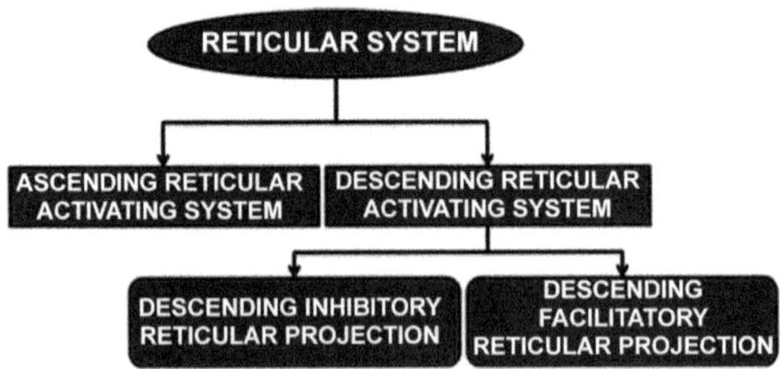

Figure 2-11 Divisions of the reticular system

Ascending reticular activating system (ARA)

The neurons form a complex network, which begins in the lower brain stem, passes through Pons, mid brain, thalamus and finally projects throughout the cerebral cortex. Indeed, the network projects into the cerebral cortex in two ways i.e. either through subthalamus or/and thalamus. This part of reticular formation plays an important role in wakefulness and general alertness (awareness). The stimulation of the ascending reticular activating system produces wakefulness by activation of the entire brain including the cerebral cortex, thalamus, basal ganglia and spinal cord. Any sensory impulse from muscle, skin, auditory, visual etc leads to the activation of the ascending reticular activating system. Once the ascending reticular activating system is activated, the activation is maintained for a long period of time. The reason is that the ascending reticular activating system activates the cerebral cortex and in turn, the cerebral cortex activates the ascending reticular activating system.

This is called a positive feedback mechanism for the maintenance of activation of the reticular activating system. The sympathetic nervous system (a division of autonomic nervous system) also activates the ascending reticular activating system.

Descending reticular activating system

This part of the reticular system controls the spinal cord. Functionally, it is divided into two types, namely descending inhibitory reticular projection and descending facilitatory reticular projection. These help in the maintenance of muscle tone, posture and movements.

Functions of the reticular formation

(i)   It regulates sleep, maintains the alertness and wakefulness cycle
(ii) It controls smooth and purposeful movements, posture and muscle tone
(iii) It controls the autonomic nervous system
(iv) It also regulates endocrine functions
(v)   It regulates the conditioned reflex
(vi) It has a role in somatic and visceral functions
(vii) It influences EEG and learning
(viii) It modulates afferent transmission

Limbic System

It is the part of the brain, which is responsible for the emotional behaviour and motivational drive. It is also termed as the emotional brain. Like reticular formation, this area is also defined functionally. There are a large number of different brain regions that function together to control the emotional functions of the humans and all those brain regions are included in the limbic system. The structures of the limbic system are located deep within the brain, beneath the cerebral cortex and above the brainstem. The major parts of the limbic system include the mammillary bodies of the hypothalamus, septum, paraolfactory area, amygdala, hippocampus, some portions of basal ganglia, limbic cortex, epithalamus and anterior nucleus of the thalamus. The emotional behaviour controlled by the limbic system includes reward, punishment, rage (during excessive punishment, a person assumes defensive posture with wide open eyes), fear, and sexual drive. Moreover, it also controls memory and olfaction (Figure 2-12). The role of different regions of the limbic system may be explained below:

1. **Hypothalamus:** The hypothalamus is a small part of the brain i.e. just 1% of total brain mass and is located just below the thalamus on both sides of the third ventricle. It controls vegetative and behavioural functions. All the functions controlled by the hypothalamus except for behavioral functions are termed as vegetative functions and these are discussed in the hypothalamus paragraph in section 4.

   Emotional Behavioural functions:

   (i) The stimulation of the periventricular nucleus leads to fear and punishment reactions

   (ii) The stimulation of lateral hypothalamus can lead to rage and fighting phenomenon

   (iii) The stimulation of ventromedial hypothalamus causes tranquillity

   (iv) Some portions of the hypothalamus can also lead to sexual drive

2. **Amygdala:** Amygdala comprises of an almond shaped cluster of nuclei, located deep in the temporal lobe of the brain and constitutes an important part of the limbic system. It is much more developed in men than in women. It operates at the semiconscious level and helps in control the behaviour of the person. Basolateral The basolateral nucleus is the major nuclei of the amygdala, which is helpful for emotional behaviour. The emotional functions of amygdala include the following:

   (i) When amygdale is stimulated electrically, the animals respond with aggression, fear and rage.   The removal   of amygdale makes the animal tame and does not respond to feared moments or   situations that would have caused rage before.

   (ii) It helps in the formation and storage of memories associated with emotional events.

3. **Basal Ganglia:** Since the limbic system interacts with nuclei of basal ganglia, therefore, it may be considered as a part of the limbic system. This comprises of several nuclei in each cerebral hemisphere and discussed in details above. The largest nucleus in the basal ganglia is corpus striatum and it consists of the caudate nucleus and lenticular nucleus. The lenticular nucleus is divided into putamen and globus pallidus. The mass of nerve fibres is called the internal capsule. Other structures that are part of basal ganglia are substantia nigra, red nuclei and subthalamic nuclei. The motor functions are explained above. Apart from motor functions, basal ganglia control the expression and perception of emotions and striatum plays a key role in reward processes and motivated behaviour.

4. **Hippocampus:** It is also a key part of the limbic system. It helps in the learning process. The removal of the hippocampus abolishes the short term memory. It also plays a key role in converting the short term memory in to long-term memory i.e. consolidation of memory. Moreover, it also controls the emotional behaviour as that of amygdale.

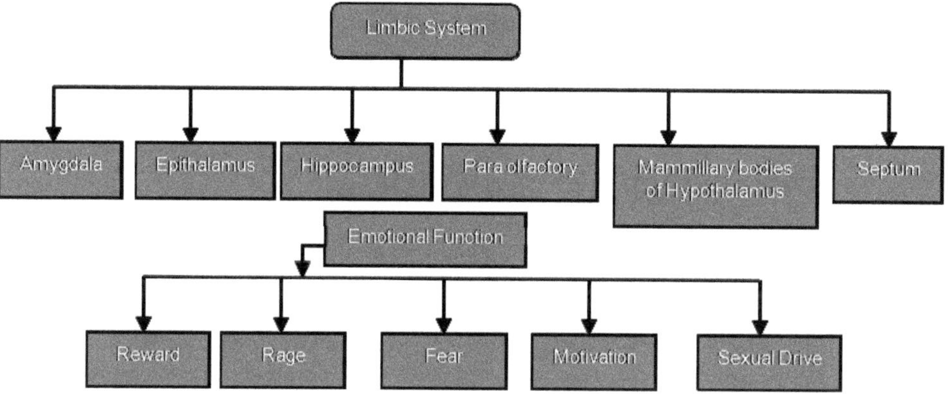

Figure 2-12 Representation of the limbic system and its functions

Blood Brain Barrier (BBB)

BBB is composed of a network of vessels that form a structural and chemical barrier between the brain and systemic circulation. It is made up of endothelial cells of the capillary wall, astrocytes and pericytes embedded in the capillary basement membrane (Figure 2-13). It functions as a selective barrier, which restricts the entry of certain

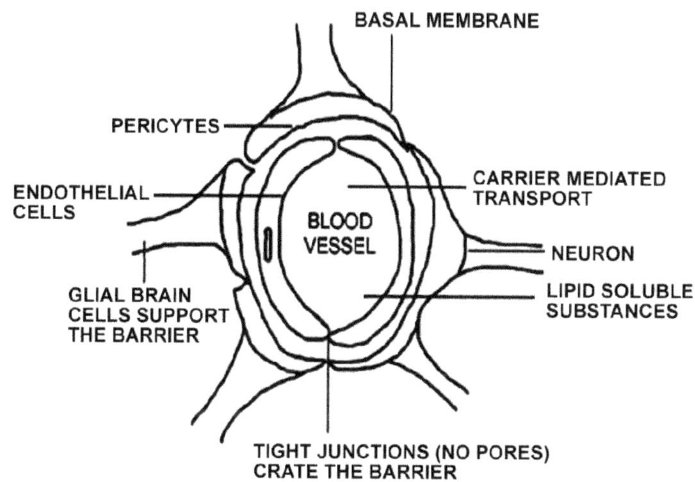

Figure 2-13 Diagram of the Blood-Brain Barrier

substances in and out of the brain. It mediates a complex system of exchange, transport and clearance. The substances that cross BBB are glucose, oxygen, CO2, H2O and lipid soluble substances. The charged molecules are not allowed to pass. The basic purpose of BBB is to protect the brain from the harmful substance and pathogens. The blood capillaries present in the brain are less leaky in nature due to tightly joined endothelial cells of blood capillaries. However, the certain parts of brain are not under BBB. These include parts of the hypothalamus, pituitary gland, some parts of medulla such as vomiting centre in CTZ (chemoreceptor trigger zone).

Electroencephalogram (EEG)

Brain cells generate action potential continuously and the addition of all these action potential consititute the brain waves. The presence of brain waves indicates the electrical activity of the brain and the electrical activity of neurons may be recorded from the surface of the brain. A record of brain waves is called electroencephalogram (EEG). There are four types of brain waves namely: alpha waves, beta waves, theta waves and delta waves (Figure 2-14) (Table 2-16).

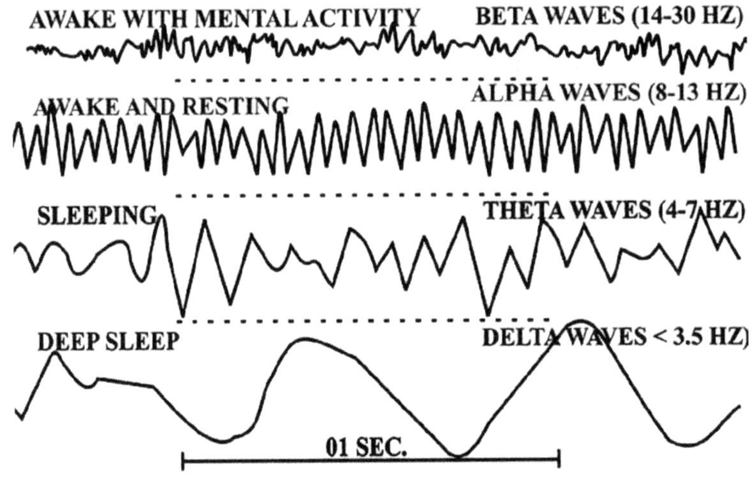

Figure 2-14 Alpha, beta, theta and delta brain waves

Table 2-16 Different types of brain waves and their characteristics in normal ECG pattern

Sr. No.	Types of waves	Frequency	Characteristics
1	Alpha Waves	8-13 Hz	Conscious, resting/relaxed mind
2	Beta waves	14-30 Hz	Conscious, active mind
3	Theta waves	4-7 Hz	Emotional stress
4	Delta waves	1-3.5 Hz	Unconscious, deep sleep, comatose

1. **Alpha Waves:** These waves occur at a frequency of 8-13 cycles per second. These waves appear in normally awake persons during the resting state. In other words, the persons are awake, but are in resting conditions. These waves disappear completely during the deep sleep.
2. **Beta Waves:** The frequency of these waves is 14-30 Hz. These waves occur during the active state of the brain.
3. **Theta Waves:** These have a frequency of 4-7 Hz. These waves appear in persons experiencing emotional stress.
4. **Delta Waves:** It includes all the waves of EEG below 3.5 Hz. These waves appear in a very deep sleep. If these occur during awake conditions, it shows the brain damage.

Human Spinal Cord

The spinal cord is a long, thin, tubular structure made up of nervous tissue, which extends from the medulla oblongata in the brainstem to the lumbar region of the vertebral column. It is the posterior part of central nervous system. Like brain, the spinal cord is also covered with protective membranes called meninges i.e. Pia mater, Arachnoid membrane and Dura mater. Three types of spaces are also present subarachnoid space, sub dural space, epidural space (explained earlier).

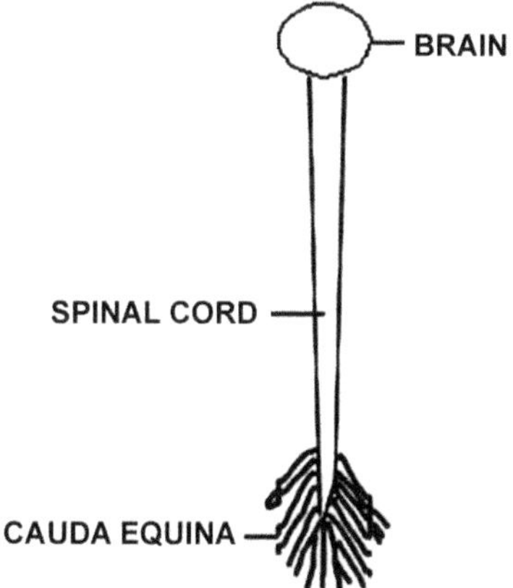

Figure 2-15 External structure of the Human Spinal Cord

External structure

It extends from the base of the brain to the second lumbar vertebra. It is about 42-45 cm long. At the end of the spinal cord, many spinal nerves branch and these branches are called Cauda equina (horse's tail) (Figure 2-15)

Internal Structure

The key structural features of the spinal cord may be described as follows:

(i) **White and grey matter:** The spinal cord consists of white matter and grey matter. The grey matter of spinal cord is shaped like a letter H or butterfly, which is surrounded by white matter. Grey matter is composed of cell bodies of neurons, neuroglia, unmyelinated axon and dendrites. The white matter consists of bundles of myelinated axons of neurons (Table 2-17).

Table 2-17 Different Divisions of Spinal Cord

Sr. No.	Grey Matter	White Matter
1	• Anterior horn • Posterior horn • Lateral grey horn	• Anterior white columns Posterior white columns • Lateral white columns

(ii) **Commissures:** The grey commissure is a thin line of gray matter, which forms the crossbar of H. It surrounds the central canal (discussed later). At the anterior side of the grey commissure, there is white commissure, which connects the white matter of right and left sides of the spinal cord.

(iii) **Central canal:** In the centre of grey commissure, there is a small space called central canal that runs throughout the spinal cord. The central canal is filled with cerebrospinal fluid, CSF. At the upper end, the central canal is continuous with the 4th ventricle. This canal extends the entire length of the spinal cord.

(iv) **Horns and Columns:** The grey matter on each side of the spinal cord is divided into horns. Therefore in each spinal cord, there are two horns i.e. anterior horn and posterior horn. Between the anterior and posterior grey horn, the lateral grey horn is present. The anterior and posterior gray horns divide the white matter into three areas: Anterior white columns, Posterior white columns and lateral white columns (Table 2-17).

(v) **Tracts:** In these white columns, three distinct bundles of nerve fibers are present, which are called tracts. The ascending (sensory) tract consists of axons that conduct nerve impulses to the spinal cord from the periphery. The descending (motor) tract consists of axons that conduct nerve impulses from the spinal cord to the periphery. From the posterior or dorsal root, the sensory nerve fibers arise and carry sensory impulses from the periphery to the spinal cord (Figures 2-16). From the anterior or ventral root, motor nerve fibers arise and carry impulses from the spinal cord to periphery (Figures 2-17) (Table 2-18).

(vi) **Neurons, Ganglia and Nerves:** In the spinal cord, three different types of neurons i.e. sensory, motor and interneuron are present. The sensory neuron is present in the dorsal/posterior root, also called as dorsal root ganglia. The motor neuron is present in the ventral/anterior root. These two neurons are interconnected with the help of interneuron.

The nerve impulse (through sensory nerve) enters from the periphery to the spinal cord and sensory information is conveyed to the sensory neuron located inside the dorsal root ganglia. Thereafter, the dorsal root nerve carries the sensory impulse from the sensory neurons and passes to interneuron. In other words, the incoming sensory nerve forms synapse with inter-neuron located in the posterior horn. Thereafter, the nerve impulse is passed from the interneuron to the motor neuron, which is located in the anterior horn. The motor nerve arises from the motor neuron (located of the anterior horn) in the form of the ventral nerve root and passes information to the periphery (Figure 2-18). All nerves arising from the spinal cord are mixed in nature i.e. they are both sensory and motor nerves and these spinal nerves arise from both sides of the spinal cord.

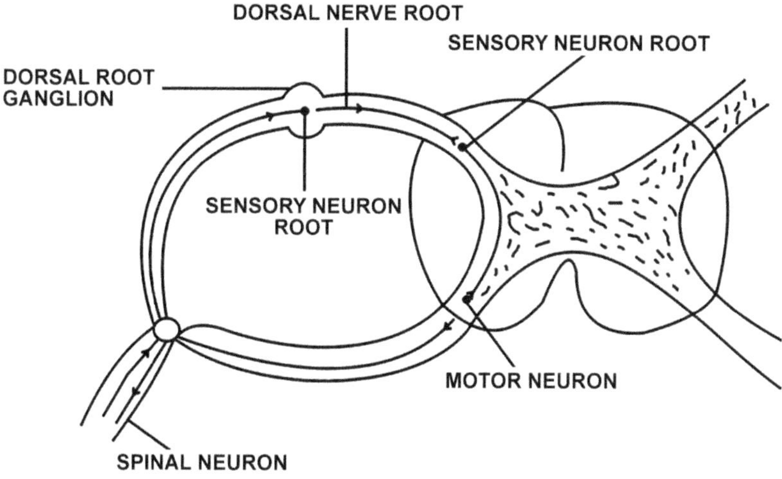

Figure 2-16 Internal structure of Human Spinal Cord (dorsal View)

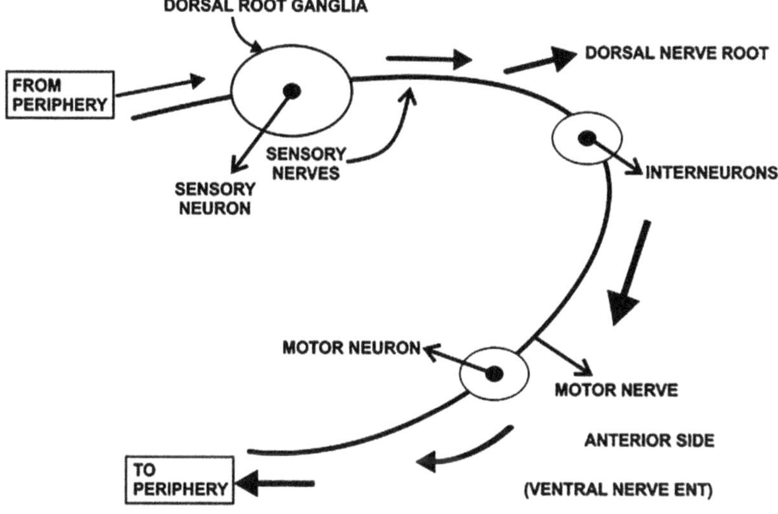

Figure 2-17 Internal structure of human spinal cord (Ventral view)

Table 2-18 Different tracts in the spinal cord, origin and functions

Sr. No.	Tract	Source	Functions
1	Ascending (sensory) tract	Posterior or dorsal root	Conduct impulses from the periphery to the spinal cord
2	Descending (motor) tract	Anterior or ventral root	Conduct impulses from the spinal cord to the periphery

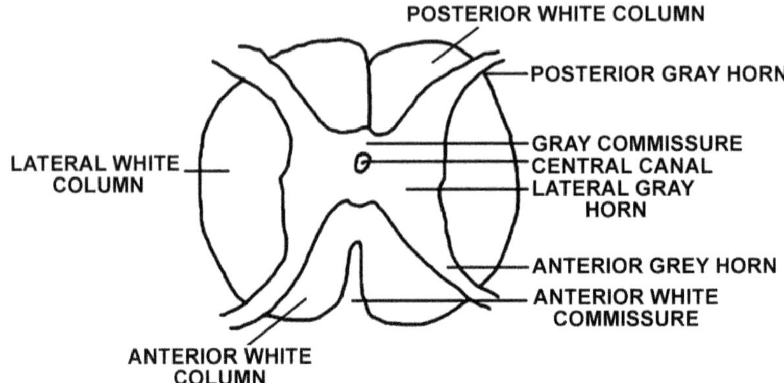

Figure 2-18 Representation of Sensory (On Posterior/Dorsal Root), Motor (Anterior/Ventral Root) and Interneurons in the Spinal Cord

Reflex Actions

The reflex actions are fast (instantaneous), predictable, automatic, involuntary response to the changes in the environment. The main purpose of reflex action is to maintain the homeostasis (balance). Some examples of reflexes include; removal of hand on touching the hot plate, changes in the size of the pupil of the eye on falling light; coughing or sneezing on the entry of irritant in throat or nose.

The reflex that involves the spinal cord are called spinal reflexes and those involve the brain are called cranial reflexes. Indeed, a cranial reflex is mediated by one of the cranial nerves and its example includes a blinking response to a bright light or to a touch to the cornea. Otherwise, most of the reflexes in the body are spinal reflexes (Figures 2-19). Reflexes may also be classified depending on their functions:

(i) **Somatic reflexes:** These reflexes cause the contraction of the skeletal muscles.

(ii) **Visceral (autonomic reflexes):** These reflexes control the smooth muscles and involve the autonomic nervous system.

Reflex Arc

A reflex action is carried a by neural pathways called as reflex arcs. In other words, it is a pathway through which reflex action occurs. It mainly consists of five components (Figure 18):

(i) **Receptor:** The distal end of the sensory neuron is called a receptor. It receives a specific stimulus, and any change in the internal or external environment, which further leads to the generation of an action potential.

(ii) **Sensory neuron:** It is present in the posterior/dorsal root of the spinal cord. The action potential is conducted from receptor to sensory neuron (located in the spinal cord) by the sensory nerves.

(iii) **Interneuron Centre:** It is a region within the spinal cord, which connects the sensory neuron and motor neuron. The integrating centre is a synapse. A reflex pathway having one synapse is called monosynaptic reflex arc. If the integrating centre is having more synapse, then reflex is called post synaptic reflex arc.

　　The integration centre functions to join the sensory neuron and motor neuron in the spinal cord. The impulses received by the sensory neuron passes to the motor neuron through integrating centre.

(iv) **Motor neuron:** It is the neuron present in the anterior/ventral root of the spinal cord. The motor nerve arises from the motor neuron.

(v) **Effector or target organ:** It is the part of the body that is controlled by the motor neuron. Motor neurons pass the information to the target organ (muscle or gland) and perform its actions.

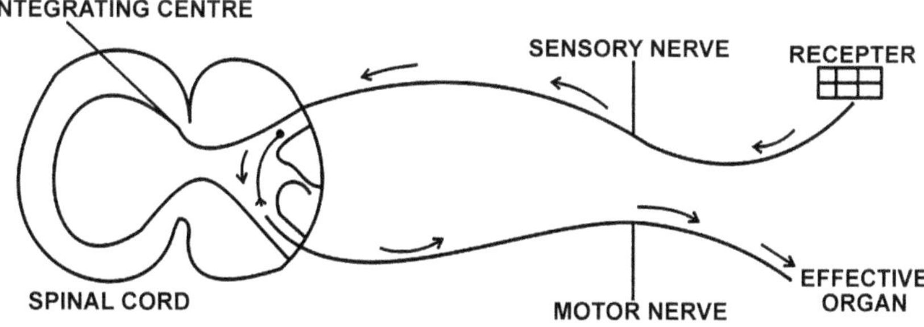

Figure 2-19 Representation of the Spinal Reflex Arc

Functions of Afferent and Efferent Nerve Tracts

Afferent nerves (Sensory Nerves)

Afferent nerves are also known as sensory nerves and these nerves carry nerve impulses from the receptors (in the periphery) to the CNS. These nerves are usually a part of the peripheral nervous system and they extend from the spinal cord (CNS) to the receptor cells located on the body surface/organs. These afferent (sensory) nerves are also paired with motor nerves (efferent nerves). When the afferent nerves send the impulse from an organ to the brain, the brain sends an impulse to the motor nerves which leads to change in the organ. For example: on touching a hot stove, an impulse is sent via afferent nerves to the brain and thereafter, efferent nerves pass the impulse to hand to remove the hand from the stove. There are different types of sensory fibers (Table 2-19):

(i) **General Somatic Afferents (Somatic sensory fibers):** These are located in the spinal nerves and occasionally, found in the cervical area. These nerves carry impulses of thermal sensation, touch, pain, pressure, and changes in the body positions from the surface of the body to the central nervous system.

(ii) **General Visceral Afferents:** These nerves carry sensory impulses (usually pain and reflex impulses) from the visceral organs, glands and blood vessels to the central nervous system. The parts of the body that are innervated by these nerves are rectum, abdomen, lungs, face, scalp, nose, mouth, and colon.

(iii) **Special Somatic Afferent:** These afferent nerves carry sensory information regarding vision, hearing and balance. These are located in the brain and ears.

(iv) **Special Visceral Afferent:** These afferent nerves are related to the gastrointestinal tract. They carry special senses of smell   and taste.

Table 2-19 Types, location and function of afferent nerves

Sr. No.	Types of afferent nerves	Location	Function
1	General Somatic Afferent	Generally found in the spinal nerves	These conduct impulses of thermal sensation, touch, pain and pressure, and changes in the body positions from the surface of the body
2	General Visceral Afferent	These nerves are present in the rectum, abdomen, lungs, face, scalp, nose, mouth, and colon.	These nerves conduct sensory impulses usually pain and reflex impulses from the viscera, glands and blood vessels to the CNS.
3	Special Somatic Afferent	These are located in the brain and ears	These afferent nerves carry information from vision, hearing and balance.
4	Special Visceral Afferent	These afferent nerves are related to the gastrointestinal tract.	They carry special senses of smell and taste.

Sensory Receptors: Within the sensory nerves, nerve cells are bundled in fibers and end in receptors that can be classified according to their function i.e. nociceptors, photoreceptors, mechanoreceptor, olfactory receptors, taste receptors and thermoreceptors (Table 2-20).

Table 2-20 Types and function of sensory receptors

Sr. No.	Types of sensory receptors	Functions
1	Nociceptors	Sense the pain
2	Photoreceptor	Response to light
3	Mechanoreceptors	Response to touch and pressure
4	Olfactory Receptors	Detect odors
5	Taste Receptors	Detect the flavors in food
6	Thermoreceptors	Detect changes in temperature

Efferent Nerves (Motor Nerves)

These nerves carry the impulses from the brain/spinal cord to the effector muscle or a gland. The motor neurons are usually present in the grey matter (ventral root) of the spinal cord or/and medulla oblongata of the brain. These are two types of motor neurons i.e. Upper and lower Motor Neurons. Lower Motor Neurons are located in the spinal cord or cranial nerves in the brain stem. Upper motor neurons are located in the cerebral cortex or brain stem. Like sensory, afferent nerve fibers, there are different types of efferent nerve fibers (Table 2-21):

(i) **General somatic efferent fibers:** These are located in the gray matter of the brain or/and spinal cord. These carry motor impulses to skeletal muscles.

Table 2-21 Types, location and function of afferent nerves

Sr. No.	Types of afferent nerves	Location	Function
1	General Somatic efferent	These are located in the gray matter of the brain and the spinal cord.	These carry motor impulses to skeletal muscles.
2	General Visceral efferent	These are located in the autonomic nervous system	These efferent fibers send motor impulses to smooth muscle, cardiac muscle and glands.
3	Special visceral efferent	These fibers emerge from the dorsal side of the facial motor nucleus	These nerves conduct motor impulses from CNS to skeletal muscles that control facial expressions and position of jaw, neck, larynx and pharynx.

(ii) General Visceral efferent fibers: These are located in the autonomic nervous system and send motor impulses to smooth muscle, cardiac muscle and glands.

(iii) Special visceral efferent fibers: These nerves conduct motor impulses from central nervous system to the skeletal muscles to control facial expressions and position of jaw, neck, larynx and pharynx.

2.2 Chapter at a Glance

Term	Description
CSF	Cerebrospinal fluid
Meninges	Three covering layers around brain and spinal cord
Subarachnoid space	Space between the pia mater and arachnoid membrane
Subdural space	Space between the dura mater and arachnoid membrane
Broca's area	Lies in frontal lobe and connected with speech
Nigrostriatal pathway	Originates from the substantia nigra and then innervates neostriatum.
Contralateral	On the opposite side
Ipsilateral	On the same side
Ballistic movements	Fast muscular movements
Corticospinal tract	Pyramidal tract
ARA	Ascending reticular activating system
Limbic System	Controls the emotional behaviour and motivational drive
BBB	Blood Brain Barrier
EEG	Electroencephalogram
Efferent Nerves	Motor Nerves
AD	Alzheimer's disease
Agonist	Ligand binds to the receptors and produces biological response
Antagonist	Ligand binds to receptor and prevents actions of agonist

Exercises

Multiple Choice Questions

1. A multipolar neuron which is located entirely within the central nervous system.
   (a) Motor neuron
   (b) Efferent neuron
   (c) Afferent neuron
   (d) Interneuron

2. Which of the following is not component of basal nuclei
   (a) Caudate nucleus   (b) Globus pallidus
   (c) Infundibulum   (d) Lentiform nucleus

3. The third ventricle is located in the
   (a) Forebrain   (b) Hind brain
   (c) Cerebellum   (d) Cerebrum

4. Blood brain barrier restricts passage of
   (a) Water   (b) Lipids
   (c) Sodium   (d) Chloride

5. A nerve impulse is first received by
   (a) Cell body   (b) Axon
   (c) Synapse   (d) Dendrite

6. Which of the following is not a lobe of a cerebrum
   (a) Parietal lobe   (b) Occipital lobe
   (c) Temporal lobe   (d) Sphenoidal lobe

7. The white matter of CNS is
   (a) Deep to gray matter   (b) Unmyelinated
   (c) Arranged in to tracts   (d) Composed of sensory fibers

8. The thalamus is located in
   (a) The telencephalon   (b) The mesencephalon
   (c) The metencephalon   (d) The diencephalon

9. The tracts of white matter that connect the right and left cerebral hemispheres are composed of
   (a) Association fibers   (b) commissural fibers
   (c) Both a and b   (d) Projection fibers

10. A neurons that carry impulses away from the CNS are
    (a) Sensory nerves   (b) Extensors
    (c) Afferent nerves   (d) Efferent nerves

Short Answer Questions

1. What are different regions of the brain?
2. What are the different coverings of the brain and spinal cord?
3. What is CSF?
4. What is the composition of CSF?
5. Name different types of ventricles of the brain.
6. What are the functions of the olfactory and parietal lobe?
7. What are afferent and efferent nerves?
8. What is the function of the cerebral cortex?
9. Write about the gray and white matter.

10. What is the spinal cord?
11. What are the functions of cerebrum?
12. Name different nuclei of basal ganglia.
13. What is BBB?
14. What is EEG?

Long Answer Questions

1. What do you mean by CSF? Explain its functions also.
2. Explain different types of spaces, fluid, and their functions.
3. Explain the four ventricles of the brain.
4. Explain the structural features of the brain.
5. Explain and draw a ventral view of human brain.
6. What are different parts of the cerebellum?
7. Explain the blood brain barrier.
8. Write a note on the structure of the spinal cord.
9. Explain about the extrapyramidal pathway and its importance.
10. What are the functions of the hypothalamus?

Bibliography

Costanzo LS. Physiology. 4th Edition. Lippincott Williams & Wilkins.

Guyton AC, Hall JE. Textbook of Medical Physiology. 11th Edition. Elsevier Saunders. 2006.

Jaggi AS, Bali A, Singh N. Pathophysiology. 1st Edition. Vallabh Prakashan. 2019.

Jain AK. Human Anatomy and Physiology for Pharmacy. 3rd Edition. Arya publications. 2017.

Lodish H, Berk A, Kaiser CA. Molecular Cell Biology. 6th Edition. W. H. Freeman & Co Ltd. 2007.

Tortora GJ, Derrickson B. Principles of Anatomy and Physiology. 15th Edition. John Wiley and Sons, Inc. 2017.

Waugh A, Grant A. Ross and Wilson Anatomy and Physiology in Health and Illness. 12th Edition. Churchill Livingstone. 2014.

Answer Key MCQs									
1.	(d)	2.	(c)	3.	(d)	4.	(b)	5.	(d)
6.	(d)	7.	(c)	8.	(d)	9.	(b)	10.	(d)

Digestive System

After completing this lesson, the Reader should be able to understand:

- *Introduction*
- *Layers of Gastrointestinal tract*
- *Neural innervations of the GIT*
- *Enteric nervous system (ENS)*
- *Automic nervous system*
- *Peritoneum*
- *Anatomy of GIT*
- *Enzymes and other Exocrine Secretions*
- *Digestion of Carbohydrates*
- *Digestion of Proteins*
- *Digestion of Fats*
- *Bile*
- *Liver*
- *Absorption of Nutrients*
- *Role of large intestine in digestion and absorption*
- *Feces and Defecation Reflex*
- *Mobility of GIT*
- *Gross and Physiological Calorific Value*
- *Diseases of GIT*

3.1   Introduction

Gastrointestinal tract (GIT) extends from mouth to anus and is involved in digestion as well as absorption of food material. There are four layers of GIT, starting from the lumen to outside. These include mucosa, submucosa, muscularis and serosa. These layers enclose the lumen and mucosa is in direct contact with lumen. For oesophagus and duodenum, the outermost layer is called as **adventitia**. However, for rest of the gastrointestinal tract, this layer is called as **serosa** (**Figure 3-1**).

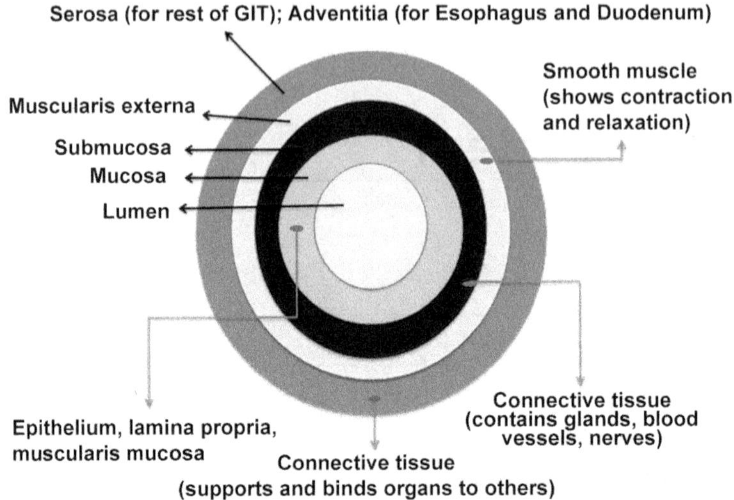

Figure 3-1 Representation of four different layers of GIT

Layers of Gastrointestinal Tract

The details of Gastrointestinal Tract layers are as follows:

1. **Mucosa:** It is innermost lining of GIT and is in contact with the lumen. It is also called mucosa membrane. It is inturn composed of a number of layers including epithelium, lamina propria, and muscularis mucosa, which perform specific functions (Table 3-1):

   (a) **Epithelium:** It is in direct contact with the lumen of GIT and it is composed of epithelial cells. The epithelial cells are of different types depending on the region of the GIT. In the mouth, pharynx, oesophagus and anal canal, it is composed of non-keratinized stratified squamous epithelium. It serves as a protective layer in these regions. However, it is composed of columnar epithelial cells in the stomach and intestine regions. Its function changes in these regions and it main functions include secretion and absorption. In this layer, both exocrine and endocrine cells are present. It means it secretes both enzymes as well as hormones. Another important point about this layer is that this layer is continuously renewed. About after every 5 to 7 days, the layer is replaced.

   (b) **Lamina propria:** This layer has important functions. It layer has blood vessels and lymphatic capillaries that help in the absorption of nutrients after digestion. It also contains MALT i.e. mucosa-associated lymphatic tissue immune cells, whose function is to provide immunity and protects from the development of disease. These immune cells are present in the tonsils, small intestine, appendix and large intestine.

(c) Muscularis mucosa: It is a thin layer and made up of smooth muscle fibres. It is folded variously in the stomach and small intestine region to increase the surface area.

2. **Submucosa:** It is the second layer of GIT after mucosa. This layer has abundant of blood vessels, lymphatic capillaries, glands and lymphatic tissue. The absorbed food material passes to blood vessels and lymphatic capillaries. Moreover, there is an extensive network of neurons called as submucosal plexus (discussed below).

3. **Muscularis:** This layer is made up of muscles, either of smooth muscle cells or skeletal muscle cells. In some parts including mouth, pharynx and oesophagus, the muscularis is composed of skeletal muscles. The skeletal muscles in this region help in voluntary swallowing. Moreover, the external anal sphincter is also composed of skeletal muscles and it helps in voluntary defecation. In rest of GIT, muscularis is composed of smooth muscles and help in involuntary contraction or relaxation of parts of GIT. These smooth muscles are arranged in two sheets: circular and longitudinal fibres. The contraction of circular and longitudinal muscles helps in peristalsis and peristaltic movements are critical for the movement of food in the forward direction. In muscularis, the second plexus of neuron called myenteric plexus is present (discussed below).

4. **Serosa:** This is the outmost layer and is present around the portions of GIT, which are suspended in the abdomino-pelvic cavity. This layer is also called visceral peritoneum.

Table 3-1 Summarised representation of different functions of four different layers of GIT

Sr. No.	Layers	Characteristic Features	Functions
1	Mucosa	Innermost layer Made up of three layers epithelium, lamina propria, muscularis mucosa	Discussed below in individual layer
	Epithelium	Innermost layer In direct contact with the lumen of GIT Made of epithelial cells Renewal of layer after every 5-7 days	Secretion of enzymes and hormones
	Lamina propria	Possess blood vessels and lymphatic capillaries	Absorption of nutrients MALT provide immunity
	Muscularis mucosa	Thin layer Made of smooth muscle fibres	Folded variously to increase the surface area
2	Submucosa	Abundant blood vessels and lymphatic capillaries Presence of submucosal plexus	Absorption of digested material Plexuses help in controlling secretions in GIT

Table 3-1 *Contd...*

Sr. No.	Layers	Characteristic Features	Functions
3	Muscularis	Made up of muscles, either smooth or skeletal muscle depending on site Smooth muscles arranged in circular and longitudinal fibres Presence of myenteric plexus	Smooth muscles help in peristalsis Skeletal muscles help in swallowing
4	Serosa	Outmost layer Present around the portions of GIT Also called visceral peritoneum	Covering of GIT organs suspended in abdomino-pelvic cavity

Neural Innervations of the GIT

About 100 million neurons are present in the GIT extending from the oesophagus to anus. These neurons help to regulate the digestive and absorptive functions of GIT. The GIT is innervated by two types of nervous system, enteric nervous system and autonomic nervous system (extrinsic set of nerves) (Table 3-2).

Table 3-2 Key differences between ENS and ANS

Sr. No.	Enteric Nervous system	Autonomic Nervous system
1.	It comprises of intrinsic set of nerves	It comprises of extrinsic set of nerves
2.	It is localized nervous system, within gut only	It is generalized nervous system that also controls gut
3.	It has Myenteric and submucosal plexuses	It is divided into sympathetic and parasympathetic nervous system

Enteric Nervous System (ENS)

It is a local nervous system, which controls the functions of GIT and it is composed of intrinsic set of nerves. Due to its extensive, local network, it is also called as brain of gut. The neurons of this enteric nervous system are arranged in the form of plexuses. There are two plexuses (Table 3-3):

(i) **Myenteric plexus (plexus of Auerbach):** This plexus is present in between the muscles of muscularis layer. The motor neurons of the myenteric plexus help to control the GIT motility and peristalsis. Indeed, it controls the strength and frequency of contraction of muscles of GIT.

(ii) **Submucosal plexus (plexus of Meissner):** This plexuses is found in the submucosa. The motor neurons of this submucosal plexus innervate the secretary cells of mucosal epithelium and control secretion in the GIT.

The interneurons of the ENS help to connect the neurons of both plexuses. The sensory neurons of the ENS innervate the mucosal epithelium and function as chemoreceptors. These neurons are activated by chemicals in foods. Moreover, these also function as stretch receptors.

Table 3-3 Key differences between two types of plexuses in the GIT

Sr. No.	Myenteric plexus	Submucosal plexus
1.	Also termed as plexus of Auerbach	Also termed as plexus of Meissner
2.	Present in between the muscles of muscularis layer	Present in the submucosa
3.	Help to control the GIT motility and peristalsis	Control secretions in the GIT

Autonomic Nervous System

The GIT is also regulated by another nervous system termed as the autonomic nervous system. It is further of two types; parasympathetic nervous system and sympathetic nervous system. There is a greater role of parasympathetic nervous system and the vagus nerve (X^{th} cranial nerve and part of parasympathetic nervous system) supply to the most of the portions of GIT. It helps to increase enzymatic secretions including salivation and gastric secretions. It also helps to promote contraction of smooth muscles, increase peristalsis and relax sphincters. It comparison, there is lesser role of the sympathetic nervous system, which acts in opposite direction to parasympathetic nervous system.

Peritoneum

It is the largest serosa membrane of the body and it has two layers. The space in between the two layers is called peritoneal cavity.

(i) **Parietal peritoneum:** It lines the walls of the abdominopelvic cavity and it is the outer layer of the peritoneum.

(ii) **Visceral peritoneum:** It is the inner layer and it directly covers the organs. It is also called as serosa.

The peritoneum is not smooth and there are five different folds (Table 3-4):

(i) **Greater omentum (fat skin):** It is the largest fold and it has a lot of adipose tissue. It can lead to weight gain and it is responsible for beer-belly (obesity of abdomen). Functionally, it has a large number of lymph nodes. It covers the transverse colon and coils of small intestine like a "fatty apron".

(ii) **Falciform ligament:** It is present over the liver and attaches the liver to anterior abdominal wall.

(iii) **Lesser omentum:** It helps in suspending stomach and duodenum in the GIT.

(iv) **Mesentery:** It attaches the small intestine to the posterior abdominal wall.

(v) **Mesocolon:** It binds the large intestine to the posterior abdominal wall.

Table 3-4 Key differences between two types of plexuses in the GIT

Sr. No.	Layers of peritoneum	Functions
1.	Greater omentum	Covers the transverse colon and coils of small intestine
2.	Falciform ligament	Present over liver and attaches it to anterior abdominal wall
3.	Lesser omentum	Helps in suspending stomach and duodenum
4.	Mesentery	Attaches small intestine to posterior abdominal wall
5.	Mesocolon	Attaches large intestine to posterior abdominal wall

There are some organs which are covered by the peritoneum only on the anterior surfaces, not on the posterior surface. These organs are called as retroperitoneal organs and these include kidneys, ascending and descending parts of colon of large intestine, duodenum and pancreas.

Anatomy of GIT

IT extends from mouth to anus and it has been divided into different portion i.e. mouth, teeth, pharynx, oesophagus, stomach, small intestine and large intestine. It is like a long tube and with whom different glands are attached, which secrete their secretions in the lumen of GIT (Figure 3-2).

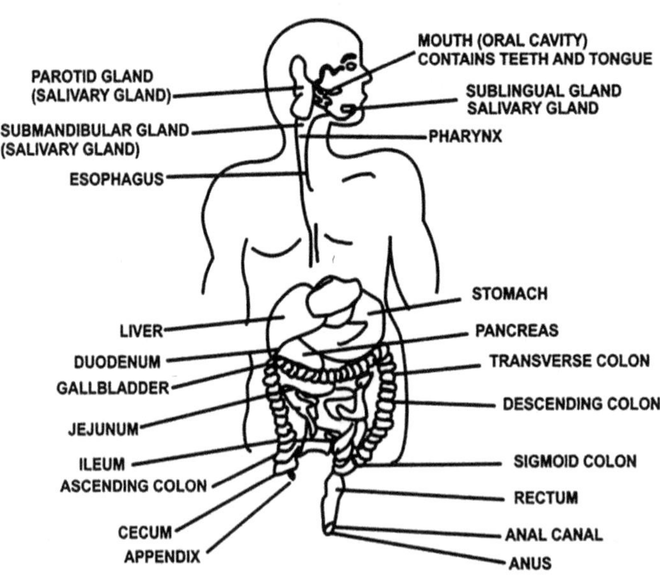

Figure 3-2 Representation of whole GIT with different structures

1. **Mouth:** The mouth is called as the oral or buccal cavity. It is formed by cheeks, hard palate, soft palates, tongue and lips. The cheeks form the lateral sides of the mouth and lips form the front part of the mouth. The hard palate is the anterior portion of roof of the mouth and it is bony in nature. It helps to separate the oral and nasal cavities. The soft palate forms the posterior portion of roof of mouth and it forms the partition between oropharynx and nasopharynx.

    Salivary glands secrete their secretions in the mouth in the form of saliva. There are three types of salivary glands and these are present in pairs in the mouth:

    (i) **Parotid gland:** It is the largest gland and present near to ear.

    (ii) **Sub-lingual gland:** It is the smallest gland and is present below the tongue.

    (iii) **Sub-mandibular gland:** It is medium sized gland and is present near the angle of mandible.

2. **Tongue:** Tongue is composed of skeletal (voluntary) muscle and covered by mucus membrane. The movement of tongue is controlled by the extrinsic and intrinsic muscles. The extrinsic muscles originate outside the tongue (attach to bones) and include hyoglossus, genioglossus and styloglossus. These help to chew the food, shape the food into round mass and force the food to back of mouth. The intrinsic muscles originate and insert inside the tongue. These include longitudinalis superior, longitudinalis inferior and these help in speech and swallowing (Table 3-5).

Table 3-5 Parts of tongue and their functions

Sr. No.	Parts	Functions
1.	Extrinsic muscles	Help to chew and shape the food into round mass and force the food to back of mouth
2.	Intrinsic muscles	help in speech and swallowing
3.	Papilae	Contain taste buds
4.	Lingual glands	Secretes mucus and lingual lipase in non-significant amount

Papilae

The dorsal (upper surface) and lateral surfaces of the tongue, there are a number of papillae. These papillae contain taste buds i.e. receptors for gestation (taste) such as for taste, salt and sour etc.

Lingual glands

The tongue also secretes some secretions containing mucus and lingual lipase. But, these are in a very small in quantity and do not play a significant role in digestion.

3. **Teeth:** Teeth are located in the sockets of alveolar processes of mandible (lower jaw) and maxillae. Externally, the alveolar processes are covered by gums or gingivae. Internally, the sockets are lined by the periodontal ligament. It is made up of dense fibrous connective tissue and helps to anchor the teeth to the socket walls.

Structurally, tooth has three parts, crown, neck and root (Table 3-6).

(i) **Crown:** It is the visible portion of the tooth. Its outer covering is enamel, which is the hardest part of the body. It is mainly composed of calcium salts, which account for about 95% of dry weight. Its inner matter is called as dentin, which comprises the major part of the teeth. It gives shape and strength to teeth. It is much harder than bones. The dentin encloses a space called pulp cavity. The pulp is present in the cavity and is composed of connective tissues, blood vessels, nerves and lymphatic vessels.

(ii) **Neck:** It is the small, constricted part and it is visible near gum.

(iii) **Root:** One or three roots help in embedding the tooth to socket. In other words, roots help to embed the teeth in the socket. The dentin and pulp is also present in neck and root. In root portion, there are narrow extensions of pulp and these are called pulp roots (root canal). In root, dentin is covered by cementum, which attaches tooth to the periodontal ligament.

Table 3-6 Different parts of teeth and their functions

Sr. No.	Parts	Features/Functions
1.	Crown Made up of three different parts	Functions described below in respective sections
	Enamel	Outer most part, hardest in nature Protective function
	Dentine	Major part of teeth Gives shape and strength to teeth
	Pulp cavity	Composed of connective tissues, blood vessels, nerves and lymphatic vessels Provides nourishment and sensory functions to teeth
2.	Neck	Small, constricted part and visible near gum
3.	Root	Help to embed the teeth in socket

Types and Number of Teeth

Teeth are of two types, deciduous or temporary teeth (primary teeth or milk teeth) and permanent teeth (Table 3-7).

Primary Teeth (Milk Teeth)

The primary teeth are 20 in number. These begin to appear around 6 month of age. In one half (upper or lower) of jaw, the different types of teeth and their number include central incisor (1), lateral incisor (1), canine (cupsid) (1), first molar (1), second molar (1). There are five teeth in one half of upper or lower jaw and therefore, total numbers of teeth are 5 x 4= 20. Five (5)= number of teeth in one half of mouth; Four (4) is total haves in the mouth (2 upper and 2 lower). The upper molars (maxillary) have three roots, while the lower molars (mandibular) have 2 roots

Permanent Teeth

These are permanent and appear after the falling of milk teeth. These are 32 in number. In one half (upper or lower) of jaw, the different types of teeth and their number include central incisor (1), lateral incisor (1), canine (1), premolars (2), molars (3). The third molar is termed as wisdom tooth. There are eight teeth in one half of upper or lower jaw and therefore, total numbers of teeth are 8 x 4= 20. Eight (8)= number of teeth in one half of mouth; four (4) is total haves in the mouth (2 upper and 2 lower).

Table 3-7 Key differences between milk and permanent teeth

Sr. No.	Milk (temporary) teeth	Permanent teeth
1.	These are temporary and fall after some time	These are permanent in nature
2.	These are 20 in number	These are 32 in number
3.	One half of jaw contains central incisor (1), lateral incisor (1), canine (cupsid) (1), first molar (1), second molar (1)	One half of jaw contains central incisor (1), lateral incisor (1), canine (1), premolars (2), molars (3)

4. **Pharynx (Throat):** It is funnel shaped tube-like structure which is common to respiration and digestion. It is connected to internal nares of nose and mouth on one side and to oesophagus and larynx on the other side. In other words, nose connects to pharynx and then to larynx. On the other hand, mouth also connects to pharynx, which is connected to oesophagus. The food passes from mouth to oesophagus through pharynx. The air passes through nose to larynx through pharynx. Thus, pharynx serves in both respiration and digestion. It is composed of voluntary muscles and is lined by mucus membrane. It has three parts:
   (i) Nasopharynx: It functions only in respiration.
   (ii) Oropharynx: It functions both in respiration and digestion.
   (iii) Laryngeopharynx: It functions both in respiration and digestion.

Oesophagus

It is a tube like structure, about 10 cm in length and lies posterior to trachea. Laryngeopharynx is continuous with oesophagus. It pierces the diaphragm through opening called esophageal hiatus and opens in the superior part of stomach. There are two sphincters in oesophagus (Table 3-8):

(i) **Upper esophageal sphincter (UES):** It is made up of skeletal muscles and lies at the junction of laryngeopharynx and upper part (starting portion) of oesophagus. Its function is to regulate the movement of food from pharynx to oesophagus.

(ii) **Lower esophageal sphincter (LES):** It is made up of smooth muscle and lies at the junction of lower end of oesophagus and superior part of stomach. Its function is to regulate the movement of food from oesophagus to stomach. In other words, its function is to allow unilateral movement of food i.e. from oesophagus to stomach. However, this sphincter closes when the contents of stomach tend to move in the backward direction i.e. towards oesophagus.

Since oesophagus is not present in the abdominal cavity, therefore, the outermost covering of oesophagus is called as adventitia, not serosa. The innermost lining of oesophagus is stratified squamous epithelium, which is also present on lips, mouth, oropharynx and laryngeopharynx. It helps to protect from abrasion, wear and tear.

Table 3-8 Key feature of pharynx and oesophagus

Sr. No.	Parts		Functions
1.	Pharynx		Passage of food and air to oesophagus and larynx, respectively
	(i)	Nasopharynx	Functions only in respiration.
	(ii)	Oropharynx	Functions in respiration and digestion
	(iii)	Laryngeopharynx	Functions in respiration and digestion
2.	(iv)	Oesophagus	Passage of food from pharynx to stomach
	(i)	Upper esophageal sphincter	Regulate the movement of food from pharynx to oesophagus
	(ii)	Lower esophageal sphincter	Regulate the movement of food from oesophagus to stomach

Deglutition

The passage of food from the mouth to stomach by act of swallowing is called as deglutition. It has 3 stages:

(i) **Voluntary stage:** In this step, the food is rolled by tongue and passed from mouth to oropharynx.

(ii) **Pharyngeal stage:** In this step, the food is passed from oropharynx to laryngeopharynx and then, to oesophagus. The presence of food in oropharynx leads to activation of sensory receptors present in the oropharynx region. These receptors convey the sensory impulses to the deglutition centre present in medulla and pons region of the brain. The returning impulses from the brain lead to closure of larynx with the help of epiglottis, which helps in preventing the passage of food to the respiratory tract. Moreover, the soft palate and uvula also move upward to close nasopharynx and help in preventing the passage of food to the nasal cavity.

(iii) Oesophageal stage: In this step, there is passage of food from oesophagus to stomach through peristalsis.

5. **Stomach:** The stomach is a J-shaped structure and present below the diaphragm. At one side, it is connected to oesophagus and at the other end, it is connected to duodenum (a part of small intestine). The stomach is divided into four main regions i.e. cardia, fundus, body, and pylorus (Figure 3-3). The cardia is connected to oesophagus and this opening is controlled by lower oesophageal sphincter. The rounded and superior portion is called as fundus and the large central portion of the stomach is called as the body. The pylorus portion connects to duodenum and this opening is controlled by smooth muscle sphincter called pyloric sphincter. In some patients, the lower pyloric sphincter fails to relax and hence, food remains in stomach. This condition is called as pylorospasm and it results in vomiting (especially in infants) to relieve pressure.

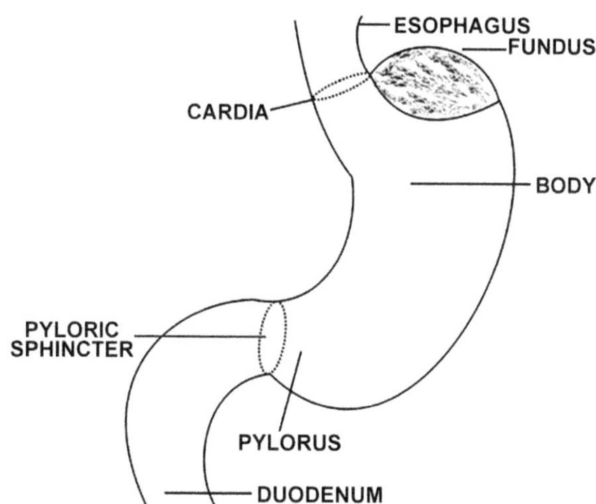

Figure 3-3 Typical structure of stomach showing its different parts

There are two curvatures, lesser curvature and large curvature. The concave border of the stomach is called the lesser curvature and the convex lateral border is called the greater curvature. The rugae are the large folds in the stomach, which can be seen by naked eye. The different types of cells of stomach with secretory functions are described in Table 3-9. The exocrine secretions of stomach are called as gastric juice and about 2-3 litre gastric juice is formed in a day. Gastric juice contains HCL, pepsinogen, intrinsic factor, mucus and gastric lipase etc. The secretion of HCL is stimulated by histamine, gastrin and acetylcholine. The chyme is a soupy liquid formed by mixing of juice with food.

Table 3-9 Exocrine and endocrine cells of stomach along with their functions

Sr. No.	Exocrine cells and functions	Endocrine cells and functions
1.	Mucous neck cells: secrete mucus	G cells: secrete gastrin in blood, which stimulates the secretion of HCL
2.	Parietal cells: secrete HCL and intrinsic factor	
3.	Chief cells: secrete pepsinogen (main), gastric lipase (less)	

6. **Pancreas:** Pancreas is a retroperitoneal gland which lies to the posterior of the greater curvature of stomach. It has three parts i.e. head, body and tail. It is about 12–15 cm long and 2.5 cm thick. Pancreas has both endocrine and exocrine functions, thus, it is also called as heterocrine gland. The most of the cells (about 99%) are acini and these are responsible for exocrine (enzymes) secretions (pancreatic juices).

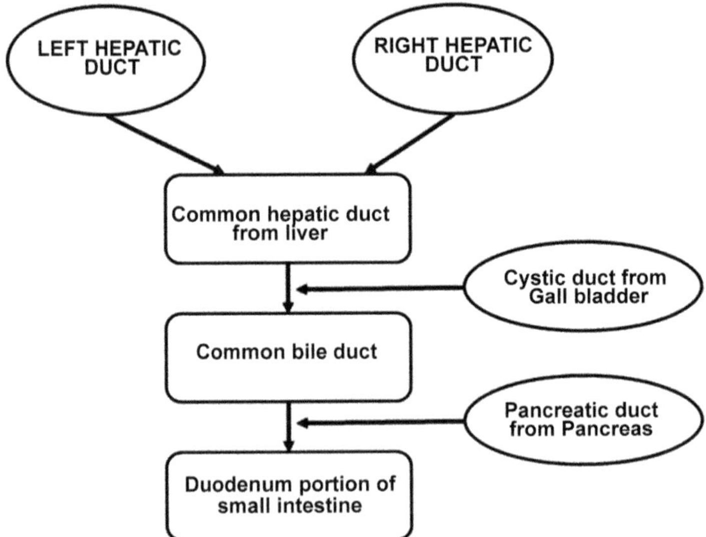

Figure 3-4 Representation of different ducts due to merging of hepatic, cystic and pancreatic ducts.

The remaining 1% cells are called as islets of Langerhans (pancreatic islets) and these are responsible for hormone (endocrine) secretion. The endocrine secretions are passed to the blood, while the exocrine secretions are passed to the small intestine. Pancreas is connected to duodenum of small intestine through hepatopancreatic ampulla (ampulla of Vater), which is guarded by a sphincter called as sphincter of oddi. Indeed, left hepatic duct and right hepatic duct from liver join to form common hepatic duct. The cystic duct arising from gall bladder merges with common hepatic duct to form common bile duct. The duct from pancreas (pancreatic duct) merges with this common bile duct to form hepatopancreatic ampulla, which is connected to duodenum portion of small intestine (Figures 3-4 and 3-5).

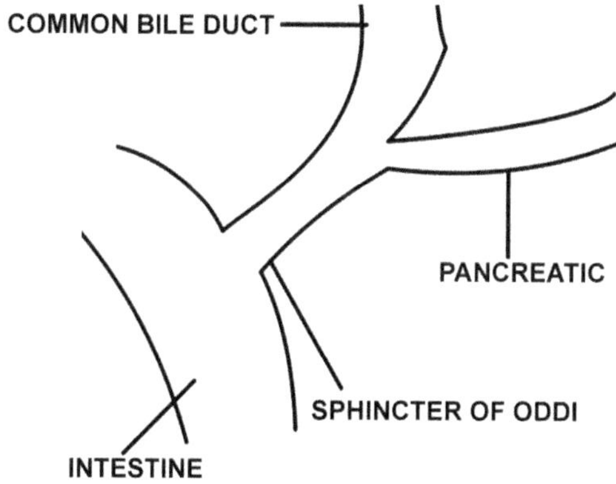

Figure 3-5 Representation of hepatopancreatic ampulla connecting with small intestine and opening controlled by sphincter of oddi.

7. **Small Intestine:** It is a very important part of the GIT as most of the digestion and absorption of food particles take place in this region. It is called as 'small intestine' because it has smaller lumen as compared to 'large intestine'. Small does not mean that it is small in length. Rather it is a very long, about 10 meter in length, which provides a very large surface area. The very long tube is accommodated in a small region because it is tightly coiled. To further enhance the absorptive functions, the surface area is further increased by the presence of circular folds, villi, and microvilli. The small intestine begins at the pyloric sphincter of the stomach and ends by joining with the large intestine.

There are a number of cells present in small intestine with different functions including absorptive cells (help in absorption of nutrients); goblet cells (secrete mucus); intestinal glands (crypts of Lieberkühn) that secrete intestinal juices called succus entericus; paneth cells (secrete lysozyme) and enteroendocrine cells (secrete hormones). These enteroendocrine cells include S cells, CCK cells and K cells, which secrete the secretin, cholecystokinin (CCK) and glucose-dependent insulinotropic peptide (GIP), respectively (Table 3-10).

Table 3-10 Representation of enteroendocrine cells, hormones and their functions

Sr. No.	Cells	Hormone	Functions
1.	S cells	Secretin	Stimulation of pancreatic secretion (major)
			Inhibition of gastric secretions (minor)
2.	CCK cells	Cholecystokinin (CCK)	Stimulation of pancreatic secretion
			Contraction of gall bladder to eject bile
			Relaxation of sphincter of Oddi to allow pancreatic juice and bile to flow into the duodenum
			Slows gastric emptying
			Induces satiety (feeling of fullness)
3.	K cells	Glucose-dependent insulinotropic peptide (GIP)	Stimulate pancreatic beta cells to release insulin

Structurally, small intestine is divided into three portions:

(i) **Duodenum:** It is the shortest part and it is connected to the pyloric sphincter of the stomach. It merges with the jejunum. The meaning of duodenum is "12". It refers to its length and width, which is equivalent to the width of 12 fingers. It also receives secretions through the hepatopancreatic duct. In this region, there are duodenal glands (Brunner's gland) that secrete alkaline mucus and help to neutralize HCL (Table 3-11).

(ii) **Jujenum:** It is about 2 metre in length and it the middle portion of the small intestine.

(iii) **Ileum:** It is the longest portion, about 2 meter in length and it is connected to cecum region of large intestine through ileocecal sphincter. Within the ileum, the aggregated lymphatic follicles called Peyer's patches are present that help in providing immunity.

8. **Large intestine:** It is the terminal portion of GIT. It is connected to ileum portion of small intestine and extends to anus. It is about 1.5 m in length and 6.5 cm in diameter. Structurally, it is divided into four portions (Figure 3-6):

(i) **Cecum:** It is attached to the ileum by ileocecal sphincter. Another small, coiled tube of about 8 cm is also attached to cecum, which is referred to as appendix or vermiform appendix. It is vestigial organ and does not perform any function in humans.

(ii) **Colon:** Cecum merges with large structure of large intestine i.e. colon. It is further divided into four regions i.e. ascending colon, transverse colon, descending colon and sigmoid colon.

(iii) **Retum:** It is about 20 cm in length and is continuous with anus.

(iv) Anus: It is the last portion of large intestine and allows the fecal matter to pass to the exterior. The opening of anus is controlled by two sphincters, external anal (made of skeletal muscle, thus voluntary in nature) and internal anal sphincter (made of smooth muscle, thus involuntary in nature). These sphincters remain close, except during defecation.

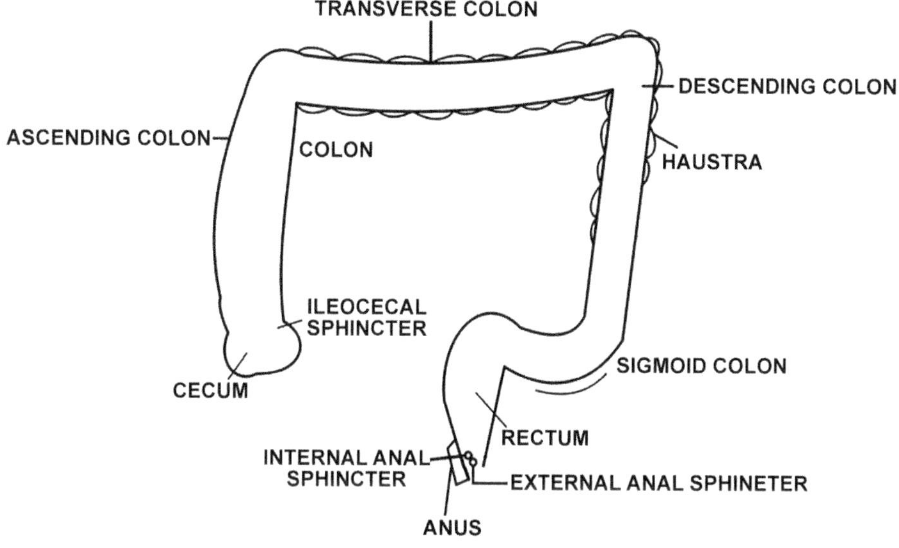

Figure 3-6 Representative structure of large intestine showing its different parts

Enzymes and Other Exocrine Secretions

The digestive function is imparted by the enzymes released from the exocrine glands of the GIT. The different secretions from exocrine glands along with their functions are represented in Table 3-11.

Table 3-11 Representation of different glands, their secretions, function and regulators

Sr. No.	Name of Organs/Glands	Secretions and Functions	Stimulants of secretions
1.	Mouth (Salivary Glands) Parotid, Sub-lingual and Sub-mandibular glands	Secretion is called saliva and it Contains Amylase (ptylin): digestion of carbohydrates Mucus: lubrication of food Chloride ions: stimulates amylase	Para sympathetic nervous system (acetylcholine) Taste, smell of food

Table 3-11 Contd...

Sr. No.	Name of Organs/Glands	Secretions and Functions	Stimulants of secretions
2.	Stomach (Gastric glands)	Gastric Juices with acidic pH (1-2) and it include the followings: HCL released from Parietal cells Make pH Acidic (1-2) Bacteria etc. die in acidic pH Helps in activation of pepsinogen to pepsin	Acetylcholine Gastrin (hormones) released from G cells Histamine
		Intrinsic factor released from Parietal cells Helps in absorption of vitamin B_{12}	
		Pepsinogen released from Chief cells Digest the proteins after its activation to pepsin	
		Gastric lipase released from Chief cells Present in infants but absent in adults Helps in digestion of fat (minor action)	
		Mucus released from mucus cells Provides a protective barrier and protect stomach from acid	
3.	Pancreas (pancreatic glands)	Pancreatic Juices, 1200-1500 ml/day with pH 7.1 to 8.2 with followings components	Food Cholecystokinin (CCK) Secretin
		Pancreatic amylase Digests carbohydrates	
		Trypsinogen Chymotrypsinogen Carboxypeptidase	Digest proteins
		Pancreatic lipase Digests fats	
		DNAase, RNAase	
		Digests nucleic acids	
		Others Water, sodium bicarbonate (provide alkaline pH), ions	

Table 3-11 Contd...

Sr. No.	Name of Organs/Glands	Secretions and Functions	Stimulants of secretions
4.	Intestine (intestinal glands; Crypts of Lieberkühn)	Intestinal secretions containing followings:	Food
		Mucus released from Goblet cells Provide Lubrication	
		Lysozyme from Paneth cells Kills microorganisms	
		Alkaline mucus from duodenal (Brunner's) glands Neutralize acidic content of gastric secretions	
		Maltase, isomaltase, sucrase, lactase and limit dextrinises Digest carbohydrates	
		Aminopeptidase, dipeptidase Digest proteins	
		Intestinal lipase Digest fats	
		Nucleosidases Digest nucleic acid	

Digestion of Carbohydrates

Starch is the major part of diet in humans. Cellulose is present in diet of ruminants e.g. cows, buffalos and it is not digested in humans due to lack of cellulose-digesting enzymes, cellulases. The digestion of carbohydrates in different parts of GIT is explained:

1. **Mouth:** The digestion of starch begins in the mouth with the help of salivary amylase. However, only a small fraction of starch is digested in mouth because food stays in the mouth for a very short period. The digestion of starch by salivary amylase stops, when food enters in the stomach because salivary amylase in inactivated at acidic pH in stomach.

$$\text{Starch} \xrightarrow[\text{Amylase}]{\text{Pancreatic}} \text{Maltose + Isomaltose + Limit dextrins}$$

Due to the formation of maltose and isomaltose, the food becomes sweet in the mouth during chewing.

2. **Stomach:** No digestion of carbohydrates takes place in stomach because of inactivation of salivary amylase in acidic pH and lack of carbohydrate digesting enzyme in gastric secretions.

3. **Small intestine:** The digestion of carbohydrates resumes in the small intestine region due to the presence of enzymes in the pancreatic juices and intestinal secretions.

Pancreatic juice

Pancreatic juice contains pancreatic amylase that acts on starch to chemically break it into smaller components.

$$\text{Starch} \xrightarrow{\text{Pancreatic Amylase}} \text{Maltose + Isomaltose + Alpha dextrin}$$

Intestinal Secretions

The enzymes present in these secretions convert smaller glucose to monomer i.e. glucose or fructose

$$\text{Maltose} \xrightarrow{\text{Maltase}} \text{2 molecules of glucose}$$

$$\text{Isomaltose} \xrightarrow{\text{Isomaltase}} \text{2 molecules of glucose}$$

$$\text{Sucrose} \xrightarrow{\text{Sucrase}} \text{Glucose + Fructose}$$

$$\text{Lactose} \xrightarrow{\text{Lactase}} \text{Glucose + Galactose}$$

$$\text{Alpha dextrin's} \xrightarrow{\text{Dextrinase}} \text{Glucose}$$

Digestion of Proteins

Proteins are made up of amino-acids and thus, different protein digesting enzymes digest to form amino acids. The various processes involved in protein digestion as follows:

1. **Mouth:** Proteins are not digested by in the mouth as there is absence of any protein digesting enzyme in saliva.

2. **Stomach:** Proteins are digested in stomach with the help of enzyme pepsin present in gastric juices.

This enzyme is present in active form i.e. pepsinogen. HCL activates the enzyme pepsinogen to form pepsin. Once pepsin is formed, it starts activating pepsinogen in an autocatalytic reaction. Pepsin acts on proteins to release peptides.

$$\text{Pepsinogen} \xrightarrow{\text{HCL}} \text{Pepsin}$$

(Inactive Enzymes)   (Active)

$$\text{Pepsinogen} \xrightarrow{\text{Pepsin}} \text{Pepsin}$$

$$\text{Autocatalytic Reaction}$$

$$\text{Proteins} \xrightarrow{\text{Pepsin}} \text{Peptides}$$

3. Small Intestine

Pancreatic Juices: The protein digesting enzymes exist in an inactive form. Therefore, these enzymes are activated to form active enzymes and then these active forms of enzymes digest proteins. Trypsinogen is acted upon by enterkinase (enzyme of small intestine) to form trypsin. Thereafter, trypsin activates trypsinogen in an autocatalytic reaction. Moreover, trypsin also activates two other protein digesting enzymes released from pancreas i.e. chymotrypsinogen, procarboxypeptidase to form chymotrypsin and carboxypeptidase, respectively. All these three enzymes act on different types of proteins to form peptides.

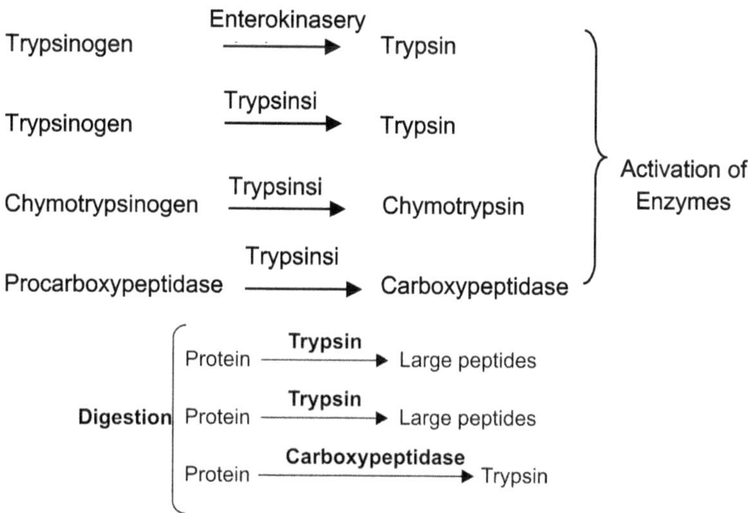

Intestinal Secretions: The protein digestion is completed by two peptidases present on the walls of small intestine i.e. aminopeptidase and dipeptidase. Aminopeptidase removes the amino acid at the amino end of the peptide. Dipeptidase cleaves dipeptides to form amino acids.

$$\text{Peptides} \xrightarrow{\text{Aminopeptidase}} \text{Amino acids + Smaller peptides}$$

$$\text{Dipeptides} \xrightarrow{\text{Dipeptidase}} \text{Amino acids}$$

Digestion of Fats

Fat is triglyceride i.e. it is made of glycerol molecule and three fatty acids (Figure 3-7). Thus, digestion of fat would yield three fatty acids and glycerol.

$$H_2C{-}OH \qquad COOH\text{-}R_1$$
$$CH{-}OH \quad + \quad COOH\text{-}R_2 \quad \longrightarrow$$
$$H_2C{-}OH \qquad COOH\text{-}R_3$$

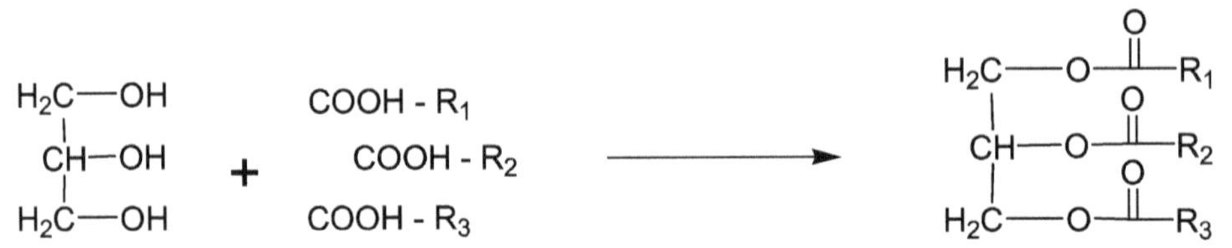

Glycerol   3 Fatty acids   Triglycerol (Fat)

Figure 3-7 Structure of fat

(i)   **In Mouth and Stomach:** The digestion of fat does not initiate in mouth or stomach because of very insignificant amounts of lingual lipase (mouth) and gastric lipase (stomach).

(ii) **Small Intestine:** The digestion starts in small intestine with the help of pancreatic lipase (major) and intestinal lipase that convert fats into fatty acids and glycerol. Since fats are not soluble in water, therefore, these cannot be directly acted upon by water soluble lipases. Accordingly, there is a need of bile salts to break larger fat globules into smaller fat molecules (about 1 µm) and this process is called as emulsification. This process of emulsification is done using bile salts (components of bile). The bile salts are the sodium and potassium salts of bile acids (chenodeoxycholic acid and cholic acid). Bile salts are amphipathic in nature i.e. bile salts have both hydrophobic (nonpolar, water insoluble, lipid soluble) and hydrophilic (polar, water soluble, lipid insoluble) portions. The hydrophobic portion of bile salts interacts with the big lipid globules, while the hydrophilic portion of bile salts interacts with the watery intestinal chyme. It leads to significant reduction in surface tension. Consequently, the large lipid globule is broken down to several small lipid globules during emulsification. Due to very small size of fat molecules (after emulsification), there is an increase in surface area and water soluble lipases can act on fat molecules to form fatty acids and glycerol (Figure 3-8).

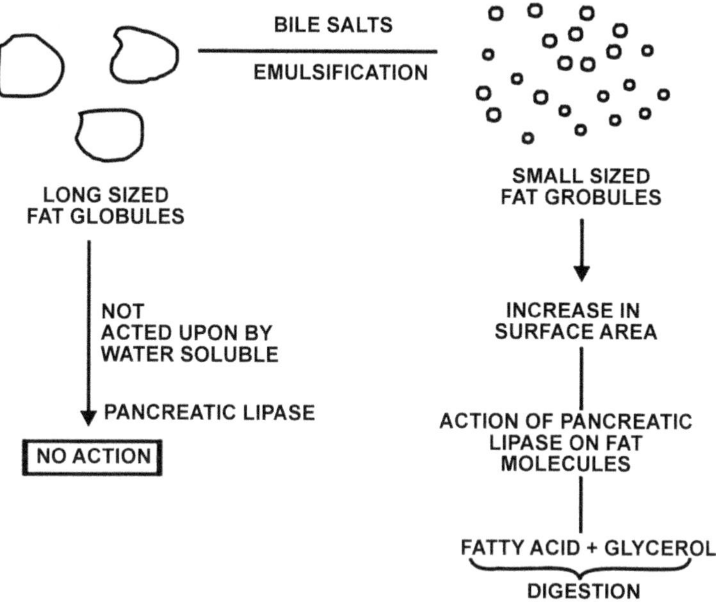

Figure 3-8 Representation of fat emulsification with the help of bile salts, which helps in its digestion with pancreatic lipase.

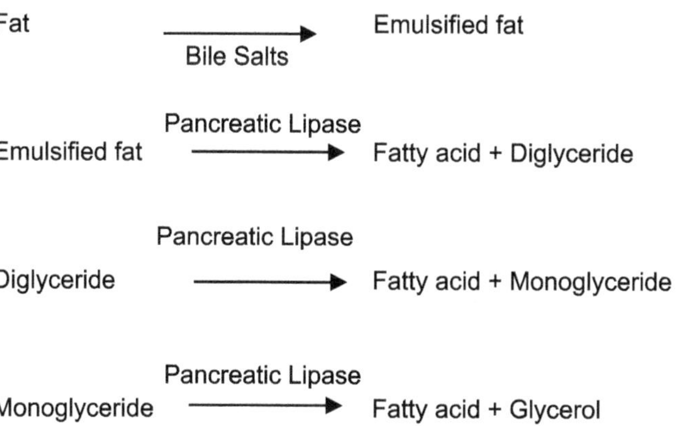

Bile

Bile is a yellowish- brown liquid which is secreted by hepatocytes of liver. After secretion, bile moves to gall bladder and it is stored in it till its release in the small intestine. About 800–1000 mL of bile is produced each daily by hepatocytes.

Composition

It consists of water, bile salts, bile pigments, cholesterol, lecithin (phospholipid) and several ions. The pH of bile is around 7.6–8.6. The main bile pigment is bilirubin, which provides colour to bile. Bile salts are sodium and potassium salts of chenodeoxycholic acid and cholic acid. The bilirubin is secreted into the bile and broken down in the intestine to form stercobilin, which provides the normal brown color to feces.

Functions of Bile in GIT

1. Bile salts help in emulsification of fat and emulsified fats are digested with lipase (Figure 3-8).
2. Bile salts also help in absorption of digested fat molecules by forming micelles (discussed below).

Liver

Liver is the largest gland and second largest organ of human body. It weighs approx. 1.2-1.8 kg and is located in the upper right corner of the abdomen.

External Structure: Liver is covered with two membranes i.e. outer membrane (also called as serous capsule) and inner membrane (Glisson's capsule). It mainly consists of four different lobes i.e. left, right, caudate, and quadrate lobes. The right lobe is 5-6 times larger than the left lobe and both are separated by falciform ligament. From the posterior side of the right lobe, the small caudate and quadrate lobe extends and gets wrap around the inferior vena cava and gall bladder, respectively. From the right and left lobe, right and left hepatic duct arises and these ducts join to form common hepatic duct. Further, from gall bladder cystic duct arises and it joins with common hepatic duct to form bile duct. From pancreas, pancreatic duct arises and it joins with bile duct to from hepatopancreatic ampulla.

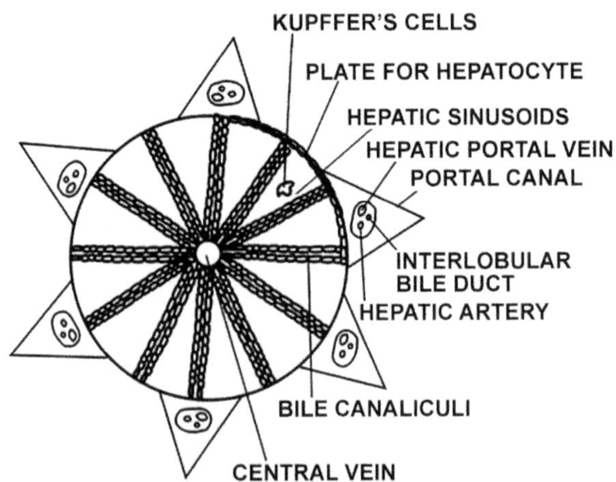

Figure 3-9 Structure of liver showing central vein along with plates of hepatocytes and portal triad.

Internal Structure

The inner membrane (Glisson's capsule) extends inward and divides the liver into number of hepatic lobules. These lobules are structural and functional units of liver. These lobules appear hexagonal and each lobule is made of liver cells called hepatocytes. The hepatocytes form plates and arranged around a central vein in radial pattern. A central vein is a hepatic vein, which is present in the centre of lobules. Hepatic sinusoids are the spaces between the plates. The sinusoids are filled with blood and blood passes through them. The sinusoids are internally lined with incomplete layer of endothelial cells. The narrow space exists between the plate of hepatic cells and endothelial cells. This space is called perisinusoidal space of disse. The network of tubular spaces between the hepatic cells is called bile canaliculi (bile capillaries) (Figures 3-9 and 3-10).

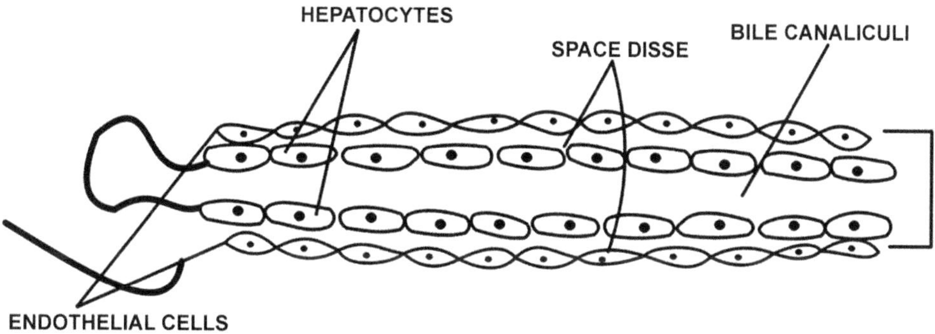

Figure 3-10 Representation of hepatocytes and endothelial cell forming hepatic plate, space of disse and bile canaliculi.

These contain bile that is secreted by the liver cells. Bile canaliculi open into small Herring's canals, which in turn open into interlobular bile duct. At the regular intervals of hepatic lobules, the portal canals are present. Portal canal contain hepatic portal vein, hepatic artery and interlobular bile duct. In hepatic sinusoids, two types of cells are present, Kupffer and fat storing cells. Kupffer cells are hepatic macrophages and their major function is phagocytosis i.e. eating worm out RBC, WBC or bacteria. The fat storing cells are also called stellate cells and their main function is storage of fats.

The blood enters the liver from two different sources i.e. hepatic artery and hepatic portal vein. The hepatic artery carrying oxygenated blood comes from aorta and enters the liver. While the hepatic portal vein carrying deoxygenated blood comes from small intestine and enters the liver. The blood is rich in nutrients absorbed from intestine. The blood from both hepatic artery and portal vein enters into sinusoids. From sinusoids, the blood enters into central vein and the blood flows from central vein to hepatic vein (Figure 3-11).

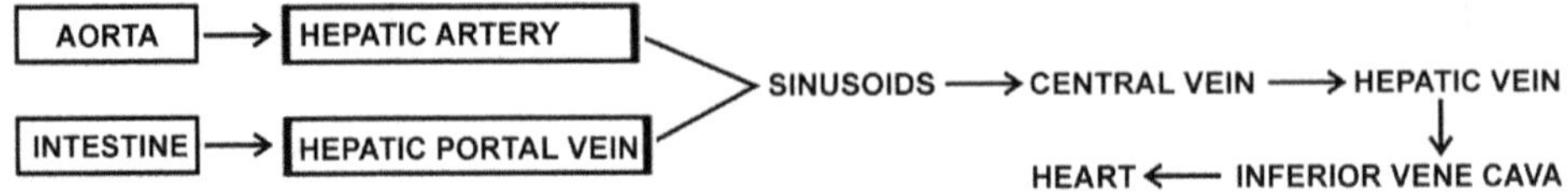

Figure 3-11 Direction of blood flow from heart and intestine to liver and from liver to heart to complete the circulation

Functions of liver

Secretion of Bile: Hepatocytes (Liver cells) secretes bile that is stored in the gall bladder. Bile helps to break down fats (emulsification) in the small intestine during digestion and also help in absorption of fatty material through micelle formation.

Synthesis of Proteins

The liver cells plays a key role in the synthesis of all plasma proteins including albumin, transferrin, globulins (except γ-globulins), lipoprotein, ceruloplasmin, α- antotrypsin, fibrinogen, prothrombins and clotting factors.

Deamination: Liver cause deamination of amino acids (i.e. removal of $-NH_2$ group) and remaining part is reused for conversion to ATP, fat or carbohydrates. It converts the harmful ammonia (results from deamination of excess amino acid) into urea and this urea is excreted via urinary system.

Detoxification: The toxic and harmful substances are converted to harmless substances in liver like drugs.

Phagocytosis of bacteria: Within the liver, blood passes through spaces called sinusoids. Kupffer's cells are special type of liver cells, which are located in the sinusoids and these carry out phagocytosis of bacteria, antigens (foreign matter) and worn out RBC.

Major centre of metabolism (Catabolism and anabolism): Liver is the major site for metabolism. Various reactions occur in liver including

Lipogenesis: Formation of fat from excessive glucose and protein

Glycogenesis: Formation of glycogen from excessive glucose

Glycogenolysis: Breakdown of glycogen to release glucose

Gluconeogenesis: Formation of glucose from non-glucose substance (amino acids)

Excretory function

The excretory product of proteins and haemoglobin i.e. urea, bilirubin and biliverdin, respectively are excreted by the liver.

Storage of vitamins and minerals

The liver store large number of chemicals which are released according to their need in the body including vitamins A, D, E, K, B_{12} and minerals such as copper and iron

Osmoregulation

The liver produces a protein angiotensinogen which in turn is broken up by renin (an enzyme produced in the kidney) to form angiotensin I. Angiotensin I is converted in to angiotensin II by angiotensin converting enzymes. Further, Angiotensin II stimulates the secretion of the hormone aldosterone from the adrenal cortex which helps in osmoregulation in maintaining proper quantity of H_2O and electrolytes in the body.

Absorption of Nutrients

Absorption is the process in which digested nutrients pass from the alimentary canal to the blood or lymph. The nutrients are absorbed in the monomeric form i.e. amino acids (derived from proteins), glucose (derived from starch), fatty acid and glycerol (derived from fats) etc. The major absorption occurs in the small intestine region due to the presence of villi and microvilli, which increase the surface area.

Absorption of Amino Acids and Glucose

Amino acids and glucose are absorbed by the secondary active transport i.e. energy is utilized for their absorption from the lumen of small intestine. In this secondary active transport, energy is used to pump three sodium ions outside the cells and two potassium ions inside the cells at basolateral membrane. Thus, there is creation of sodium gradient, which drives the movement of sodium from lumen to the cells through luminal membrane. Along with the movement of sodium, amino acid and glucose are also transported. On the luminal walls of small intestine, there is sodium-amino acid cotransporter, which allows the passage of both sodium ions and amino acids from lumen. Similarly, glucose is absorbed by sodium-glucose cotransporter, which allows the movement of both glucose and sodium ions from lumen to cell (Figure 3-12) (Table 3-12). Galactose is also absorbed in a similar way as that of glucose, but the process of galactose absorption is much faster.

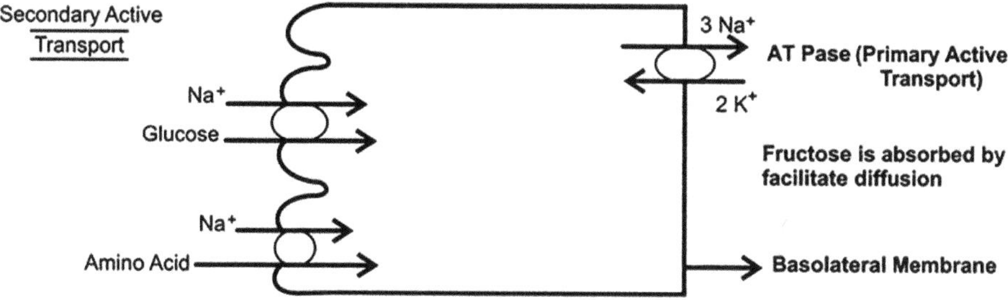

Figure 3-12 Representation of absorption of glucose and amino acids from small intestine using secondary active transport

Absorption of Fatty acids and Glycerol

These are water insoluble in nature; therefore, these cannot be absorbed directly. These are absorbed with the help of bile salts. In other words, bile salts helps in absorption of fat-soluble substances. Bile salts aggregate to form small, spherical, water-soluble droplets called micelles. Fatty substances are solubilized in the centre of these micelles. These micelles act as carries and carry fatty substances from the lumen to the intestinal cells (Figure 3-13). The fatty acid and glycerol are absorbed by intestinal cell and empty micelles are left. These empty micelles return to lumen to carry more fatty substances and this process continues. Inside the intestinal cell, the fatty acids and glycerol combine to from fat. Thereafter, these are packed by the proteins to form chylomicrons. These chylomicrons are passed to the lymphatic capillaries, called as lacteals (Figure 3-14). Thereafter, the chylomicrons are delivered by lacteals to the blood. The fat soluble vitamins are also absorbed in a similar way.

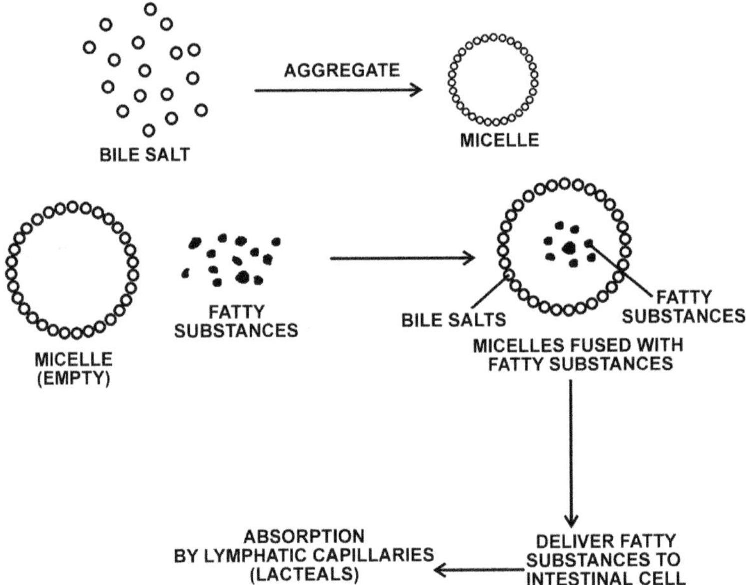

Figure 3-13 Representation of micelle formation using bile salts, which act as carriers to transport fatty material to intestinal cells.

Absorption of Water and Water-soluble Vitamins

Absorption of electrolytes and nutrient develops osmotic pressure and thus, absorption of H_2O takes place by osmosis (passive process, without ATP). Absorption of water soluble vitamin B and C takes place through diffusion. However, absorption of vitamin B_{12} requires the presence of intrinsic factor.

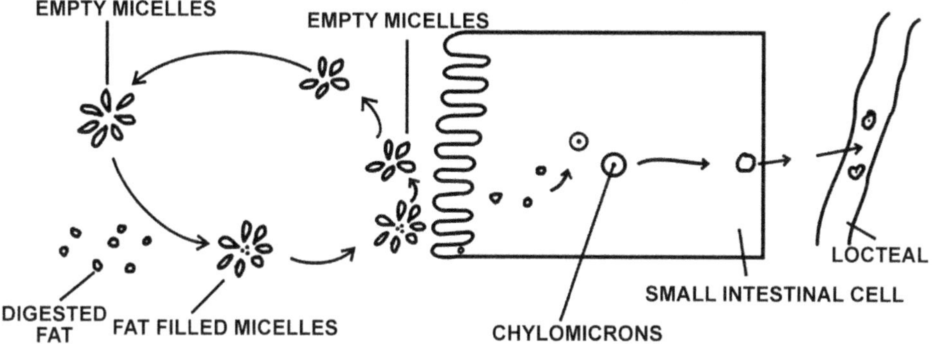

Figure 3-14 Representation of recycling of micelles transporting fatty material to intestinal cells, where fatty materials are converted to chylomicrons and thereafter, absorbed by lacteals.

Absorption of Electrolytes

Sodium ions are absorbed by sodium-amino acid cotransporters and sodium-glucose-cotransporters in an active process. Absorption of calcium is regulated by hormones i.e. its absorption is enhanced in the presence of parathormone and vitamin D.

Table 3-12 Summarized points related to absorption of different nutrients

Sr. No.	Nutrients	Region	Characteristic features
1.	Glucose	Small Intestine	Absorption using sodium-glucose cotransporter in an active process
2.	Amino Acids	Small Intestine	Absorption using sodium-amino acid cotransporter in an active process
3.	Fatty acids	Small Intestine	Absorption with the help of bile salts to form micelles, which pass to fatty substances to intestinal cell
4.	Water	Small and large Intestine	Most of absorption in small intestine in a passive manner

Role of Large Intestine in Digestion and Absorption

The key points related to functions of large intestine may be explained as below:

1. There are no digestive enzymes present in large intestine, hence there is no digestion in this region of GIT.
2. There are a number of bacteria residing in the large intestine. These bacteria perform fermentation of the remaining food and form gases in colon, which result in flatulence.

3. The resident bacteria also result in the formation of vitamin K and vitamin B, which are absorbed and used by body

4. Its major function is absorption of water. About 90% of water is absorbed in small intestine and the large intestine absorbs the remaining water. Thus, it is very important for maintaining the water balance in the body.

5. It helps in the formation of semi-solid feces. Indeed, when chyme remains in the large intestine for 3-10 hours, water is reabsorbed and semi-solid mass is formed, which is called feces. Thereafter, feces are expelled from anus.

Feces and Defecation Reflex

Feces are the waste materials and elimination of fecal material from the alimentary canal through anus is called egestion. The undigested food is passed from small intestine to large intestine by peristalsis. The undigested food passes into colon. The colon absorbs most of water and electrolytes from this food and the remaining semi-solid waste is called as feces. The color of feces is light brown due to presence of stercobilinogen and stercobilin, which are derived from bilirubin (bile pigment).

As the fecal matter passes from the sigmoid colon into rectum, there is distention of rectum. It leads to initiation of defecation relex to expel fecal matter from anus to exterior. The distention of walls of rectum leads to stimulation of

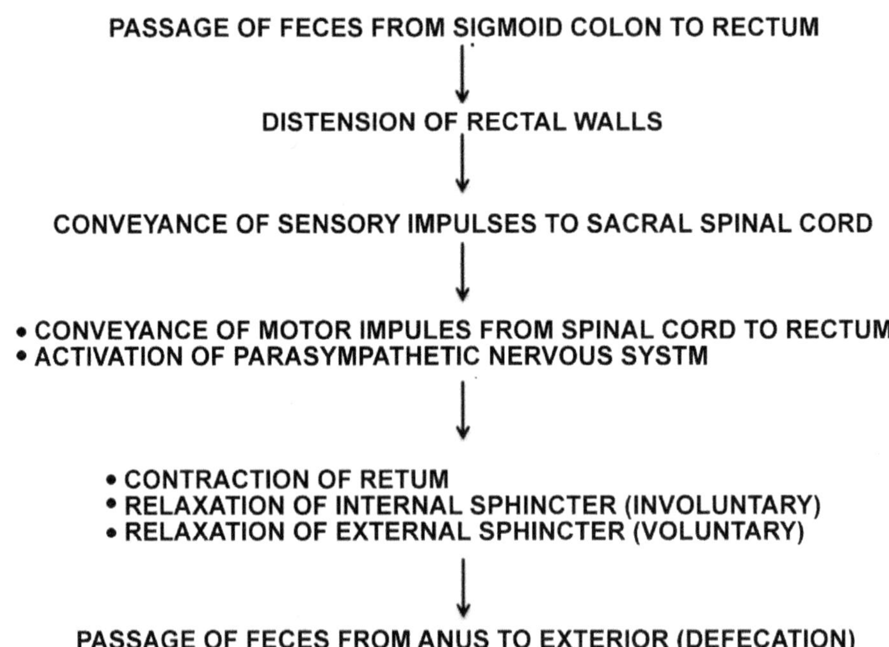

Figure 3-15 Different steps involved in defection reflex.

stretch receptors, which help in passing the sensory impulses to the sacral spinal cord. The motor impulses pass from the spinal cord to the rectum. These motor impulses along the activation of the parasympathetic nerves lead to contraction of rectum followed by voluntary contraction of abdominal muscle and diaphragm. Thereafter, there is opening of internal anal sphincter (involuntary process due to smooth muscles). External anal sphincter is voluntarily controlled and if this sphincter is relaxed, defecation occurs (Figure 3-15). However, if external sphincter is contracted, defecation is delayed and fecal matter moves backwards.

Mobility of GIT

There are significant movements in the GIT and two major types of motilities include: Peristalsis

These are the involuntary muscular movements controlled by autonomic nervous system (mainly parasympathetic nervous system) and enteric nervous system. The characteristic feature of peristalsis is the alternate contraction and relaxation, which spreads in the form of wave down the GIT. The peristaltic movements cause forward movements of food from oesophagus to   stomach and then to small intestine and large intestine.

Swallowing

It is also called deglutition and it is the process during which food present in the mouth passes from pharynx to oesophagus. It is explained in detailed above in deglutition section.

Gross and Physiological Calorific Value

Nutrients are metabolized to give energy and the energy is calculated in terms of calorie. 1 calorie is amount of energy required to raise body temperature of 1g of water by 1 degree at normal atmosphere pressure. The physiologic calorific value

Table 3-13 Key differences between two different types of calorific values

Sr. No.	Gross calorific value (GCV)	Physiological calorific value (PV)
1.	It is the amount of energy produced during combustion of 1 gm of food in calorimeter in laboratory	It is the amount of energy produced during oxidation of 1gm of food inside the body
2.	It is more than physiologic value	It is less than gross calorific value
3.	GVC for: Carbohydrates- 4.1 kcal/g Protein- 5.65 kcal/g Fat- 9.45 kcal/g	PV for: Carbohydrates- 4.0 kcal/g Protein- 4.0 kcal/g Fat- 9 kcal/g

of fat is more (almost double) than carbohydrates. It means metabolism of one molecule of fatty acid gives more energy than one molecule of glucose. The calorific value may be of two types, gross and physiological and the key differences are explained in Table 3-13.

Diseases of GIT

1. **Peptic Ulcers:** Peptic ulcer refers to a breach in mucosa in the GIT, which extends from mucosa to deep into sub-mucosa layer and sometimes, even to serosa. In erosion, there is just a superficial breach of mucosa and it remains confined in that region only (Figure 3-16).

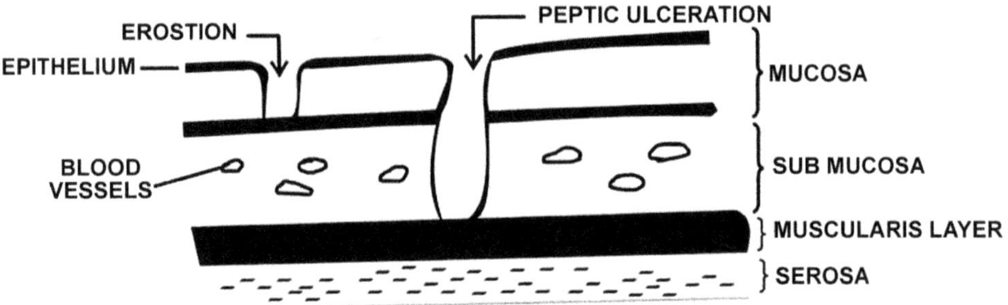

Figure 3-16 Difference in peptic ulcer and erosion

Peptic ulcers are of two types:

(i) **Duodenal Ulcers:** These ulcers are present in the duodenum portion of small intestine and these ulcers result from increased gastric emptying. Therefore, duodenum is exposed to higher gastric contents. Usually, there is a nocturnal pain, which starts 1 to 3 hours after meal. The pain is relieved by taking food (Table 3-14).

(ii) **Gastric Ulcers:** These are less common and are located on the lesser curvature of stomach. These are not due to increase in gastric secretions or HCL. Actually, the defense system of stomach is weakened and there is reduced protective covering of mucus around the stomach. In this type, pain is exaggerated by taking food (Table 3-14).

Table 3-14 Key differences between duodenal and gastric ulcers

Sr. No.	Duodenal ulcers	Gastric ulcers
1.	These are located in upper part of small intestine	These are located in stomach
2.	An increase in gastric emptying may be responsible	A decrease in mucus covering (defense) may be responsible
3.	Pain is relieved by food intake	Pain is exaggerated by food intake

2. **Inflammatory bowel disease (IBD):** Inflammatory bowel disease refers to a group of idiopathic, inflammatory conditions that are characterized by persistent inflammation of colon, rectum and/or ileum. The most common symptoms include appearance of blood and mucus in stool. There may also be a state of bloody diarrhea. There may be lower abdominal cramping, which gets very intense during the passage of stool. Abdominal pain, vomiting, diarrhea, rectal bleeding, severe cramps/muscle spasms in the region of the pelvis are the typical features of ulcerative colitis. IBD is of two types, ulcerative colitis and Crohn's disease.

   (i) **Ulcerative Colitis:** There is inflammation of the colon portion of the large intestine. Along with colon, rectum is also affected in this disease. The inflammation is restricted to the superficial mucosa of intestinal portions.

   (ii) **Crohn's Disease:** In this type, any segment of GIT may be affected, however in majority of cases; the terminal ileum of small intestine is affected. In contrast to ulcerative colitis, the entire thickness of the bowel wall may be affected in Crohn's disease. Due to the involvement of full thickness of bowel wall, there are chances of development of perianal disease eg, fistulas (a hole between different parts of the digestive tract) (Table 3-15).

Table 3-15 Key differences between duodenal and gastric ulcers

Sr. No.	Ulcerative Colitis	Crohn's Disease
1.	Inflammation of colon and rectum	Inflammation of any segment of the gut, however in majority of cases, the terminal ileum is affected
2.	Superficial mucosa of intestinal portion is affected	Entire thickness of the bowel is affected and these are transmural lesions
3.	Less chances of fistula formation	More chances of fistula as a complication
4.	Most common symptoms include blood and mucus in stool along with diarrhea	Initial symptoms include abdominal pain, particularly after eating

3. **Mumps:** In some patients, there may be swelling and enlargement of parotid glands in response to viral infection and this painful condition is called as Mumps. It generally affects children and is self-healing disease. In very severe conditions, antiviral agents may be used.

4. **Ankyloglossia:** Normally, the tongue is attached to the floor of mouth by lingual frenulum. Some persons have short or rigid frenulum and persons are not able to speak properly. These persons are called "tongue tied". A medical term for this condition is ankyloglossia.

5. **Hiatus hernia:** There is an opening called esophageal hiatus through which oesophagus pierces the diaphragm and opens in the superior part of stomach.

Sometimes, the upper part of stomach moves upwards through hiatus, i.e. above diaphragm and this condition is called as hiatus hernia.

6. **Gastroesophageal reflux disease (GERD):** There is a lower oesophageal sphincter between the lower end of oesophagus and upper end of stomach. It prevents the backward movement of gastric content from stomach to oesophagus. However in some patients, the lower oesophageal sphincter does not work and fail to close properly. As a result, the contents of stomach (HCL and enzyme) move backward towards oesophagus to produce burning sensation, which is also called as "heart burn" or gastroesophageal reflux disease (GERD).

7. **Pernicious Anemia:** In this disease, there is a deficiency of intrinsic factor due to damage to parietal cells of stomach. Therefore, vitamin B_{12} is not absorbed from GIT. The deficiency of vitamin B_{12} results in the formation of large, immature RBC (megaloblasts). The resulting anemia is called as pernicious anemia.

8. **Tonsillitis:** This is the state of infection and inflammation of palantine tonsils. It leads to sore throat. Sometimes, tonsils are removed with surgery called tonsillectomy.

9. **Appendicitis:** The inflammation of appendix is called as appendicitis and it leads to intense pain in abdomen. In this condition, surgical removal of appendix is done to prevent spreading of infection and overcome pain.

10. **Piles or haemorrhoids:** The dilation (enlargement) of veins in the anus is termed as piles. The haemorrhage can occur during defection and hence, it leads to bleeding.

11. **Gall stones:** The formation of stones in the gall bladder is called as cholelithiasis. The stones are composed of cholesterol and calcium salts. In some patients, due to excessive cholesterol and insufficient quantity of bile salts or lecithin, there is a crystallization of cholesterol to form crystals in the gall bladder. These crystals may solidify and appear like stone and these are referred to as gall stones. The presence of stones may be a very painful condition. Cholecystectomy i.e. the surgical removal of gall bladder is usually done in case of gall stone formation, if these stones cannot be removed by any other means.

12. **Jaundice:** An increase in the bilirubin concentration in the blood is called as jaundice. The bilirubin is a breakdown product of hemoglobin and excessive production of bilirubin (may be due to excessive hemolysis, breakdown of hemoglobin) may lead to jaundice. The characteristic feature of jaundice is appearance of yellow color due to excessive presence of bilirubin the body. Due to gall stone, the bile flow is obstructed the bile remains in liver and hence, diffuses into blood. This type of jaundice is called obstructive jaundice.

13. **Cholecystitis:** The inflammation of gall bladder is called cholecystitis. Sometimes, gall bladder is surgically removed and process is called cholecystectomy.

14. **Lactose intolerance:** Lactose is present mainly in milk and normally, it is digested by an enzyme lactase to form glucose and galactose. In the absence of lactase, lactose is not digested and fermentation of lactose takes place in the large intestine region due to resident bacteria. Fermentation of lactose results in the production of gas, which leads to flatulence, bloating, intestinal cramps and diarrhoea. These persons should avoid milk, instead they should consume yoghurt or curd.

15. **Peritonitis:** The inflammation of the peritoneal cavity is called as peritonitis. The bacteria may enter through the cavity either through some accidents or through surgical wounds in abdomen. The rupturing of appendix may lead to life threatening peritonitis.

16. **Ascites:** The accumulation of excess fluid in the peritoneal cavity is called ascites. It may occur during generalized edema.

17. **Protein Energy Malnutrition (PEM):** It is the malnutrition in growing children in which diet is unable to meet the demands of body. It is 2 types, Kwashiorkor and marasmus (Table 3-16).

    (i) **Kwashiorkor:** The diet may contain sufficient amount of fat and carbohydrates. However, diet is very poor in proteins. The disease develops between the age of 6 months to 3 years of age. The symptoms include reduced body growth, swollen bellies (abdomen), fading of colour of hair, reduction in resistance to fight with infection in the body, development of diarrhoea, development of edema (accumulation of fluid), swelling of body parts (due to edema), anaemia and mental retardation.

    (ii) **Marasmus:** The diet is deficient in proteins as well other nutrients like carbohydrates and fats. It generally occurs due to less diet intake. It develops in infants under age of one. It is more common than kwashiorkor. The body is lean and weak; skin becomes thin, dry and wrinkled; fat disappears from the body surface; ribs become prominent and there is no edema or swelling.

Table 3-16 Key differences between Kwashiorkor and marasmus

Sr. No.	Kwashiorkor	Marasmus
1.	There is edema and swelling	There is no edema, no swelling
2.	It occurs in the age group of 6 months to 3 years	It is more common below 1 year of age
3.	The diet has enough carbohydrates and fat. But it is poor in proteins	The diet is poor in all nutrients
4.	The diet intake is generally normal	The diet intake is very poor
5.	These symptoms are not present. Rather there is swelling of abdomen.	There is disappearance of fat, thinning of body and prominence of ribs (due to very weak body)

3.2 Chapter at a Glance

Term	Description
GIT	Gastrointestinal tract
Mucosa	The innermost lining of GIT and facing towards lumen
Enteric nervous system	The local nervous system, which controls the functions of GIT
Myenteric plexus	The group of neurons present in muscularis layer and control GIT motility, and peristalsis
Sub Submucosal plexus	Present in submucosa and control secretions in GIT
Deciduous teeth	Temporary (milk) teeth
Deglutition	The passage of food from mouth to stomach by act of swallowing
Parietal cells	Secrete HCL and intrinsic factor
Chief Cells	Secrete pepsinogen
Crypts of Lieberkühn	Intestinal glands that secrete secrete intestinal juices called succus entericus
Peyer's patches	The aggregated lymphatic follicles in ileum that provide immunity.
Emulsification	The process of breaking larger fat globules into smaller fat molecules with the help of bile salts
Glycogenesis	The formation of glycogen from excessive glucose
Glycogenolysis	The breakdown of glycogen to release glucose
Gluconeogenesis	The formation of glucose from non-glucose substance (amino acids)
Egestion	The elimination of fecal material from the alimentary canal through anus
Peristalsis	The involuntary movements in GIT that propel the food movement in forward direction

Exercises

Multiple Choice Questions

1. Which of following has highest calorific value?
    (a) fats
    (b) carbohydrates
    (c) vitamins
    (d) minerals

2. In which of following pain is relived by taking food?
   (a) Gastric ulcer
   (b) Duodenal ulcer
   (c) IBD
   (d) All the above

3. Increase in bilirubin is found in
   (a) Gall stones   (b) hemolysis
   (c) Jaundice   (d) all the above

4. Which of following is absorbed in a passive manner?
   (a) glucose   (b) water
   (c) sodium   (d) amino acid

5. Which of following has highly acidic pH?
   (a) salivary secretions   (b) oesophageal secretions
   (c) gastric secretions   (d) small intestinal secretions

6. Which of following takes place in liver problems?
   (a) increase in bleeding   (b) edema
   (c) increase in urea   (d) all the above

7. Which of following is absorbed as chylomicrons?
   (a) minerals   (b) vitamins
   (c) fats   (d) amino acids

8. Retroperitoneal organs are covered by peritoneum from
   (a) anterior side   (b) posterior side
   (c) lateral side   (d) not covered from any side

9. Which plexus is involved in controlling secretions?
   (a) Myenteric plexus   (b) plexus of Auerbach
   (c) submucosal plexus   (d) none of above

10. Which of following is released by chief cells of stomach?
    (a) Vitamin B12   (b) HCL
    (c) pepsin   (d) both a and b

Very Short Answer Questions

1. What is the role of bile salts in fat absorption?
2. What are lacteals? What are their functions?
3. How are pancreatic enzymes responsible for protein digestion activated?
4. What is physiological calorific value?
5. What is jaundice?
6. What is the role of liver in blood clotting?
7. What do you mean by peptic ulcers?
8. What is the role of parasympathetic nervous system in GIT?

9. What is the role of submucosal plexuses?

10. Write the functions of cholecystokinin.

Short Answer Questions

1. Explain the nervous system controlling GIT.
2. Explain the role of bile salts in fat digestion and absorption.
3. Explain the process of carbohydrate digestion.
4. Explain defecation reflex.
5. Explain the deglutition process.

Long Answer Questions

1. Explain the key structural features of oesophagus, stomach and large intestine.
2. Explain the structure of liver with suitable diagram along with important functions.
3. Write important enzymes and hormones released in GIT.

Bibliography

Costanzo LS. Physiology. 4th Edition. Lippincott Williams & Wilkins.

Guyton AC, Hall JE. Textbook of Medical Physiology. 11th Edition. Elsevier Saunders. 2006.

Jaggi AS, Bali A, Singh N. Pathophysiology. 1st Edition. Vallabh Prakashan. 2019.

Jain AK. Human Anatomy and Physiology for Pharmacy. 3rd Edition. Arya publications. 2017.

Lodish H, Berk A, Kaiser CA. Molecular Cell Biology. 6th Edition. W. H. Freeman & Co Ltd. 2007.

Tortora GJ, Derrickson B. Principles of Anatomy and Physiology. 15th Edition. John Wiley and Sons, Inc. 2017.

Waugh A, Grant A. Ross and Wilson Anatomy and Physiology in Health and Illness. 12th Edition. Churchill Livingstone. 2014.

Answer Key MCQs				
1. (a)	2. (b)	3. (d)	4. (b)	5. (c)
6. (d)	7. (c)	8. (a)	9. (c)	10. (c)

Energetics

After completing this lesson, the Reader should be able to understand:

- *Adenosine Triphosphate (Introduction)*
- *Formation of ATP*
- *Cellular respiration (Aerobic respiration)*
- *Anaerobic respiration*
- *Energy yield in aerobic and anaerobic respiration*
- *Functions of ATP*
- *Creatine Phosphate*
- *Formation of Creatine phosphate*
- *Elimination of Creatine Phosphate*
- *Advantages of Creatine phosphate*
- *Disadvantages of Creatine phosphate*
- *Basal Metabolic Rate (BMR)*
- *Factors affecting BMR*
- *Significance of BMR*

4.1   Introduction

Adenosine triphosphate is also known as ATP, is a biomolecule that carries energy within cells. ATP is the main energy currency of cells (**Figure 4-1**). It is an end product of photophosphorylation, cellular respiration and fermentation. ATP is used by all living things. It is also used in signal transduction pathways for cell communication and is incorporated into deoxyribonucleic acid (DNA) during DNA synthesis.

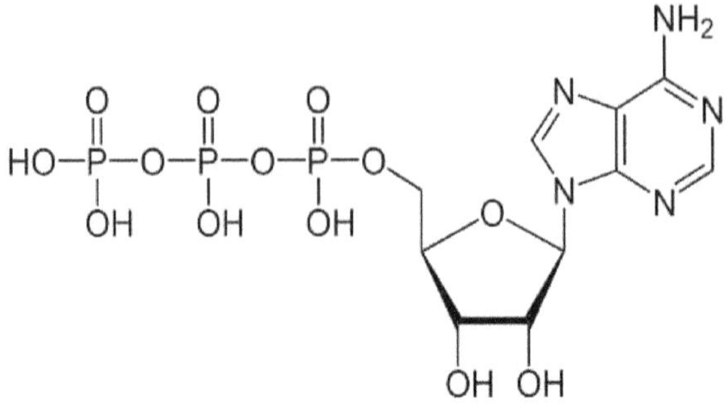

Figure 4-1 Structure of ATP

The structure of ATP is built by carbon, nitrogen, hydrogen, oxygen, and phosphorus. It is a nucleotide that contains three main structures. They are

1. Nitrogenous base, adenine
2. The sugar moiety, ribose
3. A chain of three phosphate groups bound to ribose.

The actual power source of ATP is its phosphate tail. High energy is stored in the bonds between the phosphates. This energy is needed when ATP is broken by addition of water molecule by a process called hydrolysis. Usually the outer phosphate is removed from ATP to yield energy. During this process ATP is converted into adenosine diphosphate (ADP), the nucleotide which has only two phosphates.

When a phosphate group is removed enzymatically from ATP, it leads to the formation of ADP and also releases a huge amount of energy. This energy is used by the cell in several metabolic processes and also in the synthesis of macromolecules such as proteins. There is release of further energy when a second phosphate group is removed from ATP and there is also the formation of adenosine monophosphate (AMP). If the organism doesn't need the energy, the phosphate group is added back to AMP and ADP to form ATP. This can be hydrolyzed later when energy is needed. Therefore ATP functions as a reliable energy source for cellular pathways.

Formation of ATP

ADP and phosphate ions combine in the cell to form the ATP. These reactions are carried out by a group of coenzymes. There are three important coenzymes namely,

1. Nicotinamide adenine dinucleotide (NAD)
2. Nicotinamide adenine dinucleotide phosphate (NADP)
3. Flavin adenine dinucleotide (FAD)

The structure of NAD and NADP they are similar to ATP. Both these molecules have a nitrogen-containing ring called nicotinic acid, is the chemically active part of the coenzymes. The chemically active portion is the flavin group in FAD. In the body riboflavin vitamin is used to produce this flavin group.

All coenzymes do the same work. Coenzymes accept electrons and pass them on to other coenzymes or other molecules during the process of metabolism. The removal of electrons from a coenzyme is called oxidation. On the other hand the addition of electrons to a molecule is called reduction. Hence, the reactions performed by coenzymes are called oxidation-reduction reactions. These oxidation-reduction reactions are essential to the energy metabolism of the cell. Cytochromes are one of the molecules that participates in this energy reaction. These cytochromes accept and release electrons along with the coenzymes. This system is called as electron transport system.

The formation of ATP requires a complex process called chemiosmosis. Chemiosmosis involves in the creation of a steep proton /hydrogen ion gradient. This ion gradient occurs between the mitochondria of all cells and the chloroplasts of plant cells. When a large number of protons are pumped into the membrane-bound compartments of the mitochondria, ion gradient is formed. The protons build up in the compartment and reach an enormous number. These protons are pumped, when energy is released from the electrons during the electron transport process.

After the formation of more number of protons within the compartments of mitochondria and chloroplasts, they reverse their directions and escape back across the membranes and out of the compartments. In this motion the escaping protons release their energy. This energy is utilized by the enzymes to combine ADP with phosphate ions to form ATP. By this process, the energy is trapped in the high-energy bond of ATP and the ATP molecules are made available to perform cell work. The movement of protons is chemiosmosis which is similar to the movement of chemicals (in this case, protons) across a semipermeable membrane. Because of the occurrence of chemiosmosis in mitochondria and chloroplasts, these organelles play an essential role in the cell's energy metabolism.

Cellular Respiration (Aerobic Respiration)

Cellular respiration is a process which can occur by utilizing oxygen (aerobic). In aerobic respiration oxygen is utilized in the mitochondria to break down the organic molecules like glucose and thereby to release the energy. During this process water and carbon dioxide are released as waste products. The equation is given as below,

$$C_6 H_{12} O_6 + 6 O_2 \rightarrow 6 CO_2 + 6 H_2O + ATP$$

There are 4 steps in cellular respiration,

1. Glycolysis

2. Pyruvate oxidation
3. The Krebs cycle
4. The electron transport chain.

1. **Glycolysis:** It occurs when the two pyruvic acid molecules are formed from glucose by glycolysis and diffuse into the mitochondria.

   Glucose $\rightarrow$ 2 Pyruvate + 2ATP + 2NADH

2. **Pyruvate Oxidation:** Here pyruvate molecules are oxidized to form two molecules of Acetyl CoA, which further enters in Kerb's Cycle.

   2 Pyruvate $\rightarrow$ 2 Acetyl CoA + 2NADH + 2 CO_2

3. **The Krebs cycle:** It is also known as the Citric acid cycle. In this cycle from Acetyl CoA, 2 ATP molecules, 10 energy carrier molecules and CO_2 are produced. These energy carriers will move on to the next step (Electron transport chain).

   2 Acetyl CoA $\rightarrow$ 2ATP + 4 CO_2 + 6NADH + 2FADH$_2$

4. **The Electron transport chain:** The electron transport chain is a series of chemical reactions which produces 34 ATP molecules and H_2O from the carrier molecules that were produced in the Krebs cycle.

   Hence totally 36 ATP molecules are produced in aerobic respiration.

Anaerobic Respiration

Fermentation is an Anaerobic Process. There are several forms of fermentation. Two of these forms are lactic acid fermentation and alcoholic fermentation.

1. **Lactic acid fermentation:** It occurs in animal cells if there is no oxygen available. Here pyruvic acid is converted into lactic acid. When lactic acid builds up in tissues, it causes muscle soreness. This causes the burning sensation in muscles.

2. **Alcoholic fermentation:** It occurs in some plants and unicellular organisms such as yeast and bacteria. In this process pyruvic acid is converted into ethyl alcohol and a carrier compound by liberating CO_2, which allows glycolysis to continue. This process is utilized in making bread, beer, and wine.

Energy Yield in Aerobic and Anaerobic Respiration

In aerobic respiration 36 ATP molecules are produced from each glucose molecule and in anaerobic respiration only 2 ATP molecules are produced from each glucose molecule. It shows that aerobic respiration is significantly more efficient than anaerobic respiration.

Functions of ATP

1. **Acts as energy Source:** ATP is the main energy currency of cells used for all cellular activities. Energy is released when ATP is hydrolyzed and converted to adenosine diphosphate (ADP). 7.3 kilocalories per mole or 30.6 kilojoules per mole is released when one phosphate group is removed under standard conditions. This energy carries out all reactions that take place inside the cell. ADP can also be converted back into ATP, so that the energy is available for other cellular reactions.

2. **Signal transduction:** ATP as a signaling molecule used for cell communication. Kinases are enzymes, use ATP as a source of phosphate groups to phosphorylate molecules. Kinases are important for signal transduction, which plays a role in physical or chemical signal transmission from receptors on the outside of the cell to the inside of the cell. If the signal is inside the cell, the cell can respond appropriately. Signals may be given to the cells to grow, metabolize, differentiate into specific types, or even die.

3. **DNA Synthesis:** Adenine the nucleobase is part of adenosine, a molecule that is formed from ATP and plays a role in RNA synthesis. Cytosine, guanine and uracil, are similarly formed from CTP, GTP and UTP are the other nucleobases present in RNA. Adenine is also present in DNA, and its incorporation is very similar, except ATP is converted into the form deoxyadenosine triphosphate (dATP) before becoming part of a DNA strand.

4. **ADP, AMP, and cAMP:** Adenosine diphosphate (ADP), adenosine monophosphate (AMP) and cyclic AMP (cAMP) are the other molecules that are related to ATP. In order to avoid confusion, it is important to know some differences between these molecules.

Adenosine Diphosphate (ADP)

Adenosine diphosphate (ADP), is also known as adenosine pyrophosphate (APP). It differs from ATP because it has two phosphate groups. ATP becomes ADP with the loss of a phosphate group, and this reaction releases energy. ADP is also formed from AMP. Cycling between ADP and ATP during cellular respiration gives cells the energy needed to carry out cellular activities.

Adenosine Monophosphate (AMP)

Adenosine monophosphate (AMP) is also called 5'-adenylic acid, has only one phosphate group. AMP is found in RNA and contains adenine, which is part of the genetic code. It can be produced along with ATP from two ADP molecules, or by hydrolysis of ATP. It is also formed when RNA is broken down. AMP can be converted into uric acid a component of urine and excreted.

Cyclic Adenosine Monophosphate (cAMP)

Cyclic adenosine monophosphate (cAMP) is derived from ATP and is also a messenger used for signal transduction and for activating certain protein kinases. It can be broken down into AMP. In certain cancers such as carcinoma cAMP pathways may play a role. In bacteria, it has a role in metabolism. High cAMP levels occur when a bacterial is not producing enough energy and this turns on genes that use energy sources other than glucose. Differences between ADP, AMP and cAMP are shown in **Table 4-1.**

Table 4-1   Differences between ADP, AMP and cAMP

Sr. No.	ADP	AMP	cAMP
1	Also known as adenosine pyrophosphate (APP).	Also called 5'-adenylic acid.	Derived from ATP.
2	Has two phosphate groups.	Has only one phosphate group.	Used as a messenger for signal transduction and for activation of certain protein kinases.
3	Can be synthesized from ATP.	Can be synthesized by the hydrolysis of ATP and ADP.	Can be broken down into AMP.
4	Also synthesized from AMP.	AMP can be converted into uric acid and eliminated in urine.	cAMP pathways may play a role in certain cancer.

Creatine Phosphate

Creatine phosphate is also known as Phosphocreatine is the phosphorylated form of creatine. Creatine phosphate was discovered in 1927 in muscle tissue. It is mainly seen in the skeletal muscles of vertebrates, in both free and phosphorylated forms. It plays a major role in the contraction of skeletal muscle. Creatine phosphate donates its phosphate group to ADP in presence of Creatine Kinase (CK) enzyme and forms ATP and creatine.

Creatine Kinase (CK)

$$ADP + Creatine\ Phosphate + H^+ \ \text{-----------------------}\!\!> \ ATP + Creatine$$

The creatine must be provided either from dietary sources or by endogenous synthesis to maintain the body pool of creatine phosphate. Creatine is an amino acid that plays a key role as creatine phosphate in regenerating ATP in skeletal muscle to energize muscle contraction. The enzyme creatine kinase is present in highest concentration in muscle and nerve. Oral administration of creatine kinase increases muscle stores.

Creatine phosphate is the main store of high-energy phosphates in muscle. It allows the rephosphorylation of ADP to ATP, is the immediate source of energy in muscle contraction. Metabolic processes regenerate creatine phosphate stores during rest. In normal muscle, ATP is broken down to ADP. This ADP is immediately rephosphorylated to ATP, by acquiring one phosphate moiety from creatine phosphate. Thus, creatine phosphate serves as a reservoir of ATP-synthesizing potential. Creatine phosphate is the only fuel available to regenerate ATP during fluctuations in demand. The availability of creatine phosphate limits the muscle performance during brief, high-power exercise, i.e., maximal exercise of short duration.

Formation of Creatine Phosphate

Creatine phosphate can be obtained from ingestion of meat and internal production by the liver and kidneys. It is also present in other areas of the body such as brain. *In vivo* synthesis of creatine occurs in the liver. In liver, amidine groups from arginine are transferred to glycine in presence of the enzyme glycine transaminidase to form guanidinoacetic acid. This guanidinoacetic acid is further methylated by S-adenosyl methionine in presence of guanidinoacetate methyltransferase to form creatine which is shown in **Figure 4-2**.

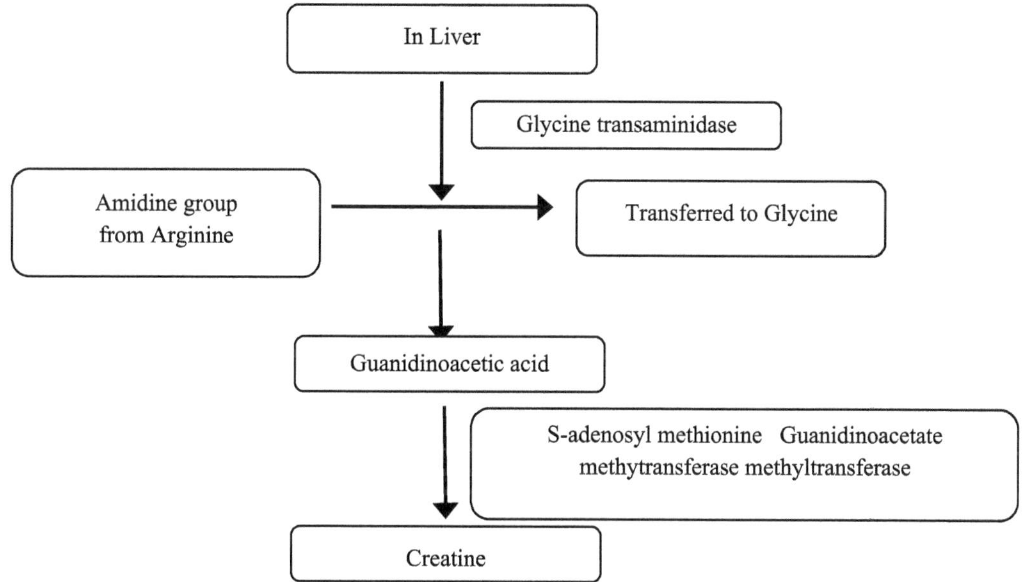

Figure 4-2 Synthesis of Creatine

The synthesized creatine is stored in storage sites example in skeletal muscle. This creatine reacts with ATP and forms creatine phosphate. Creatine phosphate is capable of donating a phosphate group to ADP to regenerate ATP. At the same time, excess ATP can be dephosphorylated during low muscle activity to convert creatine to creatine phosphate. This dual activity in synthesizing creatine phosphate from excess levels of ATP during rest and utilization of creatine phosphate to regenerate ATP shows the key utility of creatine phosphate in acting as an energy buffer in body muscle cells. Supplementation with creatine promotes the reduction of reactive oxygen species (ROS) in skeletal muscle. ROS production is increased in various pathological conditions like metabolic, neurologic, endocrine diseases and cancer. In these patients treatment with creatine has shown a significant improvement.

Elimination of Creatine Phosphate

Creatine phosphate is eliminated by kidneys. The end product of creatine degradation is creatinine. When creatinine enters the renal parenchyma it is filtered in the renal glomerulus to be excreted in the urine.

ATP is the main source of energy that body muscles use to perform contractions. During such contraction processes, ATP molecules are depleted by undergoing hydrolysis reactions and become ADP. To maintain homeostasis in muscle activity, the ATP should be supplied to the muscles regularly. Creatine phosphate synthesized within the body is capable of regenerating ATP by transferring a high-energy phosphate from itself to ADP, resulting in the formation of ATP and creatine. This kind of regeneration of ATP with creatine phosphate occurs within seconds of intense muscular or neuronal effort, acting as a quickly accessible reserve of high-energy phosphates for the recycling of ATP in body muscle cells.

Advantages of Creatine Phosphate

Studies have reported that supplementation of creatine phosphate is very effective in many people. These supplementation increases muscle mass, explosive power and muscle strength. Hence, for activities which require short bursts of energy such as football and sprinting, creatine phosphate supplementation has been used to improve the athletics performance. More over creatine phosphate is not considered as a drug by the FDA so it is used as a legal substance in athletic competitions.

Disadvantages of Creatine Phosphate

Long term studies have not done to know the effects of creatine phosphate supplementation. Some scientists speculate that with supplementation, the body may stop naturally producing creatine phosphate. More over the waste products of creatine and creatinine on the kidneys are a concern. The creatine content of urine with supplementation is 90 times greater than normal. Other side effects include nausea, gastrointestinal disturbances and increased muscle cramping. Another major disadvantage of creatine phosphate is that it is only effective for short bursts of energy. **Table 4-2** shows the advantages and disadvantages of Creatine phosphate supplementation.

Table 4-2 Advantages and disadvantages of Creatine phosphate supplementation

Sr. No.	Advantages of Creatine phosphate	Disadvantages of Creatine phosphate
1	Supplementation of creatine phosphate is very effective in many people.	Long term studies not done to know the effects of creatine phosphate supplementation.
2	The CP supplementation increases muscle mass, explosive power and muscle strength.	With supplementation the body may stop naturally producing creatine phosphate.
3	Creatine phosphate supplementation is used in athletes to improve their performance.	The waste products of creatine and creatinine on the kidneys are a concern.

Table 4-2 Contd...

Sr. No.	Advantages of Creatine phosphate	Disadvantages of Creatine phosphate
4	Creatine phosphate is not considered as a drug by the FDA. So it is used as a legal substance in athletic competitions.	Creatine phosphate supplementation causes nausea, gastrointestinal disturbances and increased muscle cramping. Moreover it is only effective for short bursts of energy.

Basal Metabolic Rate (BMR)

Basal metabolic rate (BMR) is the amount of energy utilized by the body of subject during complete mental and physical rest i.e. with comfortable room temperature and humidity, awake and sitting position, 10-12 hours post meal. BMR is the minimum energy required to maintain vital functions like the heart rate, blood circulation, respiration, maintaining body temperature, kidney function, brain and nerve function, cell growth and contraction of muscles. The average BMR of an Indian man is 1750 to 1900 Kcal/day. It can be measured as Kcal /day or kJ/square meter of body surface area /hour, which can be written as $KJ / m^2 / h$ or $KJ\ m^{-2}\ h^{-1}$.

BMR Calculation

BMR can be calculated by using the formula based on sex, age, weight and height.

Women: BMR = 655 + (4.35 × Weight in pounds) + (4.7 × Height in inches) – (4.7 × Age in years)

Men: BMR = 66 + (6.23 × Weight in pounds) + (12.7 × Height in inches) – (6.8 × Age in years)

We can convert the pounds into Kg by dividing by 2.2 and inches into cm by multiplying by 2.54.

Factors Affecting BMR

Many factors affect the BMR. They are age, sex, genetics, body temperature, emotional state, climate and circulating levels of hormones like epinephrine and nor epinephrine and those secreted by the thyroid gland (Table 4-3).

Table 4-3 Various factors affecting BMR

Sr. No.	Factors affecting BMR	Increase or decrease in BMR
1	Genetics	• Some people have high BMR • Some people have low BMR
2	Gender	• Male: BMR is high • Female: BMR is low
3	Age	Children have higher BMR than adults
4	Weight	• In Obese: BMR is high • In lean: BMR is low

Table 4-3 Contd...

Sr. No.	Factors affecting BMR	Increase or decrease in BMR
5	Body surface area	Greater body surface area, higher BMR
6	Body fat percentage	Body fat percentage is lower, BMR is higher
7	Diet	Starvation reduces BMR
8	Body temperature	Body temperature increases, BMR also increases.
9	Environmental temperature	Cold temperature increases BMR
10	Glands	<ul><li>Hyperthyroidism: BMR is high</li><li>Hypothyroidism: BMR is low</li><li>Increase in nor adrenaline release: BMR is high</li></ul>
11	Exercise	Long term exercise: BMR increases
12	Pregnancy	<ul><li>In early pregnancy: No change in BMR</li><li>In late pregnancy: BMR increases</li></ul>

1. **Genetics:** Some people are faster metabolisers and some are slower metabolisers. Indians and Chinese have a lower BMR than the Europeans. This may be due to dietary differences between them. Higher BMR exists in peoples living in tropical climates. Eg. Singapore.

2. **Gender:** BMR is generally higher in male than female. Males have greater muscle mass and a lower body fat percentage. Hence males have higher basal metabolic rate than females. Females have higher proportion of fat cells, which have lower metabolic rate than muscle cells. The BMR of females declines rapidly between the ages of 5 and 17 than that of males.

3. **Age:** BMR is inversely proportional to age, that is it decreases as age increases. Children have higher BMR than adults. As age increases the proportion of lean muscle mass decreases and the synthesis of proteins also decreases, leads to decrease in BMR. After 20 years, it drops about 2 % per decade.

4. **Weight:** BMR is directly proportional to weight. If the weight is more, the BMR is high. ex. the metabolic rate in obese women is 25% higher than that of thin women.

5. **Body surface area:** Body surface area is a reflection of height and weight. The greater the body surface area, the higher the BMR. Tall, thin people have a higher BMR than their shorter counterparts, even with the same weight, due to the greater surface area of their skin.

6. **Body fat percentage:** If body fat percentage is lower, the BMR is higher. The body fat percentage is low in males is a reason why males generally have a 10-15% higher BMR than females.

7. **Diet:** Starvation or abrupt reduction in calorie intake can dramatically reduce BMR by up to 30%. Low-calorie weight loss diets may cause BMR to drop as much as 20%. BMR of strict vegetarians is 11% lower than that of meat eaters.

8. **Body temperature:** For every increase of 0.5° C in body temperature, the BMR increases by 7 %. The chemical reactions in the body occur more fastly at higher temperatures. So in a patient with a fever of 42° C would have an increase of about 50 % in BMR.

9. **Environmental temperature:** Temperature in the environment also affects basal metabolic rate. Exposure to cold temperature causes an increase in the BMR, because to create the extra heat which is needed to maintain the body's internal temperature. A short exposure to hot temperature has little effect on the body's metabolism because it is compensated by increased heat loss. But prolonged exposure to heat can raise BMR.

10. **Glands:** Thyroxine is a hormone released by thyroid gland. It is a key regulator of BMR. It speeds up the metabolic activity of the body. If more thyroxine is produced, the BMR is increased. If too much thyroxine is produced as in thyrotoxicosis, BMR can double. If too little thyroxine is produced as in myxoedema, BMR may decrease up to 30-40 % of normal rate. Like thyroxine, adrenaline also increases the BMR but to a lesser extent. During anxiety and tension nor adrenaline is produced which also increases the metabolic rate.

11. **Exercise:** Exercise needs energy and uses it. Exercise has both long and short term effects on BMR. Long term physical exercise increases the BMR. This is due to increased overall activity of the heart and vascular system, along with other body systems and tissues.

12. **Pregnancy:** During the early stages of pregnancy BMR is not changed. But it increases in late stages of pregnancy is due to the BMR of the fetus.

Significance of BMR

1. BMR is the principal guide for diagnosis and treatment of thyroid disorders.
2. If BMR is less than 10% of the normal, it indicates moderate hypothyroidism. In severe hypothyroidism, the BMR may be decreased to 40 to 50% below normal.
3. BMR helps to know the total amount of food or calories needed to maintain body weight.
4. During starvation, under nutrition, hypothalamic disorders, Addison's disease and lipoid nephrosis the BMR is low.
5. In fever and other diseases such as diabetes insipidus, leukemia and polycythemia the BMR is high.

4.2 Chapter at a Glance

Term	Description
ATP	Adenosine tri-phosphate
ADP	Adenosine di-phosphate
AMP	Adenosine mono-phosphate
cAMP	Cyclic adenosine monophosphate
NAD	Nicotinamide adenine dinucleotide
NADP	Nicotinamide adenine dinucleotide phosphate
FAD	Flavin adenine dinucleotide
APP	Adenosine pyrophosphate
Aerobic Respiration	Cellular respiration
DNA	Deoxyribonucleic acid
CK	Creatine Kinase
ROS	Reactive oxygen species
BMR	Basal metabolic rate

Exercises

Multiple Choice Questions

1. The energy currency of cell is
   - (a) ATP
   - (b) AMP
   - (c) ADP
   - (d) All

2. The coenzymes involved in the formation of ATP are
   - (a) Nicotinamide adenine dinucleotide (NAD)
   - (b) Nicotinamide adenine dinucleotide phosphate (NADP)
   - (c) Flavin adenine dinucleotide (FAD)
   - (d) All

3. Cellular respiration is also known as
   - (a) Anaerobic respiration
   - (b) Aerobic respiration
   - (c) Phosphorylation
   - (d) None

4. Adenosine pyrophosphate (APP) is also known as
   - (a) ATP
   - (b) AMP
   - (c) ADP
   - (d) cAMP

5. _____________ plays a role in signal transduction pathway.
   - (a) ATP
   - (b) AMP
   - (c) ADP
   - (d) cAMP

6. Creatine phosphate is also known as
   - (a) Creatinine
   - (b) Phosphocreatin
   - (c) Both
   - (d) None

7. The enzyme involved in the synthesis of creatine is
   - (a) Creatine kinase
   - (b) Creatine phosphokinase
   - (c) Creatinase
   - (d) None

8. In our body creatine is synthesized in
   - (a) Liver
   - (b) Kidney
   - (c) Lungs
   - (d) Both a and b

9. The end product of creatine degradation is
   - (a) Creatine monophosphate
   - (b) Creatine diphosphate
   - (c) Creatine triphosphate
   - (d) Creatinine

10. Creatine phosphate supplementation can be used in athletics to improve their performance.
    - (a) True
    - (b) False
    - (c) Both
    - (d) None

11. BMR is the __________ energy required to maintain vital functions of body.
    - (a) Minimum
    - (b) Maximum
    - (c) Both
    - (d) Nil

12. The average BMR of an Indian man is
    - (a) 1200-1300 Kcal/day
    - (b) 1500 -1600 Kcal/day
    - (c) 1750-1900 Kcal/day
    - (d) 2000-2500 Kcal/day

13. Higher BMR exists in people living in __________ climate.
    - (a) Cold
    - (b) Tropical
    - (c) Rainy
    - (d) All

14. BMR is generally higher in
    - (a) Female
    - (b) Children
    - (c) Male
    - (d) All

15. BMR is low in
    - (a) Starvation
    - (b) Malnutrition
    - (c) Addison's diseases
    - (d) All

Short Answer Questions

1. Write about the structure of ATP.
2. Write about cellular respiration.
3. Write about anaerobic respiration.
4. Write about the energy yield in aerobic and anaerobic respiration.
5. Write the role of ATP in signal transduction.
6. Briefly write the equation of synthesis of creatine phosphate.
7. Write the sources of creatine phosphate.
8. Write the advantages of creatine phosphate.
9. Write the disadvantages of creatine phosphate.

10. Define BMR.
11. How will you calculate BMR?
12. Write the role of diet in BMR.
13. Write the role of body temperature in BMR.
14. Write the role of thyroid gland hormones in BMR.

Long Answer Questions

1. Write about the formation of ATP.
2. In detail write about ATP functions.
3. In detail write about the synthesis of creatine phosphate.
4. In detail write the advantages and disadvantages of creatine phosphate.
5. Write the significances of BMR.

Bibliography

Hulbert AJ, Else PL. Basal metabolic rate: History, composition, regulation and usefulness. Physiological and Biochemical Zoology. 2004; 77(6): 869-876.

Neupane P, Bhoju S, Thapa N, Bhattarai HK. ATP Synthase: Structure, Function and Inhibition. BioMol Concepts, 2019; 10: 1-10.

Valerie SC, Tina S. Essentials of Anatomy and Physiology. 5th edition, Philadelphia, PA: F.A. Davis Co., 2011.

Answer Key MCQs

1.	(a)	2.	(d)	3.	(b)	4.	(c)	5.	(d)
6.	(b)	7.	(a)	8.	(d)	9.	(d)	10.	(True)
11.	(a)	12.	(c)	13.	(b)	14.	(b)	15.	(d)

Respiratory System

After completing this lesson, the Reader should be able to understand:

- *Definition (Introduction)*
- *Process of Respiration*
- *Anatomy of the Respiratory System*
- *Lung Volumes and Capacities*
- *Exchange of gases*
- *Transport of gases in blood*
- *Regulation of Respiration*
- *Artificial respiration and resuscitation methods*
- *Diseases of Respiratory System*

5.1   Introduction

Definition

The respiratory system is also known as respiratory apparatus, ventilatory system which is a biological system consisting of some specific organs and structures that are used for the exchange of gases. The respiratory system plays a role in homeostasis by providing for the exchange of gases such as oxygen and carbon dioxide between the atmospheric air, blood and tissue cells. It also helps to adjust the pH of body fluids.

Process of Respiration

In the process of respiration, the body gets rid of carbon dioxide and takes in oxygen. Carbon dioxide, a waste product goes out of the body. Oxygen, which the body needs, comes in. This process occurs in three steps (Table 5-1).

Step I

The first step in this process is breathing in air, which is also known as inhaling. During inhalation air rich in oxygen enters into the body and during exhalation air rich in carbon dioxide removed from the body.

Step II

The second step is gas exchange in the lungs where oxygen is diffused into the blood and the carbon dioxide diffuses out of the blood.

Step III

The third step is cellular respiration, which produces the chemical energy that the cells in the body need, and also carbon dioxide. Finally, the carbon dioxide is breathed out of the body through the lungs.

Table 5-1 Steps involved in the process of respiration

Sr. No.	Steps of respiration	Events
1	Step I	During inhalation, air rich in oxygen enters into the body and during exhalation, the air rich in carbon dioxide removed from the body.
2	Step II	The exchange of gases takes place in the lungs, where oxygen is diffused from the lungs to the blood and carbon dioxide diffuses out of the blood to the lungs.
3	Step III	Cellular respiration produces chemical energy (ATP) and carbon dioxide. This CO_2 moves from the tissues to the lungs through the blood.

Anatomy of the Respiratory System

The respiratory system consists of the nose, pharynx (throat), larynx (voice box), trachea (windpipe), bronchi and lungs (Figure 5-1). The parts can be classified on the basis of their structure or function.

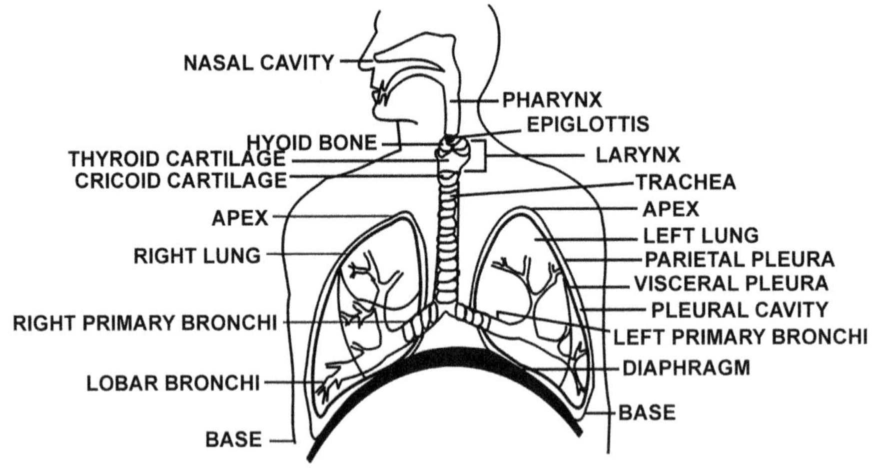

Figure 5-1 Anatomy of the Respiratory System

Structurally, the respiratory system consists of two parts.

1. **Upper respiratory Tract:** It comprises of nose, nasal cavity, pharynx and associated structures.
2. **Lower respiratory Tract:** It comprises of larynx, trachea, epiglottis, lungs, bronchi, bronchioles and alveoli.

The respiratory system also consists of the associated structures such as a thoracic cavity, diaphragm and intercostal muscles.

Functionally, the respiratory system consists of two parts **(Table 5-2)**.

1. **The conducting zone:** These comprise a series of inter connecting cavities and tubes, both outside and within the lungs. These include the nose, nasal cavity, pharynx, larynx, trachea, bronchi, bronchioles and terminal bronchioles. Their function is to filter, warm, and moisten air and conduct it into the lungs.
2. **The respiratory zone:** These comprise of the tubes and tissues within the lungs, where the exchange of gases occurs. These include the respiratory bronchioles, alveolar ducts, alveolar sacs, and alveoli. These are the main sites of gas exchange between air and blood.

Table 5-2 Differences between conducting and respiratory zone

Sr. No.	Conducting zone	Respiratory zone
1	Comprise a series of inter connecting cavities and tubes, both outside and within the lungs.	Comprise of the tubes and tissues within the lungs.
2	Nose, nasal cavity, pharynx, larynx, trachea, bronchi, bronchioles and terminal bronchioles form the conducting zone.	Respiratory bronchioles, alveolar ducts, alveolar sacs and alveoli form the respiratory zone.
3	The above organs filter, warm, and moisten air and conduct it into the lungs.	These are the main sites of gas exchange between air and blood.

Nose

The air enters and leaves the respiratory tract through the nose. Nose may be divided into different structures and these include

(i) **External nose:** It is the part of the nose visible on the face. It is made up of bone and hyaline cartilage and these structures are covered with muscle and skin. The bony frame work of external nose is formed by the frontal bone, nasal bones and maxillae. Hyaline cartilage forms the cartilaginous framework of the external nose and connected to skull bones by fibrous connective tissue. It allows the air to enter when we breathe and allows the particle to enter for the perception of smell and taste.

(ii) External nares: The external nose has two openings called the external nares or nostrils. The tiny hairs present inside the nostril prevent the entry of dust particles.

(iii) Nasal Cavities: There are two nasal cavities which are present within the skull, separated by the nasal septum. Nasal septum is a bony plate made up of ethmoid bone and vomer. The ciliated epithelium forms the inner most lining of nasal mucosa, with goblet cells that secrete mucus. Anteriorly, the nasal cavity merges with the external nose, and posteriorly it joins with the pharynx through two openings called internal nares or conchae. The lateral wall of each nasal cavity has three conchae bones of shelf-like or scroll-like projections (Figure 5-2 and Table 5-3).

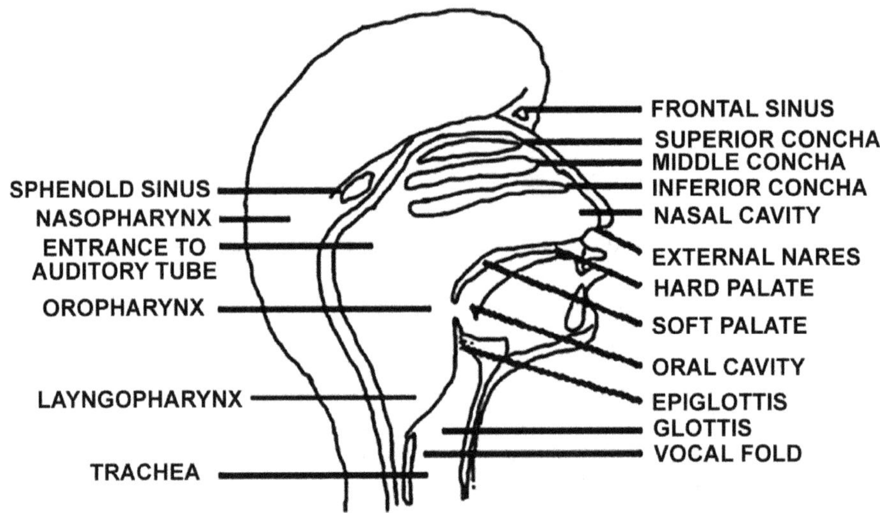

Figure 5-2 Structure of Nose

The surface area of the nasal mucosa is increased by these conchae. The paranasal sinuses ducts drain mucus and the nasolacrimal ducts drain tears into the nasal cavity. The paranasal sinuses are cavities in cranial and facial bones, lined with mucous membrane that are continuous with the lining of the nasal cavity. Besides producing mucus, the paranasal sinuses serve as resonating chamber for sound as we speak or sing. The air which passes through the nasal cavity is warmed and humidified, so that the air that reaches the lungs is warm and moist. The mucus traps the bacteria and particles of air pollution. The cilia present in the nasal cavity continuously sweep the mucus toward the pharynx. Most of this mucus is usually swallowed or spit out, and most of the bacteria present will be destroyed by the hydrochloric acid present in the gastric juice. Olfactory receptors are present in the upper nasal cavity that detects vaporized chemicals that have been inhaled. The olfactory nerves pass through the ethmoid bone to the brain.

Table 5-3 Parts of nose and their functions

Sr. No.	Parts	Functions
1	External nose	• Allows the air to enter when we breathe. • Allows the particle to enter for the perception of smell and taste.
2	External nares	• It prevents the entry of dust particles.
3	Nasal Cavities	• The air entering the body is warmed, moisturized and filtered before it reaches the lungs.

Pharynx

The pharynx or throat is a muscular tube of about 13 cm long that commences at the internal nares and extends to the cricoid cartilage. Cricoid cartilage is the most inferior cartilage of the larynx, which is also known as voice box. The pharynx lies posterior to nasal and oral cavities, superior to larynx and anterior to the cervical vertebrae. Its wall is composed of skeletal muscles and is lined with a mucous membrane. The pharynx is kept patent (open) by the relaxed skeletal muscles. The contraction of this skeletal muscles helps in swallowing. The pharynx functions as a passageway for air and food, provides a resonating chamber for speech sounds, and houses the tonsils, which involves in immunological reactions against microorganisms. Pharynx can be divided into three parts nasopharynx, oropharynx, and laryngopharynx (Table 5-4).

Nasopharynx

It is the uppermost portion, present behind the nasal cavities. Nasopharynx is blocked by the soft palate which elevates during swallowing and thereby prevents food or saliva from going up. On the posterior wall of the nasopharynx is the adenoid or pharyngeal tonsil, a lymph nodule that contains macrophages. Two eustachian tubes open into the nasopharynx and extend upto the middle ear cavities. The eustachian tubes permit air to enter or leave the middle ear thereby allowing the eardrums to vibrate properly. The nasopharynx is a passageway for air only, but the oropharynx and laryngopharynx serves as both an air and food passageway, although not for both at the same time.

Oropharynx

Oropharynx lies posterior to the oral cavity and extends from the soft palate to the level of hyoid bone. Its mucosa is stratified squamous epithelium, continuous with that of the oral cavity. Anteriorly it opens into larynx and posteriorly into esophagus. It serves both respiratory and digestive functions, as a common passageway for air, food and drink.

Laryngopharynx

It is the inferior portion of the pharynx, which is also known as hypopharynx. It begins at the level of the hyoid bone. Inferiorly, it opens into the esophagus posteriorly and the larynx anteriorly. Like oropharynx, laryngopharynx has both respiratory and digestive pathway and is lined by non keratinized stratified squamous epithelium.

Table 5-4 Parts of pharynx and their functions

Sr. No.	Parts	Functions
1	Nasopharynx	Passage way for air
2	Oropharynx	Passageway for air and food
3	Laryngopharynx	Passageway for air and food

Larynx

The larynx is also called as the voice box that connects the laropharynx with the trachea. The name larynx indicates one of its functions that is speaking. The other function of the larynx is as an air passageway between the pharynx and the trachea. The larynx is made of nine pieces of cartilage. The thyroid cartilage, epiglottis, cricoid cartilage are single pieces and the arytenoid, cuneiform, and corniculate cartilages are paired connected by ligaments. The arytenoid cartilage is the most important one because it influences the changes in position and tension of the vocal folds and thereby speech.

Cartilage is a flexible tissue that prevents collapse of the larynx. On the other hand, the esophagus is a collapsible tube, except when food is passing through it. Thyroid cartilage is the largest cartilage of larynx which one can feel on the anterior surface of their neck. The uppermost cartilage is epiglottis. The larynx is elevated and the epiglottis is closed over the top, during swallowing to prevent the entry of saliva or food into the larynx. The mucosa of the larynx is ciliated epithelium, whereas for the vocal cords it is stratified squamous epithelium. The vocal cords are present at the sides of the glottis, so that the air passes freely into and out of the trachea during breathing. The intrinsic muscles of the larynx pull the vocal cords across the glottis, and exhaled air vibrates the vocal cords to produce sounds during speaking, which can be turned into speech. It is also possible to speak while inhaling. Vagus and accessory nerves are the motor cranial nerves that are connected to the larynx for speaking. Usually for most of the people, the speech area is present in the left cerebral hemisphere (Figure 5-3).

Trachea

The trachea or windpipe is a tubular structure for the passage of air. It is about 12 cm long and 2.5 cm in diameter. It is located anterior to the esophagus and extends from the larynx to the fifth thoracic vertebra where it divides into right and left primary bronchi. The tracheal wall consists of four layers of epithelial tissue from superficial to deep. They are (1) adventitia (2) hyaline cartilage (3) submucosa and (4) mucosa. The mucosa of the trachea is made up of pseudostratified ciliated columnar epithelium and an underlying layer of lamina propria which contains elastic and reticular fibers. It provides protection against dust same as the membrane lining of the nasal cavity and the larynx. Areolar connective tissue is present in the submucosa and contains seromucous glands and their ducts.

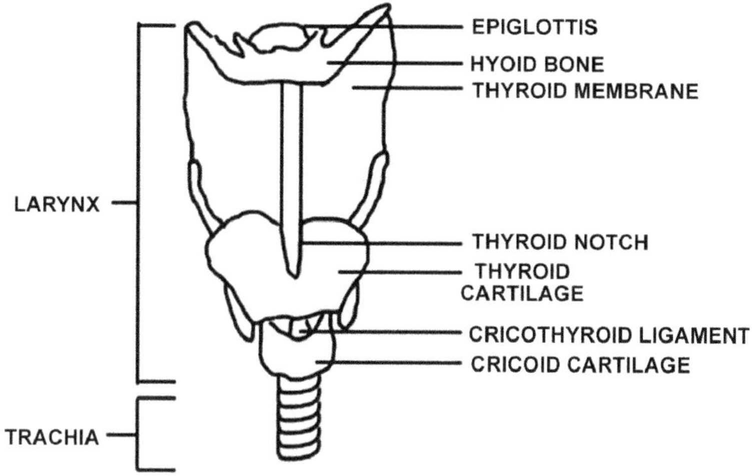

Figure 5-3 Front view of Larynx

The wall of the trachea consists of 16 to 20 "C" shaped pieces of cartilage rings that keep the trachea open. The gaps in these incomplete cartilage rings are posterior, which permits the expansion of the esophagus when food is swallowed. The patency of the trachea is maintained by the solid C shaped cartilage rings so that the tracheal wall does not collapse inward especially during inhalation and obstruct the air passageway (Figure 5-4).

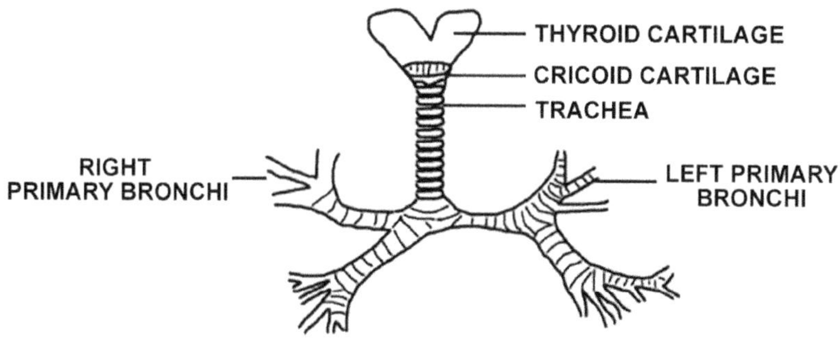

Figure 5-4 Structure of Trachea

Bronchi

At the fifth thoracic vertebra, the trachea divides into two bronchi, one is the right main bronchus that goes into the right lung and another one is the left main bronchus, which goes into the left lung. The right main bronchus is more vertical, shorter and wider than the left. Hence, an aspirated object is more prone to enter and lodge in the right main bronchus than the left. The main bronchi like the trachea contain incomplete rings of cartilage which are lined by pseudostratified ciliated columnar epithelium.

Further, the main bronchi divide to form smaller bronchi that are the lobar bronchi, one for each lobe of the lung. The right lung has three lobes and the left lung has two. The lobar bronchi in turn branch to form still smaller bronchi, called segmental bronchi that supply the specific bronchopulmonary segments within the lobes. The segmental bronchi further divide into conducting bronchioles. These conducting bronchioles in turn branch repeatedly, and the smallest ones branch into even smaller tubes called terminal bronchioles. These terminal bronchioles contain club cells, columnar, non-ciliated cells interspersed among the epithelial cells. The harmful effects of inhaled toxins, carcinogens and surfactant may be protected by these club cells. The terminal bronchioles further divide into respiratory bronchioles. The respiratory bronchioles in turn subdivide into alveolar ducts. Two or more alveoli share a common duct and forms alveolar sacs. These sacs contain alveoli.

The region of the respiratory system between the trachea and the terminal bronchi constitutes the conducting zone. On the other hand, the region from the respiratory bronchiole to alveoli forms the respiratory zone. The branching from the trachea through the terminal bronchioles resembles an inverted tree which is referred to as the bronchial tree is shown as flow chart **(Figure 5-5 and 5-6)**.

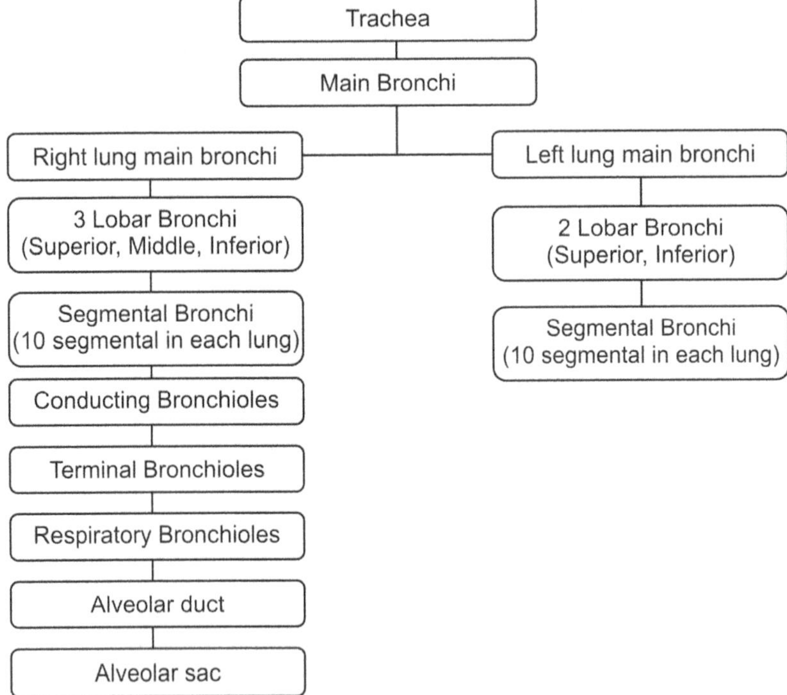

Figure 5-5 Representation of branching of the Bronchi in a flow chart

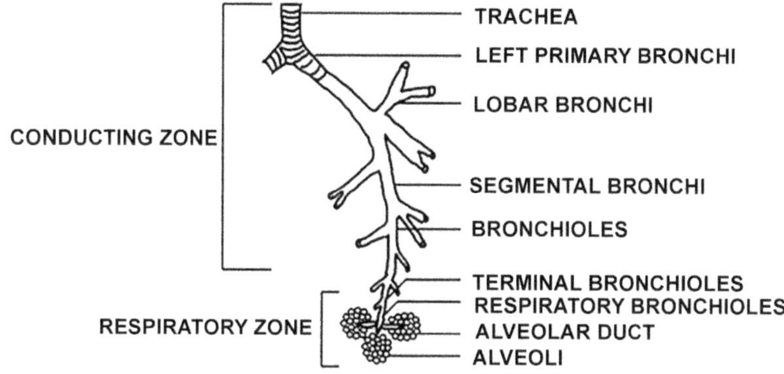

Figure 5-6 Branching of bronchi

Lungs

The lungs are 'cone shaped' organs present in the thoracic cavity, located one on either side of the heart and protected by the rib cage **(Figure 5-7)**. The left lung is slightly smaller than right because a considerable portion is occupied by the heart on the left lung. The apex of the lungs is present at the level of clavicle and base rests on diaphragm. Each lung is surrounded and protected by a double layered serous membrane called the pleural membrane. The outer layer called the parietal pleura, lines the wall of the thoracic cavity and the inner layer called the visceral pleura covers the lungs itself. Between the parietal and visceral pleura a small space is present, known as pleural cavity. This pleural cavity contains a small amount of lubricating fluid secreted by the membranes. The frictions between the pleural membranes are reduced by pleural fluid, thereby allowing them to slide easily over one another during breathing. Hilum is present at the media sternal region of lungs through which bronchi, pulmonary blood vessels, lymphatic vessels, and nerves enter and exit.

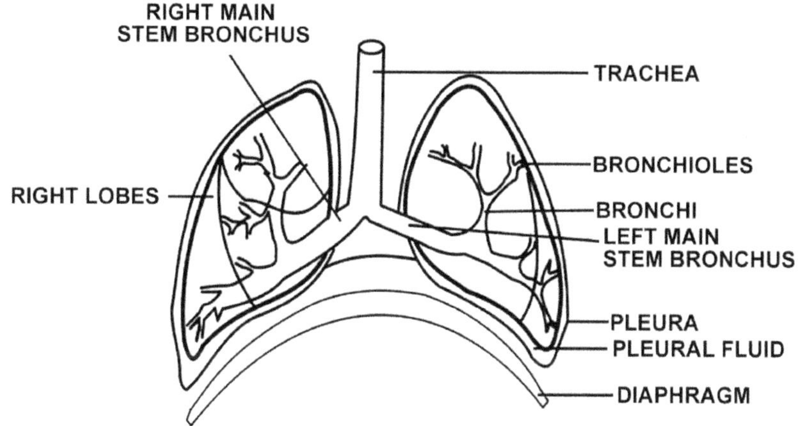

Figure 5-7 Structure of Lungs

Lobes, Fissures and Lobules

Right lung has three lobes and left lung has two lobes. These lobes are divided by fissures. There are two types of fissures, oblique and horizontal fissure. In the left lung the oblique fissure separates the superior lobe from the inferior lobe. In the right lung, the superior part of the oblique fissure separates the superior lobe from the inferior lobe. The inferior part of the oblique fissure separates the inferior lobe from the middle lobe.

Each lobe receives its respective lobar bronchus. The right main bronchus gives rise to three lobar bronchi called the superior, middle and inferior lobar bronchi, and the left main bronchus gives rise to superior and inferior lobar bronchi. These lobar bronchi then give rise to the segmental bronchi. There are 10 segmental bronchi in each lung. The segmental bronchus supplies the segment of lung is called a bronchopulmonary segment. Many small compartments are formed from the bronchopulmonary segment called lobules. Each lobule is surrounded in elastic connective tissue and contains a lymphatic vessel, an arteriole, a venule, and a branch from a terminal bronchiole. These terminal bronchioles further subdivide into minute branches called respiratory bronchioles. Alveoli are formed from their walls. These alveoli participate in exchange of gas, hence respiratory bronchioles begin the respiratory zone of the respiratory system. The epithelial lining of respiratory bronchioles changes from simple cuboidal to simple squamous as they penetrate deeply into the lungs. Respiratory bronchioles in turn subdivide into several alveolar ducts which consist of simple squamous epithelium. Two or more alveoli share a common duct and forms alveolar sacs. These sacs contain 20 to 30 alveoli and resemble the cluster of grapes.

Alveoli

In the lungs, air flows through smaller and smaller microscopic branches known as respiratory bronchioles, which connect to the alveolar ducts. There are approximately 100 alveolar sacs present at the end of each alveolar duct. These sacs contain 20 to 30 alveoli that are 200 to 300 μm in diameter. The average lung has 480 million alveoli. Alveoli are the functional units of the lungs (Figure 5-8). The walls of alveoli have two types of cells, Type I and Type II cells. The flat Type I cells are simple squamous epithelium. Elastic connective tissue is present in the spaces between the clusters of alveoli, which is important for exhalation. Macrophages are also present inside the alveoli and help to phagocytize the pathogens or other foreign material that may not have been swept out by the ciliated epithelium of the bronchial tree. Each alveolus is surrounded by a network of pulmonary capillaries. These capillaries are also made up of simple squamous epithelium, so there are only two cells between the air in the alveoli and the blood in the pulmonary capillaries, which permits efficient diffusion of gases. A thin layer of tissue fluid is essential for the diffusion of gases, because the gas must dissolve in a liquid to enter or leave a cell. The potential problem with this fluid is, that it would make the walls of an alveolus stick together internally. If it happens then the inflation would be very difficult. Pulmonary surfactant is a lipoprotein secreted by alveolar type II cells (which are also called as septal cells), prevents this problem. This surfactant mixes with the tissue fluid within the alveoli and decreases its surface tension, permitting inflation of the alveoli. Normal inflation of the alveoli permits the exchange of gases.

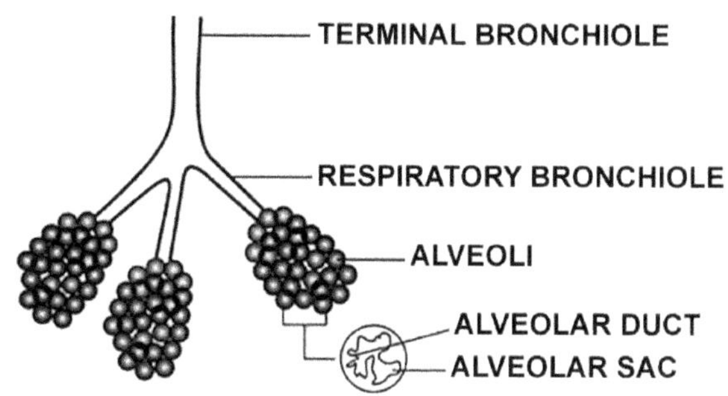

Figure 5-8 Structure of Alveoli

Diaphragm

Diaphragm is a flat muscle that is located beneath the lungs within the thoracic cavity which separates the chest from the abdomen. The diaphragm is also involved in breathing. During inspiration the air is drawn, including oxygen into the body and during expiration the gases including carbon dioxide is eliminated out. The volume of the chest cavity is increased by the contraction of diaphragm, during inspiration by drawing air into the lungs and relaxation of the diaphragm decreases the volume of the chest cavity, pushing air out during expiration **(Figure 5-9)**.

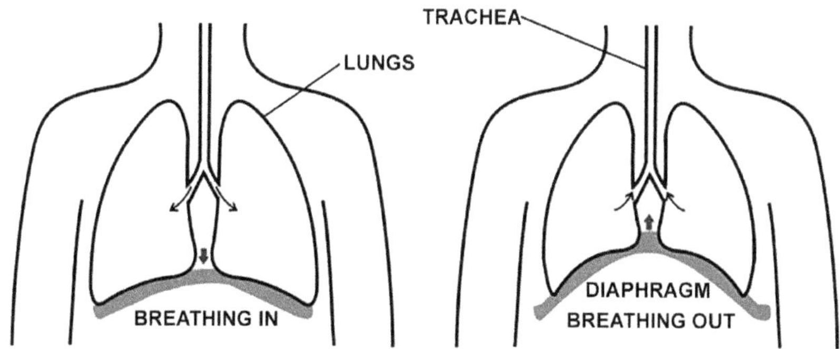

Figure 5-9 Diaphragm functioning in Breathing

Internal and external intercostal muscles

In between the ribs, the intercostal muscles are present. These muscles help in inhalation and exhalation, by contraction and relaxation. There are two types of intercostal muscles, the internal and external intercostal muscles. The internal intercostal muscles lie inside the ribcage. They draw the ribs downwards and inwards, decreasing the volume of the chest cavity and forcing air out of the lungs when breathing out. The external intercostal muscles lie outside the ribcage. They pull the ribs upwards and outwards, increasing the volume of the chest cavity and drawing air into the lungs when breathing in **(Table 5-5)**.

Table 5-5 Difference between Internal and External intercostals muscles

Sr. No.	Internal intercostal muscles	External intercostal muscles
1	Lie inside the rib cage.	Lie outside the rib cage.
2	Draw the ribs downwards and inwards, decreasing the volume of the chest cavity and forcing air out of the lungs during exhalation.	Pull the ribs upwards and outwards, increasing the volume of the chest cavity and drawing air into the lungs during inspiration.

Lung Volumes and Capacities

In an average adult, the normal rate of respiration is 12 to 20 breaths per minute.

Tidal Volume

The amount of air that moves in and out of lungs during normal inhalation and exhalation is called tidal volume. It is about 500ml. But it may decrease in few individuals due to shallow breathing (Figure 5-10 and Table 5-6).

Minute respiratory volume (MRV)

The amount of air inhaled and exhaled in one minute is called minute respiratory volume. MRV is calculated by multiplying tidal volume by the number of respirations per minute. If tidal volume is 500 mL and the respiratory rate is 12 breaths per minute, the MRV is 6000 mL, or 6 liters of air per minute. Shallow breathing usually indicates a smaller than average tidal volume, and would thus require more respirations per minute to obtain the necessary MRV.

MRV= Tidal volume × Rate of respiration / minute

MRV = 500 × 12 breaths / minute = 6L / minute

Inspiratory reserve volume

The amount of air, beyond tidal volume, that can be taken in with the forceful inspiration. Normal inspiratory reserve ranges from 2000 to 3000 mL.

Expiratory reserve volume

The amount of air, beyond tidal volume, that can be expelled with the forceful expiration. Normal expiratory reserve ranges from 1000 to 1500 mL.

Vital capacity

Vital capacity is sum of tidal volume, inspiratory reserve, and expiratory reserve. On the other way, vital capacity is the amount of air involved in the forceful inspiration followed by the most forceful expiration. Average range of vital capacity is 3500 to 5000 mL.

Residual air

The amount of air that remains in the lungs after the most forceful expiration and the average range is 1000 to 1500 mL. Residual air is important to ensure that there is some air in the lungs at all times, so that exchange of gases is a continuous process, even between breaths.

Alveolar Ventilation

The amount of air that actually reaches the alveoli and involves in exchange of gas is called alveolar ventilation. An average tidal volume is 500 mL, of which 350 to 400 mL is in the alveoli at the end of an inspiration. The remaining 100 to 150 mL of air is called anatomical dead space, the air still within the respiratory passages. Anatomic dead space is normal and everyone has it.

Physiological dead space

It is not normal, and is the volume of non-functioning alveoli that decrease exchange of gas. Diseases such as bronchitis, pneumonia, tuberculosis, emphysema, asthma, pulmonary edema, and a collapsed lung increase the physiological dead space.

The compliance of the thoracic wall and the lungs is necessary for sufficient alveolar ventilation. Thoracic compliance may be decreased by fractured ribs, scoliosis, pleurisy or ascites. Lung compliance may be decreased by any condition that increases physiologic dead space.

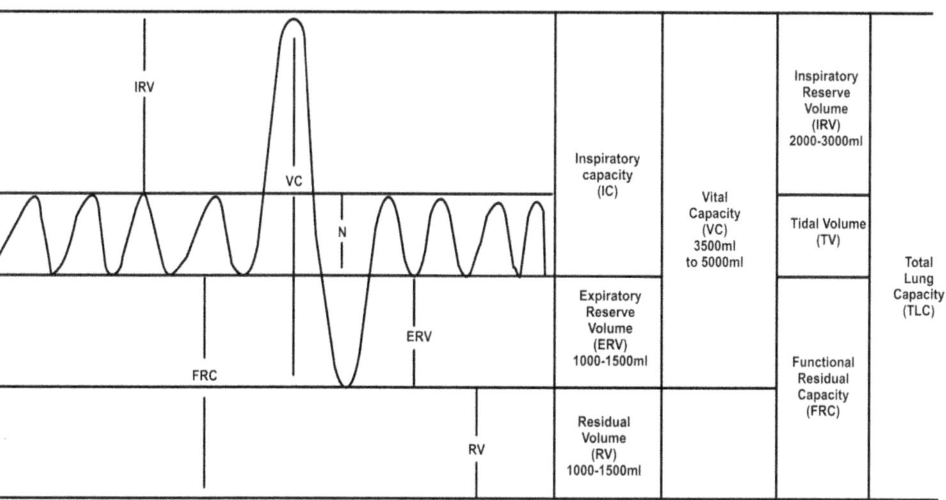

Figure 5-10 Lung Volumes and Capacities

Table 5-6 Summary of different lung volumes and capacities

Tidal Volume	Minute reserve volume	Inspiratory reserve volume	Expiratory reserve volume	Vital capacity	Residual air	Alveolar Ventilation	Anatomical dead space
Volume of air that moves in and out of lungs during normal inhalation and exhalation.	Volume of air inhaled and exhaled in one minute.	Volume of air, beyond tidal volume, that can be taken in with the forceful inspiration.	Volume of air, beyond tidal volume, that can be expelled with the forceful expiration.	Volume of air involved in the forceful inspiration followed by the most forceful expiration.	Volume of air that remains in the lungs after the most forceful expiration.	Volume of air that actually reaches the alveoli per breath.	Volume of air presents in the respiratory tract and is responsible for conducting air to the alveoli and respiratory bronchioles but do not take part in the process of gas exchange
500mL	6000mL	2000 to 3000 mL	1000 to 1500 mL	3500 to 5000 mL	1000 to 1500 mL	350 to 400 mL	100 to 150 mL
	MRV= Tidal volume X Rate of respiration / minute			Tidal volume + Inspiratory reserve volume + Expiratory reserve volume			

Mechanism of Respiration

Respiration is a process of exchange of gas in the body and it has three steps (Table 5-7).

1. **Pulmonary ventilation (Breathing):** Pulmonary ventilation is the inhalation and exhalation of air and involves the exchange of air between the atmosphere and the alveoli of the lungs.

2. **External respiration:** External respiration is the exchange of gases between the alveoli of the lungs and the blood in   pulmonary capillaries. During this process, pulmonary capillary blood receives O_2 and liberates CO_2.

3. **Internal respiration:** Internal respiration is the exchange of gases between blood in systemic capillaries and tissue cells. In this step, the blood liberates O_2 and receives CO_2 from tissues. On the other hand, cellular respiration takes place within cells and the metabolic reactions consume O_2 and glucose to produce CO_2 and ATP.

Table 5-7 Steps Involved in Respiration

Sr. No.	Steps	Events
1	Pulmonary ventilation	Exchange of air between the atmosphere and the alveoli of the lungs.
2	External Respiration	Exchange of gases between the alveoli of the lungs and the blood in pulmonary capillaries
3	Internal Respiration	Exchange of gases between the blood in systemic capillaries and tissue cells

Pulmonary Ventilation

In pulmonary ventilation, the pressure differences are created by contraction and relaxation of respiratory muscles, hence air flows between the atmosphere and the alveoli of the lungs. The respiratory center is present in medulla oblongata. The respiratory muscles such as diaphragm and intercostal muscles play a vital role in respiration. The diaphragm is a dome-shaped muscle below the lungs. When it contracts, it flattens and moves downward. The intercostal muscles are found between the ribs. There are two types of intercostal muscles, external and internal intercostal muscles. The external intercostal muscles pull the ribs upward and outward, and the internal intercostal muscles pull the ribs downward and inward. Ventilation is the result of the respiratory muscles producing changes in the pressure within the alveoli and bronchial tree.

Three types of pressure changes are important in breathing **(Table 5-8)**.

1. **Atmospheric pressure:** The pressure of the air around us is known as atmospheric pressure. At sea level, atmospheric pressure is 760 mmHg. At higher altitudes the atmospheric pressure is lower.

2. **Intrapleural pressure:** Between the parietal and visceral pleura a small space is present, called as pleural space. This space consists of serous fluid, which separates both the pleura and also exhibits some pressure. This pressure is known as intrapleural pressure. The intrapleural pressure is always slightly below atmospheric pressure (about 756 mmHg vs 760 mmHg), and hence, there is a negative pressure. The lungs have the tendency to collapse and pull the visceral pleura away from the parietal pleura. The serous fluid, however, prevents actual separation of the pleural membranes.

3. **Intra pulmonic pressure:** The pressure within the bronchial tree and alveoli is called intra pulmonic pressure. This pressure fluctuates below and above atmospheric pressure during each cycle of breathing.

Table 5-8 Types of pressure in breathing

Sr. No.	Types of Pressure	Description
1	Atmospheric Pressure	• Pressure of the air around us • 760 mmHg.
2	Intrapleural Pressure	• Pressure within the pleural space between the parietal pleura and visceral pleura • 756 mmHg. • Also called as negative pressure.
3	Intra pulmonic Pressure	• Pressure within the bronchial tree and alveoli • Fluctuates below and above atmospheric pressure.

There are three steps of pulmonary respiration; inhalation, exhalation and exchange of gases in lungs:

Inhalation

Inhalation (also known as inspiration), is the inward movement of air inside the lungs from outside atmosphere. The precise sequence of events involved in inhalation includes the following:

1. The medulla releases the motor impulses, which travel along the phrenic nerves to the diaphragm and along the intercostal nerves to the external intercostal muscles.

2. The diaphragm contracts, moves downward, and expands the chest cavity from top to bottom.

3. The ribs are pulled up and out by the external intercostal muscles, thereby expand the chest cavity from side to side and front to back.

4. As the chest cavity is expanded, the parietal pleura also expand with it. Now the intrapleural pressure becomes even more negative as a sort of suction is created between the pleural membranes.

5. The serous fluid creates the adhesion and permits the visceral pleura to be expanded too, and this expands the lungs as well.

6. As the lungs expand, intrapulmonic pressure falls below atmospheric pressure, and air enters the nose and travels through the respiratory passages to the alveoli. Until the intrapulmonic pressure is equal to atmospheric pressure entry of air continues; this is a normal inhalation.

7. Inhalation can be continued beyond normal, that is, a deep breath. This requires a more forceful contraction of the respiratory muscles to further expand the lungs, permitting the entry of more air. The summary of inhalation is shown as follow **(Figure 5-11)**.

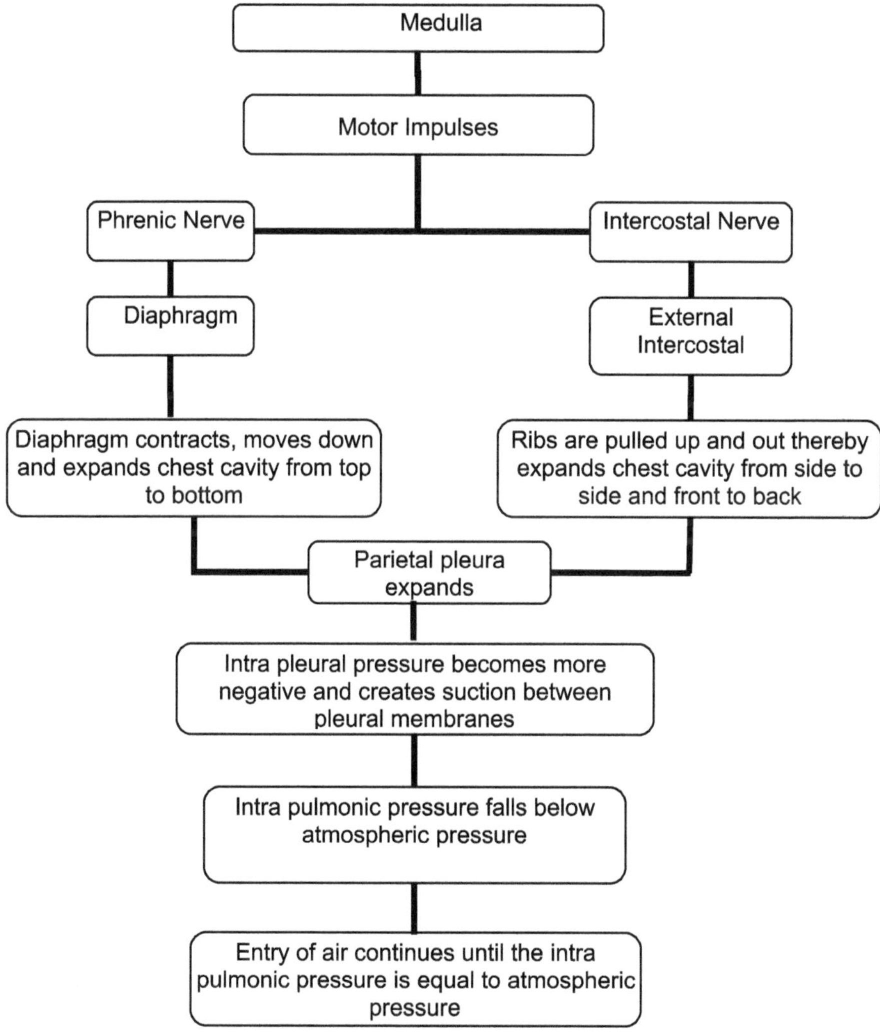

Figure 5-11 Summary of Inhalation

Exhalation is also called as expiration and it involves outward movement of air from lungs to atmosphere.

1. It begins when motor impulses from the medulla decrease and the diaphragm and external intercostal muscles relax.
2. The chest cavity becomes smaller, the lungs are compressed, and their elastic connective tissue, which was stretched during inhalation, recoils and also compresses the alveoli.
3. The intrapulmonic pressure rises above atmospheric pressure, air is forced out of the lungs until the two pressures are again equal.
4. Inhalation is an active process that requires muscle contraction. However, normal exhalation is a passive process, depending to a great extent on the normal elasticity of healthy lungs. In other words, under normal circumstances we must expend energy to inhale, but not to exhale **(Figure 5-12)**.

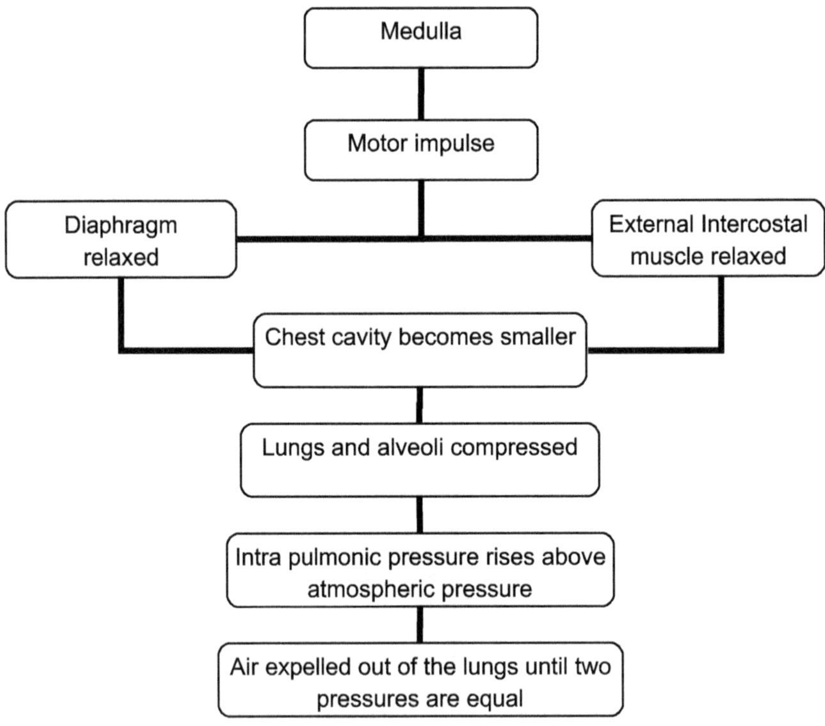

Figure 5-12 Summary of Exhalation

Exchange of gases

The exchange of oxygen and carbon dioxide takes place in the lungs and the body tissues. If the gases are exchanged between the air in the alveoli and the blood in the pulmonary capillaries are called external respiration. The exchange of gases between blood in the capillaries and the tissue of the body is called internal respiration (Table 5-9).

Table 5-9 Difference between Internal and External Respiration

Sr. No.	External Respiration	Internal Respiration
1	Exchange of gas between alveoli and blood	Exchange of gas between blood and tissues
2	Passive process	Active process

The atmospheric air consists of 78.6% nitrogen, 20.9% oxygen, 0.093% argon, 0.04% carbon dioxide, 0.06% other gases and some amount of water vapor. The exhaled air contains about 16% oxygen and 4.5% carbon dioxide. So it is clear that some amount of oxygen is retained within the body and the carbon dioxide produced by cells is exhaled. Each gas in the mixture exhibits its own pressure. This specific pressure of a gas in a mixture is called its partial pressure (Px). The total pressure of the mixture is calculated by adding all of the partial pressures. The partial pressure of gas (PGAS) is measured as mmHg.

Atmospheric pressure (760 mmHg) = PN_2 + PO_2 + PAr + PH_2O + PCO_2 + Pother gases

Partial pressure is calculated as follows,

PGAS = Percentage of the gas in the mixture X Total Pressure

Example 1: O_2 in the atmosphere

21% X 760 mmHg = 160 mmHg (PO_2)

Example 2: CO_2 in the atmosphere

0.04% X 760 mmHg = 0.15 mmHg (PCO_2)

External and Internal Respiration

Partial pressure indirectly shows concentration. It means high partial pressure denotes a higher concentration. Accordingly, a gas diffuses from an area of higher partial pressure to an area of lower partial pressure. The alveoli air has a high PO_2 and a low PCO_2. The blood in the pulmonary capillaries has a low PO_2 and a high PCO_2. Hence, oxygen diffuses from the air in the alveoli to the blood, and carbon dioxide diffuses from the blood to the air in the alveoli is called external respiration **(Figure 5-13 and Figure 5-14)**. The blood which returns to the heart has a high PO_2 and a low PCO_2 and is pumped by the left ventricle into systemic circulation.

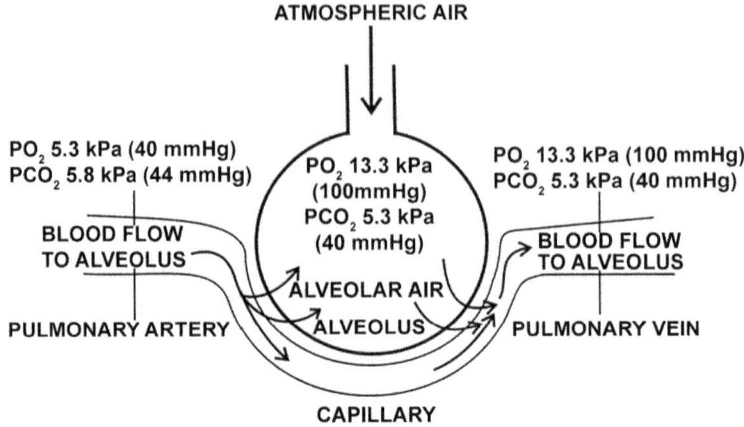

Figure 5-13 Exchange of gases – External Respiration

The arterial blood that reaches systemic capillaries has a high PO_2 and a low PCO_2. The body cells and tissue fluid have a low PO_2 and a high PCO_2 because cells continuously utilize oxygen in cell respiration and produce carbon dioxide in this process. Hence in internal respiration, diffusion of oxygen from the blood to tissue and diffusion of carbon dioxide from tissue fluid to the blood take place. Now the blood that reaches systemic veins to return to the heart has a low PO_2 and a high PCO_2 and is pumped by the right ventricle to the lungs to participate in external respiration.

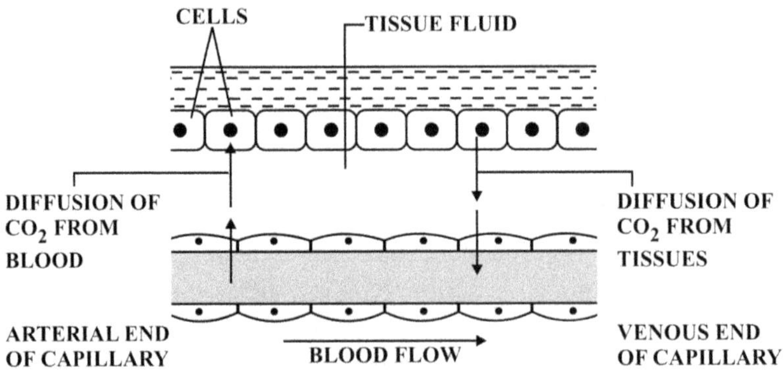

Figure 5-14 Exchange of gases – Internal Respiration

Transport of gases in blood

Oxygen transport: Molecular oxygen is carried in blood in two ways:

1. Dissolved in plasma
2. Bound to hemoglobin within red blood cells.

Oxygen is poorly soluble in water, so only about 1.5% of the oxygen transported is carried in the dissolved form. Oxygen is transported in blood as oxyhemoglobin. Some amount of oxygen is dissolved in blood plasma and it creates the PO_2 values. But it is of only about 1.5% of the total oxygen transported and not enough to sustain life. The mineral iron is part of hemoglobin is responsible for the oxygen-carrying capacity.

$$O_2 + Hemoglobin \rightarrow Oxyhemoglobin$$

In the lungs PO_2 is high, so oxygen binds with hemoglobin. This is an unstable bond, and breaks when the blood passes through tissues with low PO_2; thereby the oxygen is released to the tissues. If the oxygen concentration is lower in the tissue, the hemoglobin will release more amount of oxygen. This ensures that active tissues receive as much oxygen as possible to continue cell respiration e.g. exercising muscles. High PCO_2 (actually a lower pH) and a high temperature are the other factors that increase the release of oxygen from hemoglobin.

The percent of oxygen saturation of hemoglobin (SaO_2) is a measure of blood oxygen. If the PO_2 increases, the SaO_2 will also increase and on the other hand if the PO_2 decreases, the SaO_2 will also decrease though not as rapidly. If PO_2 is 100 then SaO_2 will be 97% in systemic arteries and if PO_2 is 40 in veins then SaO_2 will be 75%. It shows that the venous blood still has bit of oxygen. When this blood flowed through very active tissue, the hemoglobin will release more amount of oxygen. This reserve of oxygen in veins provides active tissues with the oxygen they need.

Carbon dioxide transport

The transport of carbon dioxide is somewhat complicated. Normally body cells produce about 200 ml of CO_2 per minute and the same amount excreted by the lungs. Blood transports CO_2 from the cells to the lungs in three forms.

1. **Dissolved in plasma (7–10%):** The smallest amount of CO_2 is transported simply dissolved in plasma.
2. **Chemically bound to hemoglobin (20%):** In this form, dissolved CO_2 is bound to hemoglobin and carried in the RBC as carbaminohemoglobin.

   $CO_2 + Hb$ (Hemoglobin) $\rightarrow HbCO_2$ (carbaminohemoglobin)
3. **As bicarbonate ion in plasma:** Most of the carbon dioxide is carried in the plasma in the form of bicarbonate ions. When carbon dioxide enters the blood, it diffuses into red blood cells. The RBC contains the enzyme carbonic anhydrase. This enzyme catalyzes the reaction of carbon dioxide and water to form carbonic acid.

   $CO_2 + H_2O \rightarrow H_2CO_3$ (Carbonic acid)

The carbonic acid is unstable and dissociates into H^+ and HCO_3^-

$H_2CO_3 \rightarrow H^+ + HCO_3^-$ (Bicarbonate ion)

Then these bicarbonate ions diffuse out of the RBC into the plasma, leaving the hydrogen ions (H^+) in the RBC. This leads to accumulation of more H^+ ions and makes the RBC more acidic, but hemoglobin acts as a buffer to prevent this acidosis. In order to maintain an ionic equilibrium, chloride ions (Cl^-) from the plasma enter into the RBC. This is called the chloride shift. When the blood reaches the lungs, an area of lower PCO_2, these reactions are reversed and CO_2 is re-formed and diffuses into the alveoli to be exhaled. Table 5-10 shows the transport of gases in blood.

Regulation of Respiration

Two types of mechanisms regulate the respiration.

1. Nervous regulation
2. Chemical regulation.

Any changes in the rate or depth of respiration are ultimately brought about by nerve impulse. Hence nervous mechanism is considered as first in regulation of respiration.

Table 5-10 Transport of gases in blood

Sr. No.	Transport of gases in blood	
	Oxygen	Carbon dioxide
1	Oxygen is poorly soluble in water	Carbon dioxide is freely soluble in water
2	Transported in two forms. a. As dissolved in plasma b. As oxyhemoglobin	Transported in three forms. a. As dissolved in plasma b. As Carbaminohemoglobin c. As bicarbonate ions
3	Mostly in blood O_2 is carried in the form of Oxyhemoglobin.	Most of the CO_2 is carried in the form of bicarbonate ions in blood.

Nervous regulation

The respiratory center is located in the medulla oblongata and pons, which are parts of the brain stem. The respiratory center is made up of three types of neurons, two present in the medulla and one in the pons. The inspiration center and expiration center are present within the medulla. The inspiration center generates impulses in rhythmic spurts. These impulses travel along nerves to the respiratory muscles to stimulate their contraction. The result is inhalation **(Figure 5-15)**. When the lungs inflate the baroreceptors in lungs detect this stretching and generate sensory impulses to the medulla. These impulses depress the inspiration center. This is called the Hering-Breuer inflation Reflex. This reflex also prevents over inflation of the lungs.

When the inspiration center is depressed, there is a decrease in impulses to the respiratory muscles. So these muscles relax and cause exhalation. Now the inspiration center becomes active again to begin another cycle of breathing. If there is a need for forceful exhalations, such as during exercise, the inspiration center activates the expiration center, which generates impulses to the internal intercostal and abdominal muscles.

The two respiratory centers in the pons work with the inspiration center to produce a normal rhythm of breathing. The inhalation is prolonged by the apneustic center and is interrupted by impulses from pneumotaxic center, which contributes to exhalation. Inhalation lasts for 1 to 2 seconds in normal breathing, followed by a slightly longer exhalation, producing the normal respiratory rate range of 12 to 20 breaths per minute.

There are various factors that may affect the respiration and these include

1. Respiration is affected by emotions like sudden fright may bring a gasp or a scream, and anger increases the respiratory rate. During these situations, impulses from the hypothalamus modify the output from the medulla. The cerebral cortex plays a role to change the respiration rate while talking, singing, breathe faster or slower, or even to stop breathing for 1 or 2 minutes. These changes cannot be continued for a longer time, and the medulla will eventually resume control.

2. Reflexes like coughing and sneezing remove irritants from the respiratory tracts. The medulla contains the centers for both of these reflexes. Sneezing is stimulated by an irritation of the nasal mucosa and coughing is stimulated by irritation of the mucosa of the pharynx, larynx, or trachea. The reflex action is same for both. An inhalation is followed by exhalation with the glottis closed to build up pressure. Then the glottis opens suddenly and the exhalation is explosive. A cough directs the exhalation out the mouth, while a sneeze directs the exhalation out the nose.

3. Hiccup is also a reflex due to spasms of the diaphragm. The hic sound occurs when the inhalation is stopped and the glottis snaps shut. The stimulus may irritate the phrenic nerves or nerves of the stomach. Excessive alcohol is an irritant that can cause hiccups.

4. Yawning is another respiratory reflex. Yawning may occur due to lack of oxygen or accumulation of carbon dioxide but the exact reason is unknown.

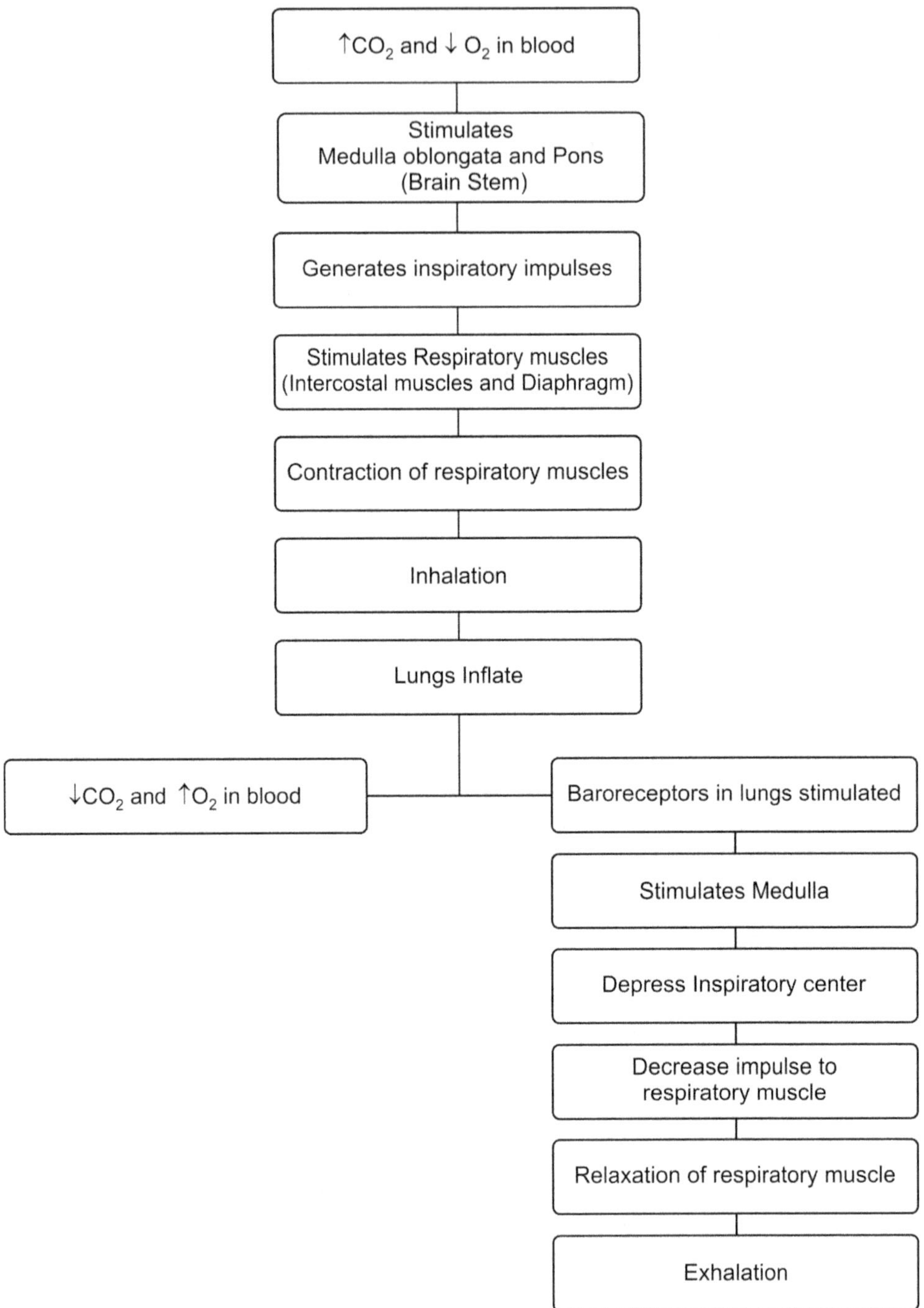

Figure 5-15 Flow Chart Showing Nervous Regulation of Respiration

Chemical regulation

Chemical regulation of respiration is stimulated when there is decrease in O_2, pH and increase in CO_2 level in blood. Chemoreceptors detect the changes in the concentration of blood gases and pH. These chemoreceptors are located on carotid artery, aortic arch and medulla. A decrease in oxygen level in the blood (hypoxia) is detected by the chemoreceptors in the carotid and aortic arteries. These receptors generate the sensory impulses which travel along the gloss pharyngeal and vagus nerves to the medulla, thereby increasing respiratory rate or depth or both. This response will bring more air into the lungs so that more oxygen can diffuse into the blood to correct the hypoxic state.

When carbon dioxide is present in excess amount in the blood (hypercapnia) lowers the pH of blood. This carbon dioxide reacts with water to form carbonic acid (a source of H^+ ions). This excess CO_2 makes the blood more acidic. The chemoreceptors present in medulla are very sensitive to changes in pH, especially when it decreases. The excess CO_2 lowers blood pH, the medulla responds by increasing respiration. This is not only for the purpose of inhaling, but also increases exhalation to expel more CO_2 and to raise the pH back to normal (Figure 5-16).

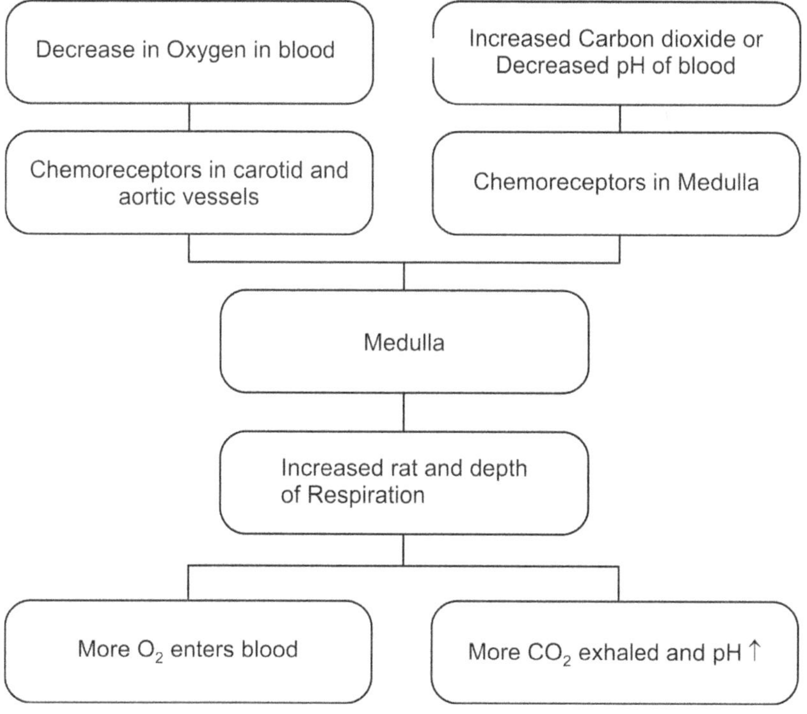

Figure 5-16 Flow Chart Showing Chemical Regulation of Respiration

Which Gas is a Major Regulator for Respiration?

Among the two respiratory gases, which is the more important as a regulator of respiration? Our guess might be oxygen, because it plays a vital role in energy production in cell respiration. However, oxygen is not a major regulator of oxygen. Rather, carbon dioxide is the major regulator of respiration, and the reason is that carbon dioxide affects the pH of the blood. An excess of CO_2 causes the blood pH to decrease that is become acidic a process that must not be allowed to continue. Therefore, any increase in the blood CO_2 level is immediately compensated by increasing breathing to exhale more CO_2.

In certain circumstances, oxygen becomes the major regulator of respiration. In severe chronic pulmonary diseases such as emphysema, the exchange of both oxygen and carbon dioxide is decreased. The decrease in pH caused by accumulation of CO_2 is corrected by the kidneys, but the blood oxygen level keeps decreasing. The oxygen level may fall very low, thereby; it provides a very strong stimulus to increase the rate and depth of respiration.

Artificial respiration and resuscitation methods

Artificial respiration (AR) is also known as artificial ventilation, forcing the air into the lungs of the person who has stopped the breathing, usually by blowing through their mouth or nose to keep him/her alive and to help start breathing again.

Two main methods of artificial respiration are there.

1. Manual methods
2. Instrumental methods

Manual methods

(a) **Schafer's Method:** The subject is laid in prone position and a small pillow is placed underneath the chest and epigastrium. Turn the head to one side. The operator kneels down by the side of the subject facing towards his head. Two hands of the operator are placed on two sides of the lower part of the chest and then the operator slowly puts his body weight leaning forwards and pressing upon the loins of the subject. Now the intra-abdominal pressure rises, there by the diaphragm is pushed up and air is forced out of the lungs.

This is followed by the release of pressure by coming back to the original erect position of the operator. It leads to decrease in abdominal pressure, diaphragm descends and air is drawn in. These movements should be repeated about twelve times a minute. By this method the total pulmonary ventilation is of 6,500 ml per minute, and this is sufficient for complete aeration of blood.

Advantages

1. It is prone position, so mucus and water from abdomen and lungs can be easily drained.
2. It is very simple method and non tiring can be done for a longer time.
3. This method can be used even if the patient has injuries at thorax and back **(Table 5-11)**.

Disadvantages

1. It is unphysiological one where inspiration is passive and expiration is active.
2. Cannot be used if the patient has abdominal injury.

(b) **Sylvester's Method:** In this method the subject is placed in supine position. The operator stands or kneels near the head and holds the two arms of the subject. Then the operator raises the subject's hands above his head and then folds the hands back upon the chest, compressing the chest wall at the same time.

These type of movements increases and decrease the thoracic cavity, thereby drawing in and pushing out air from the lungs. This is the most commonly used method in the operation theatre or in other accidents. Here the tongue of the subject should be pulled out and the mucus from the mouth cavity should be wiped out from time to time.

Advantages

1. Both inspiration and expiration is active, so good ventilation is obtained.

Disadvantages

1. The patient is in supine position, so no drainage of mucus and water from mouth and lungs.
2. Since it is a tiring procedure, assistance is needed.
3. Cannot be used if there is rib or thoracic fracture (Table 5-11).

(c) **Holger-Nielson Method:** The subject is placed in prone position with the arms abducted at the shoulders and elbows remaining flexed. The head is turned to one side and rests on the hands. The mouth is cleaned by wiping the mucus and fluid. In front of the subject the operator kneels down facing towards the head. Two hands are placed on the back of the chest with the thumbs and fingers spread apart.

Now the operator puts his body weight leaning forward upon the subject's back. This leads to compression of the chest and in expiration. The subject's arms forwards by holding them above the elbows. This helps in natural inspiration. This process should be repeated for about 10-12 times a minute.

Advantages

1. It is prone position, so mucus and water from abdomen and lungs can be easily drained.
2. Can be used if there is any abdominal injury.
3. Both inspiration and expiration are active, so good ventilation is obtained.

Disadvantages

1. Since it is tiring method, needed assistance.
2. Cannot be used if there is injury to scapula.

(d) **Mouth-to-Mouth Method:** Here the subject is laid in the supine position with extended head. The operator should sit by the side of the subject's head. The lower jaw of the subject should be held by one thumb and index-finger and clamps the nostrils with the other thumb and index-finer. The operator then keeps his mouth over the subject's mouth and exhales forcibly which causes inflation of the lungs and thorax. The operator then takes off his mouth and the process is repeated 10-20 times per minute. It is positive-pressure breathing.

Advantages

1. Expired air is blown into the mouth of the patient, which contain CO_2, which stimulate patient respiratory centre.
2. Inspiration is active and expiration is passive which is physiological one.
3. Best method of AR in new born.

Disadvantages

Since it is a supine position, water and mucus may drain into lungs and cause infection.

(e) **EVE's Rocking Method:** The patient is tied on a stretcher. At an angle of 45° the head and feet are alternately tilted. Per minute eight or nine movements are carried out, each movement for 7 seconds, 4 seconds head down and 3 seconds feet down. When head is down, the weight of the abdominal viscera presses against the diaphragm, so that air is pushed out of the lungs leads to expiration. When the feet are down, diaphragm descends and air is drawn into the lungs leads to inspiration.

Table 5-11 Methods of manual AR, their advantages and disadvantages

Sr. No.	Method	Advantages	Disadvantages
1	Schafer's Method	• It is prone position, so mucus and water from abdomen and lungs can be easily drained. • It is very simple method and non-tiring can be done for a longer time. • This method can be used even if the patient has injuries at thorax and back.	• It is unphysiological one where inspiration is passive and expiration is active. • Cannot be used if the patient has abdominal injury
2	Sylvester's Method	• Both inspiration and expiration is active, so good ventilation is obtained.	• The patient is in supine position, so no drainage of mucus and water from mouth and lungs. • Since it is a tiring procedure, assistance is needed. • Cannot be used if there is rib or thoracic fracture.
3	Holger-Nielson Method	• It is prone position, so mucus and water from abdomen and lungs can be easily drained. • Can be used if there is any abdominal injury. • Both inspiration and expiration are active, so good ventilation is obtained.	• Since it is a tiring method, needed assistance. • Cannot be used if there is injury to scapula.

Table 5-11 *Contd...*

Sr. No.	Method	Advantages	Disadvantages
4	Mouth-to-Mouth Method	• Expired air is blown into the mouth of the patient, which contain CO2, which stimulate patient's respiratory center. • Inspiration is active and expiration is passive which is physiological one. • Best method of AR in new born.	• Since it is a supine position, water and mucus may drain into lungs and cause infection.
5	EVE's Rocking Method	• Most useful in children and infants. • Unskilled person can perform it.	• Less superior when compared to other manual methods.

Instrumental Method

Machineries are used instead of a human operator. The advantage is that it can be done for good length of time, whereas the human operator is likely to be fatigued.

The machines work on two principles

(i) Negative-pressure breathing by alternately compressing and relaxing the chest wall

(ii) Positive-pressure breathing by introducing air or oxygen directly into the lungs-intermittently or continuously.

    (a) Drinker's Method: Here the patient is placed in an airtight chamber, the head remaining outside. The pressure in the chamber is alternately lowered and raised by mechanically driven pumps. When the pressure is lowered the chest swells up and air is drawn into the lungs. The chest becomes compressed and air is pushed out when the pressure is raised.

    By this way, artificial ventilation may be continued for longer time. This method is very useful in cases where prolonged artificial respiration is necessary, such as in morphine poisoning, in paralysis of the respiratory muscles, as in poliomyelitis, pneumothorax etc.

    (b) Bragg Paul's Method: In this method a rubber bag is wrapped round the chest wall of the subject. By pumps, pressure in the bag is alternately raised and lowered thereby compressing and relaxing the chest wall alternately. In this way respiration is carried out. It is of four types.

        (i) Continuous Insufflation Method: This method is used in subjects who need to undergo operation requiring opening of the thorax. None of the above methods are applicable here. A thin flexible tube is inserted into the trachea as far as its bifurcation and a constant stream of oxygen with or without 5% CO_2 is passed into the lungs so that lungs remain slightly distended. Hence it is possible to maintain respiration without any movement of the subject.

(ii) **Intermittent Inflation Method:** This method is used to maintain the respiration of animals during experiments. In this method, a cannula is introduced into trachea and tied. By means of a pump warm moist air is driven into the lungs. After each blast, the lung collapses and air is expelled through a side tube in the cannula. A very elaborate apparatus is used when artificial gas mixtures used.

(iii) **Tank respirator:** In this method the patient's body is placed inside the tank and his head is protruded through a flexible but airtight collar. A motor-driven leather diaphragm that moves back and forth with sufficient excursion to raise and lower the pressure within the tank was placed opposite to the patient's head. Positive pressure is produced around the body by inward movement of leather diaphragm and causes expiration. Outward movement of leather diaphragm produces negative pressure and causes inspiration.

(iv) **Resuscitator:** The resuscitator forces the air pass through the mask that is placed on the patient's face into the lungs during the positive pressure cycle and then either allows air to flow out the lungs during the remainder of the cycle or pull the air out by negative pressure. It has safety valve which prevents the positive pressure from rising normally about +14 mm Hg and the negative pressure from falling below -9 mm Hg.

Artificial respiration plays a vital role in newly born babies, whose respiration is delayed.

Artificial respiration in new born babies

(i) Hold the baby upside down to allow more blood to go to the brain and pat on the back.

(ii) Put the child alternately in warm and cold water which stimulate reflex respiration.

(iii) CO_2 is pumped through the nostrils or mouth into the lungs of the child. This is done by forcibly blowing through the mouth of the child after closing its nostrils. Now the CO_2 tension of blood is raised, which stimulate the respiratory center. Mouth-to-mouth resuscitation is quite effective in infants.

Diseases of the Respiratory System

Obstructive Lung Diseases

In obstructive lung diseases, there is an obstruction in the respiratory airways. Therefore, there is a limitation on the amount of air that may be exhaled. The air comes out of lungs more slowly than normal. Even at the end of full exhalation, a high amount of air remains in the lungs. The hallmark of obstructive lung diseases is the decreased expiratory flow rate and forced expiratory volume (FEV1).

However, the forced vital capacity (FVC) is nearly normal. Thus, the FEV1/FVC ratio is reduced and becomes less than 0.7. The common examples of obstructive lung diseases include asthma, chronic obstructive lung diseases (COPD), bronchiectasis and cystic fibrosis.

Restrictive Lung Diseases

There is a restriction on lung expansion and lungs cannot expand as in normal persons. There is stiffness in the lungs and thus, there is reduction in both FVC and FEV1. As a result, the ratio of FEV1/FVC is near normal. The common examples of restrictive lung diseases include acute or chronic interstitial lung diseases, pneumoconiosis, sarcoidosis and Idiopathic Pulmonary Fibrosis (IPF).

Bronchial Asthma

It is a chronic inflammatory disorder, which is characterized by reversible air way obstruction due to abnormal bronchial hyperactivity or hyper-responsiveness to a stimulus (mostly allergic). It is characterized by three important features including 'inflammation', 'hyper-reactivity to a stimulus' and 'reversible bronchospasm'. Asthma may be precipitated by various agents ranging from allergens to infection, drugs (aspirin), emotions (stress, anxiety) or exercise. Allergic asthma is the most common type of asthma. Clinically, there are by episodes of dyspnea (difficult respiration) and associated wheezing. Wheezing is a characteristic symptom of asthma and is defined as high pitched whistling sound produced due to turbulent airflow through the obstructed airways. Apart from wheezing, patients may complaint of tightness in chest and burning sensation.

Chronic Obstructive Lung Diseases (COPD)

It has two types, emphysema and chronic bronchitis.

Emphysema

It is characterized by permanent enlargement of airspaces of lungs due to widespread destruction of alveolar walls. Due to this, there is a significant reduction in total surface area of alveoli and thus, there is impairment in exchange of gases. Cigarette smoking and deficiency of alpha 1-antitrypsin are important cause of development of emphysema. Shortness of breath is the most common symptom of emphysema. Other symptoms include cough, wheezing and severe weight loss. There is prolonged expiration, and patient sits in a forward in hunched-over position, and attempts to squeeze the air out of lungs with effort. The long term complications include development of pulmonary hypertension, which then leads to right sided heart failure.

Chronic Bronchitis

It is state which is characterized by presence of persistent productive cough for at least 3 consecutive months in at least two consecutive years. Therefore, bronchitis is defined by clinical symptoms, while emphysema is defined anatomically. The clinical symptoms include prominent cough and production of sputum. The chronic obstruction leads to development of significant COPD, which is characterized by hypercapnia, hypoxia and cyanosis.

5.2 Chapter at a Glance

Term	Description
Homeostasis	Maintenance and regulation of the stability and constancy by cell, tissue and organ which is needed to function properly.
Conducting zone	Comprise a series of inter connecting cavities and tubes, both outside and within the lungs.
Respiratory zone	Comprise of the tubes and tissues within the lungs.
Cricoid cartilage	The most inferior cartilage of the larynx, which is also known as voice box.
Nasopharynx	Passage way for air
Oropharynx	Passageway for air and food
Laryngopharynx	Passageway for air and food
Parietal pleura	Lines the chest wall
Visceral pleura	Covers the lungs
Pleural cavity	Space between parietal and visceral pleura
Pulmonary surfactant	Lipoprotein secreted by alveolar type II cells
Diaphragm	A flat muscle that separates chest from abdomen
Internal intercostal muscles	Lie inside the rib cage.
External intercostal muscles	Lie outside the rib cage.
Tidal volume	Amount of air in one normal inhalation and exhalation.
Minute respiratory volume	Amount of air inhaled and exhaled in 1 minute.
Alveolar ventilation	Amount of air that reaches the alveoli and involves in exchange of gas is called alveolar ventilation.
Pulmonary ventilation	Exchange of air between the atmosphere and the alveoli of the lungs.
External Respiration	Exchange of gas between alveoli and blood
Internal Respiration	Exchange of gas between blood and tissues
Intrapleural Pressure	Pressure within the pleural space between the parietal pleura and visceral pleura
Intra pulmonic Pressure	Pressure within the bronchial tree and alveoli
Oxyhemoglobin	The complex of oxygen with hemoglobin
Carbaminohemoglobin	The complex of carbon dioxide with hemoglobin
Artificial respiration	Forcing the air into the lungs of the person who has stopped the breathing

Exercises

Multiple Choice Questions

1. Respiratory center is located in
   (a) Medulla oblongata
   (b) Hypothalamus
   (c) Cerebrum
   (d) Cerebellum

2. Lungs are covered by which layer?
   - (a) Parietal
   - (b) Pleural
   - (c) Pericardium
   - (d) Myocardium

3. Exchange of gas take place in this part during respiration.
   - (a) Diaphragm
   - (b) Trachea
   - (c) Pharynx
   - (d) Alveoli

4. Larynx opens into pharynx by?
   - (a) Thyroid
   - (b) Alveoli
   - (c) Glottis
   - (d) None

5. Instrument used to measure the amount of air inhaled and exhaled during respiration.
   - (a) Spirometer
   - (b) Density meter
   - (c) Lactometer
   - (d) Hygrometer

6. The respiratory pigment present in human is
   - (a) Melanin
   - (b) Haemocyanin
   - (c) Calamine
   - (d) Hemoglobin

7. Tidal volume in man is
   - (a) 100ml
   - (b) 300ml
   - (c) 200ml
   - (d) 500ml

8. Intra pleural pressure is
   - (a) 760 mmHg
   - (b) 756 mmHg
   - (c) Both
   - (d) None

9. Carbon dioxide is transported in blood as
   - (a) Oxyhemoglobin
   - (b) Carboxyhemoglobin
   - (c) Carbabinohemoglobin
   - (d) All

10. Mechanisms that regulate respiration
    - (a) Nervous regulation
    - (b) Chemical regulation
    - (c) Both a and b
    - (d) None

Short Answer Questions

1. Write the parts and functions of nose.
2. Define conducting and respiratory zone.
3. Write the parts and functions of pharynx.
4. Name the receptor responsible for smell and its location.
5. Mention the different layers of trachea.
6. Give a note on location of lungs.
7. Write the types of cells present in alveoli.
8. What is the role of pulmonary surfactant?
9. Write the difference between internal and external intercostal muscles.

10. Define anatomical dead space.
11. Write the difference between internal and external respiration.
12. Define artificial respiration.
13. Write a note on artificial respiration in new born babies.
14. Name the manual methods of artificial respiration.
15. Name the instrumental methods of artificial respiration.

Long Answer Questions

1. Write short notes on trachea.
2. Write short note on lungs its lobes, fissures and lobules.
3. Explain about the steps involved in the process of respiration.
4. Explain about the steps involved in breathing.
5. In brief write about the pressure changes of respiration.
6. Discuss about the transport of O_2 in blood.
7. Discuss about the transport of CO_2 in blood.
8. Write about the nervous regulation of respiration.
9. Write about the chemical regulation of respiration.
10. Explain the manual methods of resuscitation.

Bibliography

Chatterjee CC, Human Physiology, Vol-I, 11th edition. Medical Applied Agency, Calcutta, 2016.

Tortora GJ, Derrichson B, John Wiley and Sons. Principles of Anatomy and Physiology, 15Th edition, Hoboken, NJ:John Wiley and Sons, Inc., 2017.

Valerie SC, Tina S. Essentials of Anatomy and Physiology. 5th edition, Philadelphia, PA: F.A. Davis Co., 2011.

Answer Key MCQs

1. (a)	2. (b)	3. (b)	4. (c)	5. (a)
6. (d)	7. (d)	8. (b)	9. (c)	10. (c)

Urinary System

Learning Objective

After completing this lesson, the Reader should be able to understand:

- *Urinary system (Introduction)*
- *Functions of the Urinary system*
- *Anatomy of the Urinary system*
- *Formation of urine*
- *Transportation of urine, storage, and elimination*
- *Micturition and Micturition reflex*
- *Characteristics of Urine*
- *Role of kidneys in Acid-Base balance*
- *Renin-Angiotensin-Aldosterone System*
- *Disorders of Kidney*

6.1   Introduction

The urinary system is one of the excretory systems of the body. The main function of it is formation and excretion of urine and thereby maintains the body homeostasis. The waste substances like urea, ammonia, and creatinine are produced by the body cells. These substances need to be removed from the body otherwise they may accumulate to toxic levels. The kidneys form the urine and along with urine, these toxic substances are also eliminated. The major work of the urinary system is done by the kidneys. The other parts of the urinary system act as passageway and storage of formed urine.

Functions of Urinary System

The functions of the urinary system are as follows:

1. **Maintenance of ionic composition of blood:** The kidneys maintain the concentration of several ions in the blood, mainly sodium ions, potassium ions, calcium ions, chloride ions and phosphate ions.

2. **Maintenance of blood pH:** The kidneys eliminate hydrogen ions into the urine and conserve bicarbonate ions in the blood. These activities help to maintain blood pH.

3. **Maintenance of blood volume:** The blood volume was maintained by the kidneys by absorbing or excreting the water in the urine. An increase in blood volume increases blood pressure and a decrease in blood volume decreases blood pressure.

4. **Maintenance of blood pressure:** The blood pressure is also maintained by the kidneys by synthesizing the enzyme renin. This renin activates the renin–angiotensin–aldosterone system. An increase in renin level causes an increase in blood pressure and vice versa.

5. **Maintenance of blood osmolarity:** A constant osmolarity of blood is maintained by the kidneys, by regulating loss of water and loss of solutes in the urine.

6. **Synthesis of hormones:** Two hormones are synthesized by the kidneys namely calcitriol and erythropoietin. Calcitriol is the active form of vitamin D and helps to regulate the calcium homeostasis whereas; erythropoietin stimulates the synthesis of red blood cells.

7. **Maintenance of blood glucose level:** The kidneys can utilize the amino acid glutamine in gluconeogenesis, i.e. the synthesis of new glucose molecules like the liver. This glucose is released into the blood to maintain a normal blood glucose level.

8. **Elimination of waste substances:** The kidneys eliminate the waste substances which don't have any useful function in the body through the urine. The waste products like ammonia, urea, bilirubin, creatinine and uric acid are produced during the metabolic reactions in the body are eliminated through urine. Ammonia and urea are produced from the deamination of amino acids. Bilirubin is formed from the catabolism of hemoglobin. Creatinine is formed from the breakdown of creatine phosphate in muscle fibers and uric acid is formed from the catabolism of nucleic acids. Other wastes excreted in the urine are foreign substances from the diet, such as drugs and environmental toxins.

Anatomy of Urinary System

The urinary system consists of the following parts summarized in **Table 6-1**.

Table 6-1 Parts of the Urinary system and their functions

Sr. No.	Parts of Urinary System	Functions
1	Two Kidneys	Filter and clean the blood.
2	Two Ureters	Tube like structure that take urine from kidneys to the bladder.

Table 6-1 Contd...

Sr. No.	Parts of Urinary System	Functions
3	One Bladder	Acts as a reservoir and stores urine until eliminated.
4	One Urethra	An opening through which urine is eliminated from the body.

Kidneys

One pair of reddish, bean-shaped kidneys is located in the upper abdominal cavity on either side of the vertebral column, behind the peritoneum. Each kidney is about 10–12 cm long, 5–7 cm wide, and 3 cm in thickness and weighs about 135–150 g. The upper portions of the kidneys rest on the lower surface of the diaphragm and are enclosed and protected by the lower rib cage. The right kidney is slightly lower than the left because the liver occupies some space on the right side superior to the kidney (Figure 6-1). The kidneys are covered by a fibrous connective tissue membrane called the renal fascia, which helps to hold the kidneys in place. Each kidney has hilum, on the medial side through which the renal blood vessels, lymphatic vessels, nerves, and ureters pass.

Each kidney is surrounded by three layers of tissues. They are,

1. Renal capsule
2 Adipose capsule
3. Renal fascia

Renal capsule is the innermost layer. It is a smooth sheet of irregular connective tissue that is continuous with the outer layer of the ureter. It acts as a barrier against trauma and maintains the shape of the kidney.

Adipose capsule is the middle layer, protects the kidney from trauma and holds it firmly in the abdominal cavity.

Renal fascia is the outer most layer. It anchors the kidney to the surrounding structures and to the abdominal wall.

The longitudinal section of the kidney shows two regions.

1. Renal cortex - A superficial, light red region.
2. Renal medulla - A deep, darker reddish brown region.

The renal medulla has many cone-shaped structures called renal pyramids. The wider base of each pyramid faces the renal cortex and its narrow apex, called renal papilla faces towards the renal hilum. The medulla is divided into two zones – outer cortical zone and inner juxtamedullary zone. The portions of the renal cortex that extends between renal pyramids are called renal columns.

The renal cortex and renal pyramids of renal medulla form the functional portion of the kidney. Nephrons are the microscopic functional units of kidney and each kidney has about one million nephrons. These nephrons form the urine and drain it into large papillary ducts, which extend through the renal papillae of the pyramids. These papillary ducts drain into cup-like structures called major and minor calyces. Nearly 8 to 18 minor calyces and 2 to 3 major calyces are present in each kidney. The filtrate which enters the calyces becomes urine because no further reabsorption can occur. Finally, the urine drains from the major calyces into a single large cavity called renal pelvis and passed through the ureter to the urinary bladder **(Figure 6-2)**.

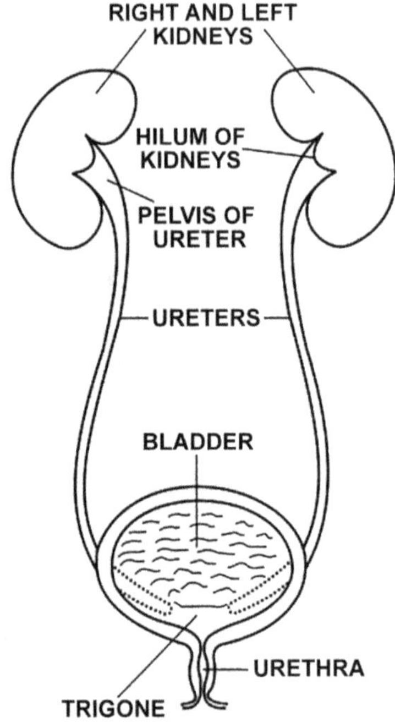

Figure 6-1 Anterior view of the Urinary System

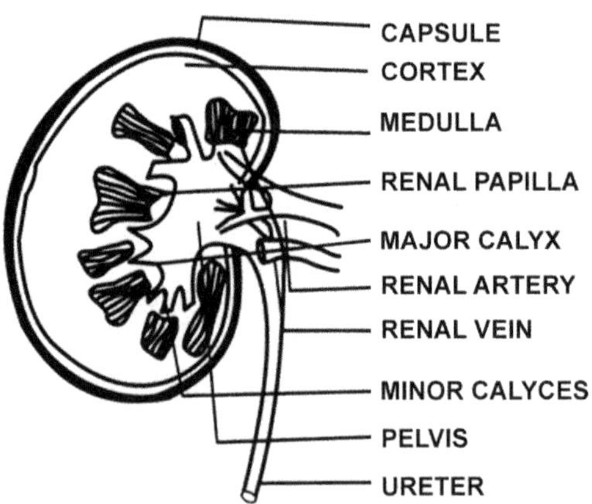

Figure 6-2 Longitudinal section of Right kidney

Structure of Nephron

Nephrons are the structural and functional units of the kidney. Each kidney has approximately one million nephrons **(Figure 6-3)**. Each nephron has two parts. They are

1. Renal corpuscle where plasma is filtered
2. Renal tubule into which the filtered fluid or glomerular filtrate passes.

Renal corpuscle

The renal corpuscle has two components. One is a tuft of the capillary network which is also called glomerulus and another is Bowman's capsule, which is also known as a glomerular capsule. The glomerulus is formed by the tuft of afferent and efferent arterioles. The Bowman's capsule is a double-walled epithelial cup that surrounds the glomerular capillaries. Plasma is filtered through the glomerular capsule, and then the filtered fluid passes into the renal tubule.

Renal tubule and collecting duct

The renal tubule has three parts,

1. Proximal convoluted tubule
2. Loop of Henle
3. Distal convoluted tubule.

The renal corpuscle and convoluted tubules lie within the renal cortex. The loop of Henle extends into the renal medulla, makes a hairpin turn and then returns to the renal cortex. The distal convoluted tubules of several nephrons open into a single collecting duct. These collecting ducts unite and converge into many large papillary ducts, which in turn drain into minor calyces. The collecting and papillary ducts extend from the renal cortex through the renal medulla into the renal pelvis. In a nephron, the proximal and distal convoluted tubules are connected by Henle's loop. The first part of the Henle's loop begins at the point where the proximal convoluted tubule takes its final turn downward. It starts in the renal cortex and extends downward into renal medulla, where it is called the descending limb of the loop of Henle. The Loop of Henle is divided into four parts. They are a thick and thin-walled descending limb of the loop of Henle and thin and thick-walled ascending loop of Henle. This loop of Henle makes the hairpin turn and returns to the renal cortex where it terminates at the distal convoluted tubule and is known as ascending limb of the loop of Henle. The distal convoluted tubules of several nephrons empty their content into collecting duct. Then several collecting ducts unite to form a papillary duct which empties urine into a calyx of the renal pelvis.

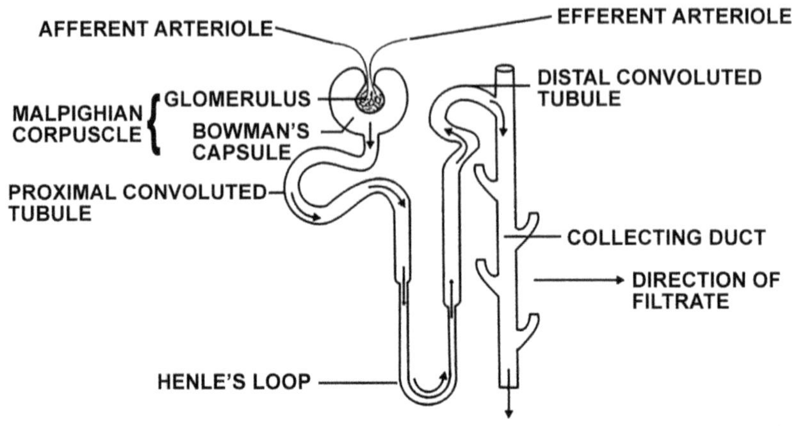

Figure 6-3 Structure of Nephron

There are two types of nephrons **(Table 6-2)**:

1. Cortical nephrons
2. Juxtamedullary nephrons.

Table 6-2 Difference between the cortical and Juxtamedullary nephrons

Sr. No.	Cortical nephron	Juxtamedullary nephron
1	80 – 85 % are cortical nephrons	10 – 15 % are juxtamedullary nephrons
2	Renal corpuscles lie in the outer portion of the renal cortex.	Renal corpuscles lie deep in renal cortex.
3	Loop of Henle is short. Lie mainly in the cortex and penetrates only into the outer region of the renal medulla.	Loop of Henle is long that extends to the deepest region of the medulla. This loop of Henle has two parts: a thin ascending limb followed by a thick ascending limb.
4	Receive blood supply from peritubular capillaries that arise from efferent arterioles.	Receive blood supply from peritubular capillaries and from the vasa recta that arise from efferent arterioles.

Formation of Urine

Urine is formed by three steps. They are,

1. Glomerular filtration
2. Tubular reabsorption
3. Tubular secretion

Glomerular filtration

It is the first step in urine formation. The blood pressure forces plasma, which has dissolved solute molecules and small proteins through the glomeruli and into Bowman's capsule. This fluid is called glomerular filtrate or renal filtrate. This filtrate moves into the glomerular capsule and then into the renal tubule. The blood pressure in the glomeruli is somewhat high 60 mmHg, when compared with that of other blood capillaries. The pressure in Bowman's capsule is very low and its inner layer is highly permeable. Hence approximately 20% to 25% of the blood that enters glomeruli becomes renal filtrate in Bowman's capsule. The blood cells and larger proteins are not filtered in glomeruli, so they remain in the blood. Waste products are dissolved in plasma which are eliminated as renal filtrate and useful materials such as nutrients and minerals are also present in renal filtrate but they are reabsorbed.

The glomerular filtration rate (GFR) is defined as the amount of filtrate formed by the kidneys in 1 minute. The average GFR is 100 to 150 mL per minute. The rate of blood flow through the kidney determines the GFR. If blood flow increases, the GFR increase and more filtrate if formed. On the other hand, if blood flow decreases, GFR decreases and low filtrate is formed. There by urine output also decreases.

Tubular reabsorption

Tubular reabsorption takes place in the renal tubules. In 24 hours the kidney forms 150 to 180 liters of filtrate and normal urinary output is 1 to 2 liters. Hence it is clear that most of the renal filtrate does not become urine. Approximately 99% of filtrate is reabsorbed back into the blood and only 1% of the filtrate is eliminated as urine. Nearly most of the reabsorption and secretion take place in the proximal convoluted tubules because these cells have microvilli which increase the surface area. The distal convoluted tubules and collecting tubules are also important sites for the reabsorption of water.

Mechanisms of Reabsorption

Various substances from the filtrate are reabsorbed by many mechanisms are shown in the **Table 6-3**.

1. **Active transport:** The renal tubule cells use ATP to transport the useful materials from the filtrate into blood. These useful materials are glucose, vitamins, amino acids and ions. The renal tubules have a threshold level for the reabsorption of the above substances. This means there is a limit for the removal of these substances from the filtrate. For example the renal threshold value for glucose is 180 mg/dl.

The reabsorption of calcium ions is increased by parathyroid hormone. The parathyroid gland secretes parathyroid hormone if the calcium level in the blood decreases. The reabsorption of the calcium ions by the kidneys is one of the mechanisms by which the blood calcium level is raised back to normal.

The hormone aldosterone secreted by the adrenal cortex, increases the reabsorption of Na^+ ions and the excretion of K^+ ions. Apart from regulating the blood levels of sodium and potassium ions, aldosterone also affects the blood volume.

2. **Passive transport:** Many of the negatively charged ions are reabsorbed into the blood followed by the reabsorption of positive ions, because unlike charges attract. Example: Chloride, potassium, calcium, magnesium ions, urea and water.

3. **Osmosis:** The reabsorption of water follows the reabsorption of minerals especially Na^+, Cl^- and glucose. The reabsorption of water with solutes in the tubular fluid is called obligatory water reabsorption. This is because the water is obliged to follow the solutes when they are absorbed. This type of water reabsorption occurs in the proximal convoluted and descending limb of the loop of Henle, because these parts of the nephron are always permeable to water.

4. **Pinocytosis:** Some proteins are too large can't be reabsorbed by active transport. So they are adsorbed to the membranes of the cells of the proximal convoluted tubules. The cell membrane then sinks inward and folds around the protein to take it in. Usually, all the proteins in the filtrate are reabsorbed and none is eliminated in urine.

Table 6-3 Mechanisms of reabsorption of different substances from renal filtrate

Sr. No.	Mechanism of reabsorption	Substances reabsorbed
1	Active transport	Glucose, vitamins, amino acids, sodium ions and calcium ions.
2	Passive transport	Chloride, potassium, calcium, magnesium ions, urea and water.
3	Osmosis	Water, glucose, sodium and chloride.
4	Pinocytosis	Proteins.

Tubular secretion

Tubular secretion changes the composition of urine. In tubular secretion, substances are actively secreted from the blood into the filtrate in renal tubules.

Waste substances, such as ammonia, creatinine and the metabolic products of medications may be secreted into the filtrate to be eliminated in urine. Hydrogen ions may also be secreted by the tubule cells to maintain the normal pH of blood.

Hormones that influence the reabsorption of water and ions

Various hormones influence the reabsorption of water and ions from the filtrate into blood (Table 6-4). Aldosterone is secreted by the adrenal cortex in response to high blood potassium level, low blood sodium level or to a decrease in blood pressure. When aldosterone stimulates the reabsorption of sodium ions, water also reabsorbed along with it into the blood. This helps to maintain normal blood volume and blood pressure (Figure 6-4).

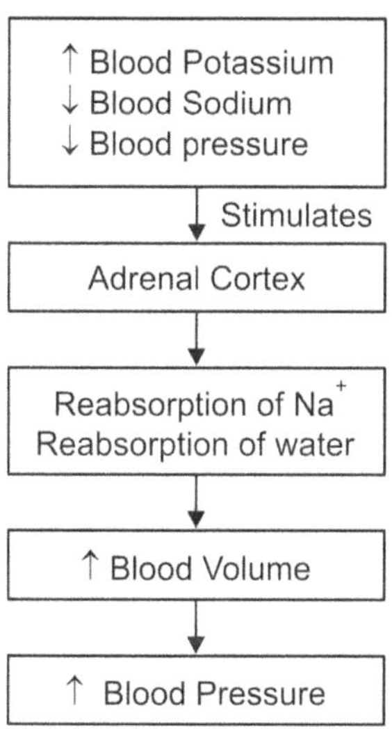

Figure 6-4 Role of aldosterone in controlling blood pressure

Atrial natriuretic peptide (ANP) which is an antagonist of aldosterone is secreted by the atria of the heart. It is secreted when the atrial walls are stretched by high blood pressure or high blood volume. ANP decreases the reabsorption of sodium ions by the nephrons and being excreted in filtrate along with water. Thereby ANP lowers the blood volume and blood pressure **(Figure 6-5)**.

Antidiuretic hormone (ADH) is released by the posterior pituitary when the amount of water in the body decreases. This ADH acts on the distal convoluted tubule and collecting ducts and reabsorbs the water from the filtrate. This helps to maintain the normal blood volume and blood pressure and also helps the kidneys to produce urine that is more concentrated than body fluids. If the amount of water in the body increases, the secretion of ADH stops and the nephrons will reabsorb less water. Now the urine becomes diluted and water is eliminated until its concentration in the body returns to normal **(Figure 6-6)**.

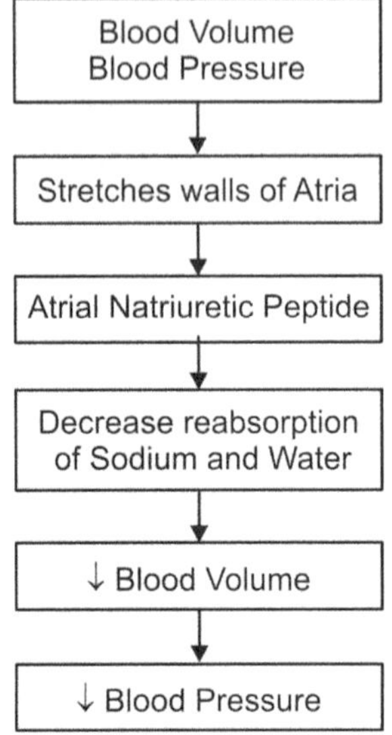

Figure 6-5 Role of ANP in controlling blood pressure

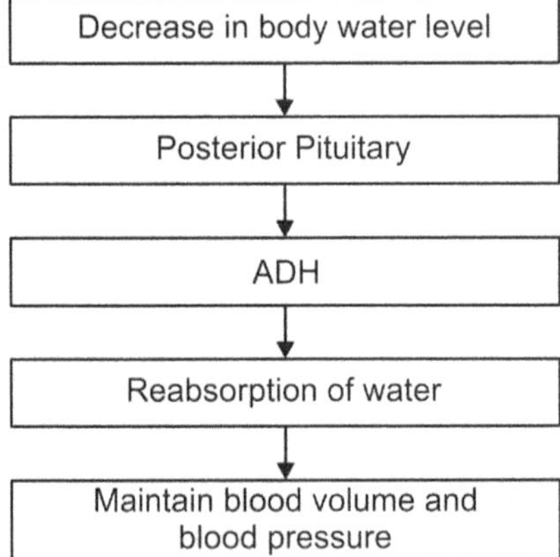

Figure 6-6 Role of ADH in controlling blood pressure

Parathyroid hormone increases the reabsorption of calcium ions from the filtrate into the blood and excretion of phosphate ions into the filtrate.

Table 6-4 Hormones that influence the reabsorption of water and ions.

Sr. No.	Gland	Hormone	Function
1	Adrenal cortex	Aldosterone	• Increases sodium reabsorption • Increases water reabsorption
2	Atria of the heart	Atrial natriuretic peptide	• Decreases reabsorption of sodium • Decreases reabsorption of water
3	Posterior pituitary	Antidiuretic Hormone	• Increase reabsorption water from the filtrate.
4	Parathyroid gland	Parathyroid hormone	• Increases reabsorption of calcium ions • Increases excretion of phosphate ions.

Transportation of Urine, Storage, and Elimination

The nephrons form the urine. This urine is drained by the collecting ducts of nephron into papillary ducts. These papillary ducts, in turn, drain the urine into minor calyces. These minor calyces join and become major calyces. These major calyces unite to form the renal pelvis. From the renal pelvis, urine first drains into the ureter and then into the urinary bladder. Then the urine is eliminated from the bladder through the urethra. It is shown in **(Figure 6-7)**.

Ureters

Each ureter extends from the hilum of the kidneys to the urinary bladder. The ureter exhibits the peristalsis movement and pushes urine towards the urinary bladder. Peristaltic waves from the renal pelvis to the urinary bladder vary in frequency from one to five per minute, depending on how fast urine is being formed.

The ureters are of 25 to 30 cm in length and are thick-walled, narrow tubes of 1 mm to 10 mm in diameter. Like kidneys the ureter is retroperitoneal. The ureters open into the urinary bladder. As the urinary bladder fills with urine, the pressure within it compresses the openings into the ureters and prevents the backflow of urine. The walls of the ureter are composed of three layers of tissue. The innermost coat is mucosa, is a mucous membrane with transitional epithelium and an underlying lamina propria of areolar connective tissue. The intermediate coat is muscularis, is composed of inner longitudinal and outer circular layers of smooth muscle fibers. The superficial coat is adventitia, a layer of areolar connective tissue containing blood vessels, lymphatic vessels, and nerves.

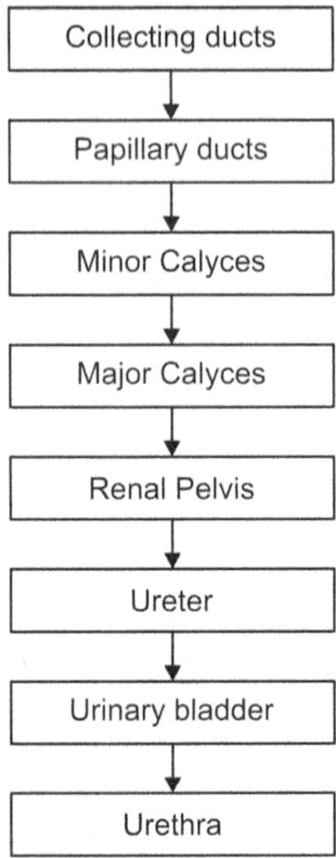

Figure 6-7 Flow chart showing transportation of urine

Urinary bladder

The urinary bladder is a muscular sac below the peritoneum and behind the pubic bones. In women the bladder is inferior to the uterus and in men, it is superior to the prostate gland. The bladder acts as a reservoir for accumulating urine. If once it attains the maximum volume the bladder contracts and eliminates urine. Transitional epithelium forms the mucosa of the bladder, permits the expansion without tearing the lining. When the bladder is empty, the mucosa looks wrinkled and forms folds. These folds are called rugae which permits the expansion. On the floor of the bladder is a triangular area known as trigone. This trigone is not having the rugae and doesn't expand. The smooth muscle layer in the wall of the bladder is called the detrusor muscle. This muscle is in sphere form. When it contracts it becomes a small sphere and its volume diminishes. Around the opening of the urethra the muscle fibers of the detrusor form the internal urethral sphincters which are involuntary (Figure 6-8).

Urethra

Urethra is an opening which carries urine from the bladder to the exterior. The external urethral sphincter is made up of skeletal muscle, is under voluntary control. In women, the urethra is 2.5 to 4 cm long and is anterior to the vagina. In men, the urethra is 17 to 20 cm long. The first part of the urethra just outside the bladder is called as prostatic urethra, because it is surrounded by the prostate gland. The next part of the urethra is the membranous urethra, around which is the external urethral sphincter. The longest portion of urethra is known as cavernous urethra, which passes through the cavernous tissue of penis. The male urethra carries both urine and semen.

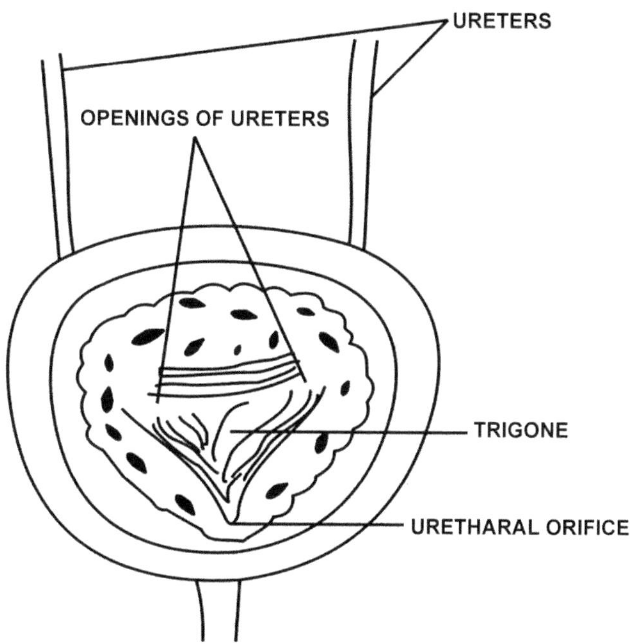

Figure 6-8 Structure of Urinary Bladder

Micturition and Micturition Reflex

Discharge of urine from the urinary bladder is called as micturition. Micturition reflex is also known as urination reflex or voiding. It is a spinal cord reflex over which voluntary control may be exerted. The stimulus for the micturition reflex is, stretching of the detrusor muscle of the urinary bladder. The bladder can hold up to 800 mL of urine or even more, but the reflex is activated much before the maximum volume is reached. When the urine volume reaches 200 to 400 mL, this leads to the stretching of detrusor muscle of the bladder. This stretching is sufficient to generate sensory impulses. These sensory impulses travel to the spinal cord. Now the motor impulses return along parasympathetic nerves to the detrusor muscle causing the contraction of urinary bladder. At the same time the, the internal urethral sphincter relaxes. If the external urethral sphincter is voluntarily relaxed, urine flows into the urethra and the bladder is emptied. By voluntary contraction of the external urethral sphincter, urination can be prevented. But if the bladder continues to fill and be stretched, voluntary control is no longer possible. **Figure 6-9** shows the flow chart of Micturition.

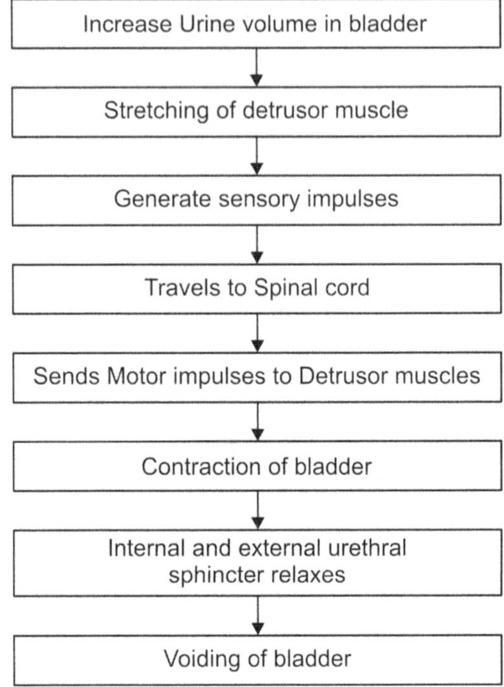

Figure 6-9 Flow chart of Micturition

Characteristics of Urine

The characteristics of urine include the physical and chemical properties which are often evaluated as part of urine analysis **(Table 6-5)**.

Table 6-5 Characteristics of normal urine

Sr. No.	Characteristics	Description
1	Amount	1.5 to 2 liters per day. Highly variable on excessive water loss and excessive fluid intake.
2	Color	Straw or amber. Darker means more concentrated.
3	Specific gravity	1.010 to 1.025 a measure of the dissolved material in urine
4	pH	Ranges from 4.6 to 8. Average 6.0. Diet has great impact on pH.
5	Constituents	95% water and 5% salts and waste products.
6	Nitrogenous wastes	Urea – From amino acid metabolism Crceatinine – From creatine phosphate metabolism Uric acid – From nucleic acids metabolism

Amount

Normal urinary output per day is 1.5 to 2 liters. Many factors may significantly affect the output. Excessive sweating or loss of fluid through diarrhea will decrease urine output to conserve body water (oliguria). On the other hand excessive intake of fluid will increase urine output (Polyuria). Consumption of alcohol will also increase urine output because alcohol inhibits the secretion of ADH and the kidneys will reabsorb less water.

Color

Urine is pale yellow in color. Concentrated urine is deeper yellow in color than dilute urine. Freshly excreted urine will be clear in appearance.

Specific gravity

The specific gravity of urine ranges from 1.010 to 1.025. It is a measure of the dissolved materials in urine. The specific gravity of water is 1.000, means that there are no solutes present. Hence higher the specific gravity value indicates presence of more dissolved material. The specific gravity of urine is an indicator of the concentrating ability of the kidneys.

Potential of Hydrogen (pH)

The pH of urine ranges from 4.6 to 8.0 with an average of 6.0. Diet has the greatest impact on urine pH. A vegetarian diet causes the urine more alkaline, whereas the high protein diet causes the urine more acidic.

Constituents

Urine has approximately 95% of water. It is the solvent for the excretion of waste products and salts. Usually salts are not considered as waste products because they may be utilized by the body when needed. However the excess amount of salts will be excreted in urine.

Nitrogenous wastes

These waste substances contain nitrogen. Liver produce urea when excess amino acids are deaminated to liberate energy. Creatinine is formed from the metabolism of creatine phosphate, an energy source in muscles. Uric acid is obtained from the metabolism of nucleic acids like DNA and RNA. Other non-nitrogenous waste products which are excreted in urine are urobilin and metabolites of drugs. Urobilin is formed from the hemoglobin of senile RBCs.

Role of Kidneys in Acid – Base Balance

The kidneys are the primary organs responsible for maintaining the pH of the blood and tissue fluids within normal ranges. They play a key role to compensate the pH changes with respect to body metabolism or the result of diseases and thereby make the necessary corrections. This regulatory function of the kidneys is somewhat complex. If body fluids are too acidic, the kidneys will secrete more H^+ ions into the renal filtrate and will return more bicarbonate ions (HCO_3^-) into the blood. This will help to increase the pH of blood to the normal value. On the other hand when the body fluids become alkaline, the kidneys will return the H^+ ions to the blood excrete bicarbonate ions in urine. This will help to lower the pH of blood back to normal.

Naturally the body fluids are more acidic. The cells of the renal tubules can secrete H^+ ions or ammonia in exchange for Na^+ ions and by doing so; influence the absorption of other ions. Hydrogen ions are obtained from the reaction of CO_2 and water. With this hydrogen ion, an amine group from an amino acid combines to form ammonia. The tubular cells secrete the hydrogen ions and ammonia into the renal filtrate and two Na^+ are reabsorbed in exchange. In this filtrate the hydrogen ion and ammonia from NH_4 which reacts with a chloride ion to form ammonium chloride (NH_4Cl) that is excreted in urine. As the Na^+ ions returned to the blood, bicarbonate ions follow. In this two hydrogen ions have been excreted in urine and two sodium ions and two bicarbonate ions have been returned to the blood. These reactions prevent the body fluids from becoming too acidic. The acid – base is also maintained by the phosphate buffer system.

Phosphate buffer system

This buffer system consists of two components. They are, sodium dihydrogen phosphate (NaH_2PO_4) which is a weak acid and sodium monohydrogen phosphate (Na_2HPO_4) which is a weak base. The following reactions take place if a potential pH change is created by strong acid.

$$HCl + Na_2HPO_4 \rightarrow NaCl + NaH_2PO_4$$

(Strong acid)   **(Weak acid)**

The strong acid reacts with sodium monohydrogen phosphate to produce a salt NaCl that has no effect on pH and a weak acid that has a little effect on pH. If a potential pH change is created by a strong base, the following reaction takes place.

$$NaOH + NaH_2PO_4 \rightarrow H_2O + Na_2HPO_4$$

(Strong base)   **(Weak base)**

The strong base reacts with sodium dihydrogen phosphate to form water, which has no effect on pH and a weak base that has little effect on pH. The cells of the kidney tubules can eliminate excess hydrogen ions by forming Na_2HPO_4, which is excreted in urine. The retained sodium ions are returned to the blood along with bicarbonate ions.

Renin-Angiotensin-Aldosterone System

If there is decrease in blood volume and blood pressure, the juxtaglomerular cells of kidney secrete renin enzyme into the blood. Release of renin from the juxtaglomerular cells of kidney is also stimulated by the sympathetic system. Renin converts angiotensinogen into angiotensin I which is a 10 amino acid peptide. This angiotensin I is converted into angiotensin II by angiotensin converting enzyme. This angiotensin II affects the renal physiology in the following ways.

1. It contracts the afferent arterioles and there by decreases the glomerular filtration rate.
2. It enhances the reabsorption of Na^+, Cl^- and water in the proximal convoluted tubule by stimulating the activity of Na^+-H^+ antiporters.
3. It stimulates the adrenal cortex to release aldosterone hormone which in turn stimulates the reabsorption of Na+, Cl- and secrete more K+ ions. This Na+ and Cl- reabsorption also stimulates the reabsorption of more amount of water. This leads to increase in blood volume and blood pressure **(Figure 6-10)**.

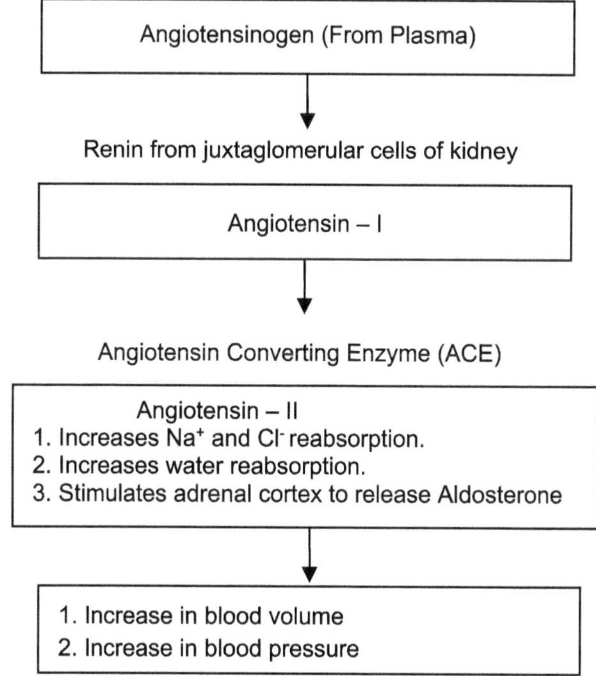

Figure 6-10 Renin-Angiotensin-Aldosterone System

Disorders of Kidney

Renal Calculi

Renal calculi are also called as kidney stones. These stones are the crystals of the salts that are generally present in urine. Very high concentration of salt in urine may lead to precipitation of the salt and formation of crystals. The size of the crystals may range from 10 to 20 mm in diameter. The kidney stones are made up of calcium oxalate, uric acid or calcium phosphate. These stones are normally formed in the renal pelvis. The reasons for stone formation are decreased fluid intake or over ingestion of minerals, which leads to the formation of very concentrated urine, in which the salts precipitate and forms the stones. When these stones from the kidney enter into the ureter it may cause intense pain and bleeding. Treatment of the kidney stone includes surgical removal of the stones or disintegration of stones by shock wave lithotripsy. The shock waves crush the stones into small pieces which will be eliminated through the ureter without damaging it.

Urinary tract infections

These infections may occur in any part of the urinary tract. Usually it is caused by the microorganisms of sexually transmitted diseases or by the bacteria that are part of the normal bacterial flora of colon. In women, the urethra and anus are in close proximity. Thereby the colon bacteria may gain access to the urinary tract. If sterile techniques are not followed in the use of urinary catheters in hospitalized or bed ridden patients may also leads to urinary tract infections.

Glomerulonephritis

It is an inflammation of the glomeruli of the kidney. The most common cause is an allergic reaction to the toxins produced by streptococcal bacteria that have recently infected any part of the body, especially the throat. Here the glomeruli became inflamed, swollen and filled with blood that the filtration membranes allow blood cells and plasma proteins to enter the filtrate. It results in elimination of erythrocytes and plasma proteins through urine. If the glomeruli are permanently damaged means it leads to chronic renal failure.

Nephrotic syndrome

It is a condition characterized by proteinuria that is protein in urine and hyperlipidemia that is high blood levels of cholesterols, phospholipids and triglycerides. Increased permeability of filtration membrane causes proteinuria in which proteins especially albumin is excreted in urine. Loss of albumin results in hypoalbuminemia that is low concentration of albumin in blood. It may also lead to the formation of edema around the eyes, ankles, feet and abdomen.

Renal Failure

Renal failure is a decrease of glomerular filtration. It is of two types.

1. Acute renal failure
2. Chronic renal failure

Acute renal failure (ARF)

The kidneys stop working almost entirely. The main features of ARF are suppression of urine flow characterized either by oliguria where daily urine output between 50 mL to 250 mL or by anuria daily urine output less than 50 mL. Causes include low blood volume, decreased cardiac output, damaged renal tubules, kidney stones, non-steroidal anti-inflammatory drugs and some antibiotics. Renal failure causes multiple problems. There is edema due to salt and water retention and metabolic acidosis due to inability of the kidneys to excrete acidic substances. Blood concentration of urea found to be increased due to its impaired elimination. Potassium levels also increases, which can lead to cardiac arrest. Anemia may also occur as the kidneys are not producing enough erythropoietin. Kidneys play a role in the conversion of vitamin D to calcitriol, which is essential for the absorption of calcium. Hence ARF may lead to osteomalacia.

Chronic renal failure (CRF)

It is a progressive and irreversible decline in glomerular filtration rate (GFR). CRF may occur due to chronic glomerulonephritis, pyelonephritis, polycystic kidney diseases etc. CRF develops in three stages.

1. **Stage I: Diminished renal reserve:** 75% of the functioning nephrons are destroyed. At this stage the person may have no signs or symptoms because the remaining nephrons enlarge and take over the function of the lost nephrons.

2. **Stage II: Renal insufficiency:** Once 75% of the nephrons lost, the person enters the second stage, called renal insufficiency, characterized by decrease in GFR and increased blood levels of nitrogen containing wastes and creatinine.

3. **Stage III: End stage renal failure:** The final stage is called end stage renal failure. It occurs when 90% of the nephrons are lost. At this stage GFR diminishes to 10 to 15 % normal, oliguria is present and blood levels of nitrogenous wastes and creatinine increases further. People with end stage renal failure need dialysis treatment and may need kidney transplantation.

Urinary bladder cancer

This type of cancer usually occurs in people over 50 years of age and is three times more likely to develop in males than females. Blood in urine is the primary sign of the disease. People experience painful and frequent urination. If the disease is identified in the early stage it can be treated properly. Fortunately 75% of bladder cancers are confined to the epithelium of the urinary bladder and can be removed easily by surgery. This cancer usually occurs in who smoke cigarettes, works in leather, dye, rubber, aluminum industries as well as in paint industries.

6.2 Chapter at a Glance

Term	Description
Gluconeogenesis	Formation of glucose from non carbohydrate substances
Renal fascia	Fibrous connective tissue membrane that covers the kidney
Nephron	Microscopic functional unit of kidney
Glomerulus	Tuft of blood capillaries
Bowman's capsule	Expanded end of renal tubule that encloses the glomerulus
Glomerular filtration rate	Amount of filtrate formed by the kidneys in 1 minute
ANP	Atrial natriuretic peptide
ADH	Antidiuretic hormone
Rugae	Folds present in urinary bladder
Micturition	Discharge of urine from the urinary bladder
Renal calculi	Kidney stones
UTI	Urinary tract infection
Glomerulonephritis	Inflammation of the glomeruli of the kidney
Proteinuria	Protein in urine
Renal failure	Decrease in glomerular filtration

Exercises

Multiple Choice Questions

1. Loop of henle reabsorbs
   (a) Water (b) Potassium
   (c) Sodium (d) Glucose

2. Calcium homeostasis is maintained by
   (a) Erythropoietin (b) Calcitriol
   (c) Renin (d) All

3. The structural and functional unit of kidney is
   (a) Neuron (b) Nephron
   (c) Both (d) None

4. Which hormone involved in the regulation of water –salt balance of blood?
   (a) ADH (b) ANP
   (c) Aldosterone (d) Calcitonin

5. Which hormone promotes the excretion of potassium ions and the reabsorption of sodium ions?
   (a) Aldosterone (b) ADH
   (c) Renin (d) ANP

6. This posterior pituitary hormone reabsorbs the water into blood from filtrate.
   (a) ADH   (b) Aldosterone
   (c) Renin   (d) ANP

7. Which of the following is not considered a component of kidney stones?
   (a) Uric acid   (b) Calcium phosphate
   (c) Calcium oxalate   (d) Bicarbonate

8. Angiotensin I is converted into Angiotensin II in presence of
   (a) ACE   (b) Angiotensinase
   (c) Kinase   (d) All

9. Each kidney contains approximately about
   (a) One million nephrons   (b) One thousand nephrons
   (c) One trillion nephrons   (d) One billion nephrons

10. The two major regions of the kidneys are
    (a) Renal and nephritic pyramids
    (b) Major and minor calyces
    (c) Medulla and Cortex
    (d) None

Short Answer Questions

1. Name the hormones and its functions synthesized by kidney.
2. Name the waste products that are eliminated by the kidneys.
3. Write the parts and functions of urinary system.
4. Name the structural and functional unit of kidney. Write the difference between the cortical   and Juxtamedullary nephrons.
5. Write the steps involved in urine formation.
6. Write the role of ANP and ADH in the reabsorption of water.
7. Define micturition and Micturition reflex.
8. Write a short note on urinary bladder.
9. Write a note on urinary tract infections.
10. Write a note on glomerulonephritis.
11. Describe the characteristics of normal urine in terms of appearance, amount, pH, specific   gravity and composition.
12. Write the function of rugae and detrusor muscle of urinary bladder.
13. Write a note on renal calculi.
14. Write and explain the different stages of chronic renal failure.
15. Write a note on urinary bladder cancer.

Long Answer Questions

1. Write the functions of urinary system.
2. Write the anatomy of urinary system.
3. Write a note on Micturition reflex.
4. Explain about the normal characteristics of urine.
5. Write the role of kidneys in Acid-Base balance.
6. Explain about Renin-Angiotensin-Aldosterone system.
7. Write about the disorders of kidney.
8. Explain the structure of nephron.
9. Write a note on urinary bladder.
10. Explain about the transport, storage and elimination of urine.

Bibliography

Costanzo LS. Physiology. 4th Edition. Lippincott Williams & Wilkins.

Guyton AC, Hall JE. Textbook of Medical Physiology. 11th Edition. Elsevier Saunders. 2006.

Tortora GJ, Derrichson B, John Wiley and Sons. Principles of Anatomy and Physiology, 15Th edition, Hoboken, NJ:John Wiley and Sons, Inc., 2017.

Valerie SC, Tina S. Essentials of Anatomy and Physiology. 5th edition, Philadelphia, PA: F.A. Davis Co., 2011.

Answer Key MCQs									
1.	(a)	2.	(b)	3.	(b)	4.	(c)	5.	(a)
6.	(a)	7.	(d)	8.	(a)	9.	(a)	10.	(c)

Endocrine System

Learning Objective

After completing this lesson, the Reader should be able to understand:

- *Introduction*
- *Hormones*
- *Classification of Hormones*
- *Pituitary gland*
- *Disorders of the pituitary gland*
- *Thyroid gland*
- *Disorders of the thyroid gland*
- *Parathyroid gland*
- *Disorders of the parathyroid gland*
- *Adrenal gland*
- *Disorders of the adrenal gland*
- *Pancreas*
- *Disorders of the pancreas*
- *Pineal gland*
- *Thymus*

7.1   Introduction

The glands are those organs of the body that releases many types of enzymes and hormones (Table 7-1). These glands are of two types including the exocrine glands and the endocrine glands. The exocrine glands are the glands with ducts, and they release enzymes in the body cavities. The examples of the exocrine glands include salivary glands, sudoriferous (sweat) glands and digestive glands. The endocrine glands are ductless glands and they release hormones in the blood. The examples of endocrine glands include the pituitary gland, thyroid glands, parathyroid glands, adrenal glands and the pineal gland. In addition, many organs and tissues such as the hypothalamus, pancreas, kidneys, thymus, stomach, ovaries, testes, heart, liver, placenta, small intestine and adipose tissue are not considered as the endocrine glands, but they contain different types of cells that secrete various hormones. These hormone-secreting tissues along with the endocrine glands constitute the endocrine system. The branch of science that deals with the structure and functions of endocrine glands along with the diagnosis and treatment of disorders associated with these glands are called Endocrinology (Figure 7-1).

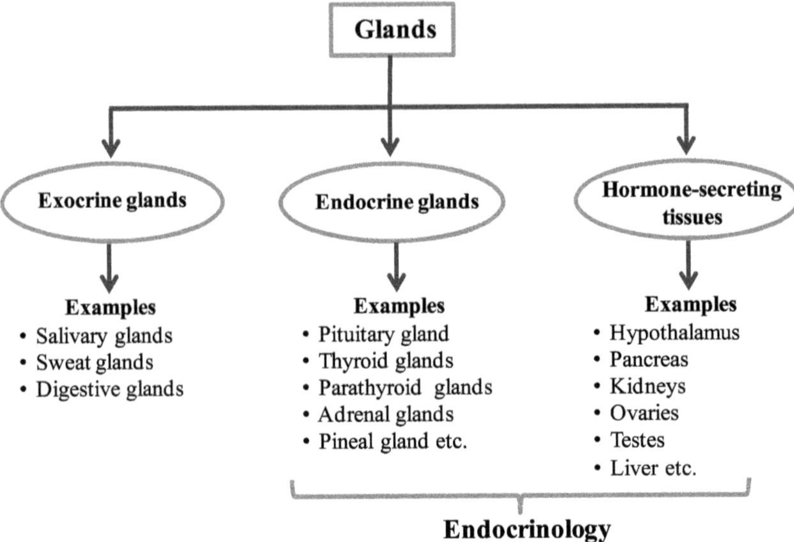

Figure 7-1 Different types of glands along with their examples

The glands can also be classified as the heterocrine glands and the holocrine glands. Heterocrine glands are those glands, which acts as an endocrine gland as well as an exocrine gland such as the pancreas. Holocrine glands act only as an endocrine gland and secrete hormones into the blood such as the adrenal gland.

Table 7-1 Key differences between the hormones and the enzymes

Sr. No.	Hormones	Enzymes
1	Hormones are released from the endocrine glands	Enzymes are released from the exocrine glands
2	The molecular weight of the hormones is less	The molecular weight of the enzymes is high
3	Hormones are used up in the reaction	Enzymes are reusable
4	Hormones may be amino acid derivatives, steroids etc.	Enzymes are always made up of proteins
5	Hormones are released in the blood	Enzymes are released in the body cavities
6	The reactions carried by hormones are irreversible	The reactions carried by enzymes are reversible

Hormones

A hormone is a mediator that is released in one part of the body but regulates the activity of various cells in other parts of the body. Hormones are of two types including the circulating hormones and the local hormones (Table 7-2).

Table 7-2 Different types of hormones and their characteristic features

	Types of hormones	Characteristic features
1	Circulating hormones	• The most common type of hormones • They pass through the secretory cells and enters the bloodstream • Examples include insulin, T_3, T_4, glucocorticoids, mineralocorticoids, etc.
2	Local hormones	• They are released from some types of cells and act locally rather than entering the bloodstream • They may act on the same cells from which they are released (called autocrines) or act on the neighbouring cells (called paracrines) • An example includes secretion of IL-2 from the T cells

The circulating hormones are the most common type of endocrine hormones that pass from the secretory cells into the interstitial fluid and then moves into the blood. The examples of the circulating hormones include glucocorticoids, mineralocorticoids, insulin, T_3, T_4 etc. Unlike the circulating hormones, the local hormones do not enter the bloodstream. They are released from some types of cells and may act on the same cells from which they are released (called autocrines) or act on their neighbouring cells (called paracrines). An example of a local hormone is the secretion of interleukin-2 (IL-2) from T cells (a type of white blood cells) that act on nearby immune cells to activate the immune response (paracrine response) or the same T cells for their proliferation (autocrine response) (Figure 7-2).

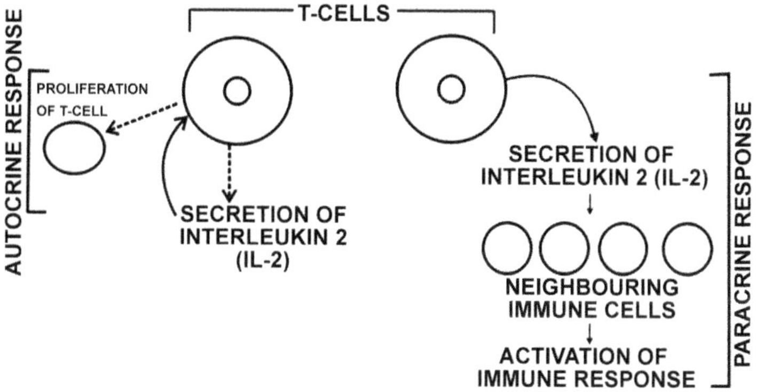

Figure 7-2 Autocrine and paracrine response of interleukin-2 (IL-2)

Additionaly, several mediators act as both neurotransmitters (mediators of the nervous system) and hormones (mediators of the endocrine system) such as norepinephrine. The latter is released as a neurotransmitter from the sympathetic postganglionic neurons and as a hormone from the chromaffin cells of the adrenal gland medulla. The differences between the neurotransmitters and the hormones are summarized in Table 7-3.

Table 7-3 Summarization of key differences between the hormones and the neurotransmitters

Sr. No.	Hormones	Neurotransmitters
1	Hormones are released from the endocrine glands	Neurotransmitters are released from the axons of the neurons
2	Hormones are mediators of the endocrine system	Neurotransmitters are mediators of the nervous system
3	They act far from their site of release by binding to the receptors present on the target cells	They act close to their site of release by binding to the receptors present on the postsynaptic membrane
4	They act on almost every type of cells	They act on specific muscles and glands
5	Actions of the hormones are slower	Actions of the neurotransmitters are very fast
6	The response of hormones is a long-lasting response	They produce a response for a brief period
7	Examples include cortisol, aldosterone, T_3, T_4, calcitonin etc.	Examples include acetylcholine, epinephrine, dopamine, serotonin etc.

General characteristics of the Hormones

1. Hormones are synthesized and released by the endocrine glands.
2. They are circulated in the blood and their site of action is far away from the site of release.
3. The chemical nature of the hormones varies. They may be amino acid derivatives, polypeptides, steroids and so on.
4. Hormones are effective in very low concentration.
5. Hormones act on almost every type of cells in the body and regulate their activities.
6. Like neurotransmitters, the hormones bind to the specific receptors present on their target cells to produce actions. Thus, they are also called chemical messengers.
7. The hormones produce a slow but a long-lasting response.
8. The release of hormones in a lesser or higher quantity than that of normal range produces many types of disorders.
9. The release of hormones from the endocrine glands is regulated in many ways e.g. via a negative-feedback mechanism, via a positive-feedback mechanism etc.

Classification of Hormones

Chemically, hormones are classified into two types including lipid-soluble hormones and water-soluble hormones. Apart from the different chemical makeup of lipid-soluble and water-soluble hormones, they are also significantly different based on their functions.

A. **Lipid-soluble hormones:** The lipid-soluble hormones include steroid hormones, thyroid hormones and nitric oxide (NO). These hormones have different functions based on their chemical structure. They are transported in the blood by binding to a special kind of proteins called transport proteins. These transport proteins increase the blood solubility of lipid-soluble hormones by converting them temporarily into the water-soluble hormones. After reaching their target cells, these hormones are detached from the protein-hormone complex and produce their actions in a free form.

Steroid hormones are derived from cholesterol and different functional chemical groups attached to the core structure of cholesterol constitute various steroid hormones with unique individual functions. Examples of steroid hormones include glucocorticoids and mineralocorticoids. Thyroid hormones are the products of tyrosine (an amino acid) and iodine. The attachment of iodine to tyrosine molecules increases the lipid-solubility of thyroid hormones. Examples of thyroid hormones include triiodothyronine (T_3) and tetraiodothyronine (T_4). Nitric oxide (NO) gas is both a neurotransmitter and a hormone, whose synthesis is catalysed by an enzyme called nitric oxide synthase (Table 7-4).

B. **Water-soluble Hormones:** The water-soluble hormones include amine hormones, peptide and polypeptide hormones and eicosanoid hormones. Unlike lipid-soluble hormones, these water-soluble hormones do not bind to the transport proteins and are circulated in a free form in the watery blood plasma. Amine hormones are the derivatives of certain amino acids that include catecholamines such as epinephrine, norepinephrine and dopamine (derivatives of tyrosine), histamine (a derivative of histidine) and serotonin (a derivative of tryptophan). Peptide and polypeptide hormones are the combinations of few (usually 3-49) to large (usually 50-200) number of amino acids. Oxytocin and vasopressin are peptide hormones while insulin and human growth hormone (hGh) are polypeptide hormones. The eicosanoid hormones are the derivatives of arachidonic acid (a fatty acid made up of 20 carbons), which are important local hormones. These hormones may also act as circulating hormones. Prostaglandins (PGs) and leukotrienes (LTs) are examples of eicosanoid hormones (Table 7-4).

Table 7-4 Chemical classification of the hormones

Sr. No.	Types of Hormones	Examples
	Lipid-soluble hormones	
1	Steroid hormones	Glucocorticoids; Mineralocorticoids
2	Thyroid hormones	Triiodothyronine (T_3); Tetraiodothyronine (T_4)
3	Nitric oxide (NO) gas	Nitric oxide
	Water-soluble hormones	
1	Amine hormones	Catecholamines (epinephrine, norepinephrine and dopamine); Histamine; Serotonin
2	Peptide and polypeptide hormones	Oxytocin; Vasopressin
3	Eicosanoid hormones	Prostaglandins (PGs); Leukotrienes (LTs)

Mechanism of Hormone action

The mechanism of hormone action depends on both the types of hormones as well as their target cells because various target cells respond differently to the same hormone. For example, insulin stimulates the synthesis of glycogen and triglycerides by acting on different kinds of cells including liver cells and adipose cells, respectively. The mechanism of different types of hormones i.e. lipid-soluble hormones and water-soluble hormones are described in the following paragraphs:

A. **Mechanism of lipid-soluble Hormones:** Lipid-soluble hormones such as steroid hormones and thyroid hormones produce their effects by binding to the receptors present in the cytoplasm or the nucleus of target cells. These hormone molecules diffuse from the blood into the target cells by crossing the lipid bilayer of the plasma membrane, where they bind to specific receptors and activate them. This activation of receptor-hormone complex alters the gene expression of specific genes that leads to transcription of the DNA into the mRNA, which further encodes for the synthesis of new proteins. The formation of these new proteins is responsible for the typical response of lipid-soluble hormones (Figure 7-3).

B. **Mechanism of water-soluble hormones:** Water-soluble hormones such as amine hormones, peptide hormones and eicosanoid hormones do not cross the lipid bilayer of the plasma membrane due to their chemical nature (negligible lipid-solubility). Therefore, water-soluble hormones (also called the first messengers) produce their response by binding to the receptors that protrude from the surface of target cells, called surface receptors. The resultant receptor-hormone complex activates the plasma membrane protein called G protein, which in turn activates adenylate cyclase. The activated adenylate cyclase converts ATPs into the cyclic AMPs (cAMP; also called the second messenger) that activate one or more protein kinases, which are present either in the cytoplasm of a target cell or bound to the plasma membrane. These activated protein kinases then lead to the phosphorylation of numerous cellular proteins along with their activation or deactivation. This modulation of cellular proteins produces various responses in the body, which are manifested as the physiological response of water-soluble hormones (Figure 7-4).

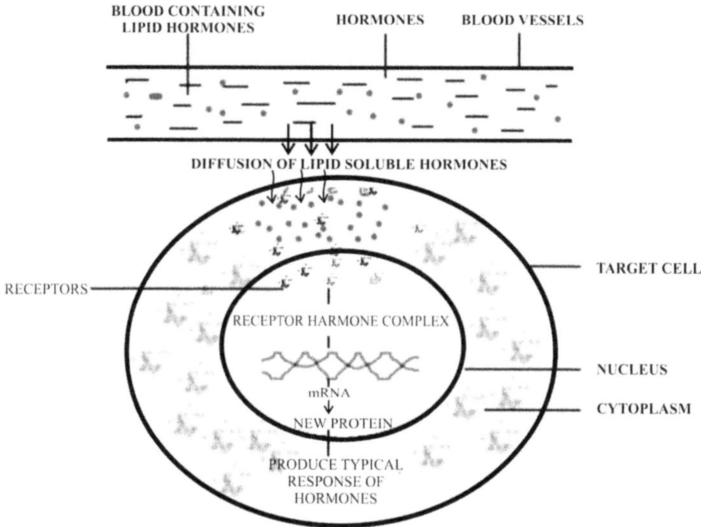

Figure 7-3 Mechanism of lipid-soluble hormones

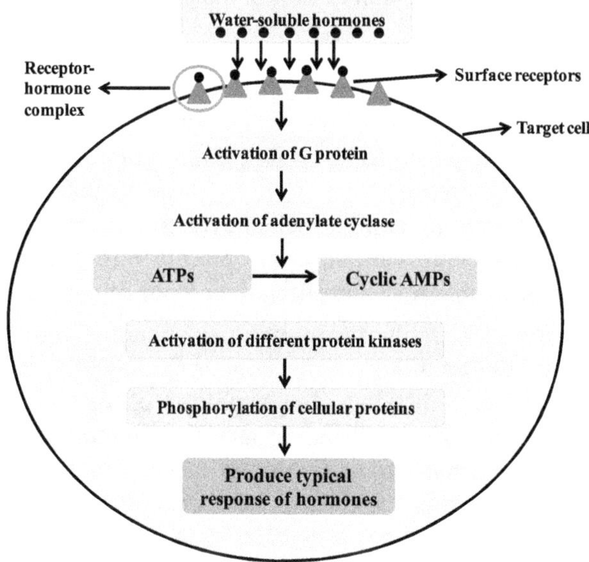

Figure 7-4 Mechanism of water-soluble hormones

Pituitary Gland

The pituitary gland or hypophysis is a pea-shaped gland that is located inside the hypophyseal fossa of the sella turcica of the sphenoid bone. It measures about 1.0-1.5 cm in diameter. The pituitary gland is controlled by the hypothalamus and is attached to the latter by a stalk called the infundibulum. Anatomically, the pituitary gland is divided into two parts including the anterior pituitary (anterior lobe) and the posterior pituitary (posterior lobe), which have entirely different structures and functions (Figure 7-5). The pituitary gland is also called a 'Master endocrine gland' because it secretes various types of hormones that further control the functions of other endocrine glands such as the thyroid gland and the adrenal gland.

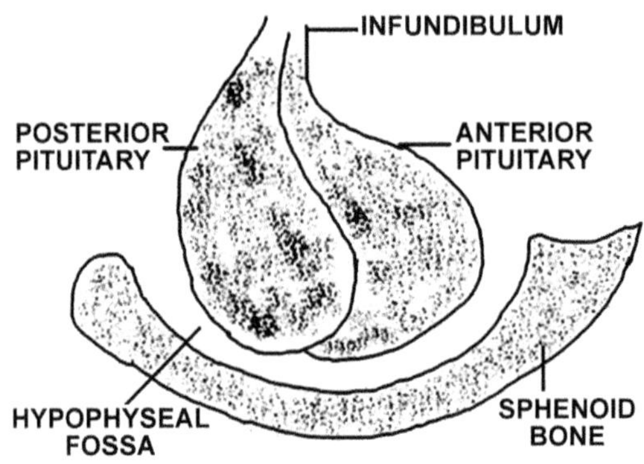

Figure 7-5 The external view of the pituitary gland

One more part (third part) of the pituitary gland called pars intermedia (intermediate lobe) is present during the birth of a child but it gets degenerated during human fetal development and does not exist as a separate lobe in adults. However, during its degeneration, some of its cells migrate into the adjacent parts of the pituitary gland i.e. anterior and posterior. These remnants cells of the pars intermedia secrete a hormone called melanocyte-stimulating hormone (MSH) (Figure 7-6). The target receptors of MSH are present on melanocytes (a type of skin cells). MSH is responsible for controlling the colour of the skin.

A. **Anterior Pituitary:** The anterior pituitary or adenohypophysis is comprised of about 75% of the total weight of gland. Anatomically, it consists of two parts including the pars distalis, a larger portion of the anterior pituitary and the pars tuberalis that form a sheath around the infundibulum. Functionally, the anterior pituitary consists of five types of cells including somatotrophs, thyrotrophs, gonadotrophs, lactotrophs and corticotrophs (Figure 7-7). These cells synthesize and release seven different hormones, which in turn stimulate other endocrine glands to secrete various hormones that have diverse functions in the body such as growth and reproduction. The anterior pituitary hormones that act on other endocrine glands are known as tropic hormones or tropins. The secretion of hormones from different types of anterior pituitary cells is stimulated by releasing hormones and suppressed by inhibitory hormones (Table 7-5). The releasing and inhibitory hormones are released from the hypothalamus, which makes an important link between the nervous system and the endocrine system.

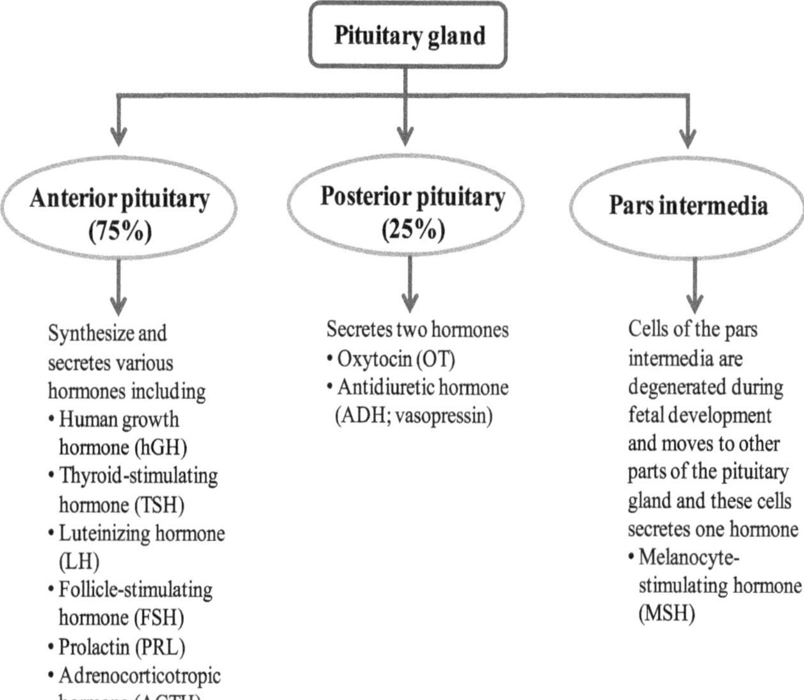

Figure 7-6 The different parts of the pituitary gland and hormones released from those parts

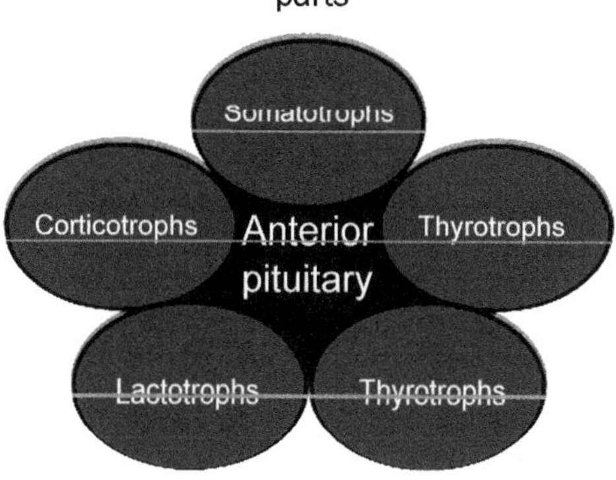

Figure 7-7 The cells of the anterior pituitary

Regulation of secretion of the anterior pituitary hormones

The release of anterior pituitary hormones is controlled in two ways. First, the neurosecretory cells of the hypothalamus secrete five releasing-hormones and two inhibiting-hormones, which stimulate and suppress the secretions of anterior pituitary hormones, respectively. The summarization of these releasing and inhibiting hormones is given in Table 7-5. Second, the secretions of anterior pituitary hormones from thyrotrophs, gonadotrophs and corticotrophs are also regulated by other hormones, which are released from their target glands via a negative feedback mechanism. The target gland hormones inhibit the release of anterior pituitary hormones when their levels are high in the blood. For example, Adrenocorticotropic hormone (ACTH) stimulates the adrenal gland cortex to release glucocorticoids such as cortisol. The elevated blood levels of cortisol decrease the release of ACTH and corticotropin-releasing hormone (CRH) by suppressing the activity of anterior pituitary corticotrophs and hypothalamic neurosecretory cells, respectively (explained later in this chapter).

I. **Somatotrophs:** The somatotrophs are the most abundant cells present in the anterior pituitary that secretes a hormone called somatotropin or human growth hormone (hGH). The hormone is released in more concentration in growing children. The main physiological function of hGH is to stimulate the cells of various tissues such as liver, skeletal muscles, cartilage and bones to synthesize and secrete the small protein hormones called insulin-like growth factors (IGFs) or somatomedins (Table 7-5). The functions of these somatomedins include:

1. IGFs help in the growth and multiplication of cells. They also increase the uptake of amino acids into the cells, thus stimulates the synthesis of proteins. Moreover, they also decrease the breakdown of proteins and the use of amino acids for ATP production.

2. Due to the protein-synthesis actions of IGFs, hGH accelerates the growth of skeletal muscles in teenagers before the onset of puberty. In adults, these hormones help in the maintenance of mass of muscles and bones. Moreover, they also promote the tissue repairing and healing of injuries.

3. IGFs enhance the process of lipolysis in adipose tissues that leads to an increase in the availability of fatty acids for ATP production.

4. IGFs decreases the use of glucose by various body cells for ATP production by decreasing its uptake. In the case of glucose scarcity, this action of IGFs spares the glucose so that it is available to neurons for ATP production.

Regulation of secretion of human growth hormone (hGH): The somatotrophs release hGH in bursts, every few hours. The release of this hormone is higher, especially during sleep. The secretory activity of somatotrophs is controlled by two hypothalamic hormones including growth

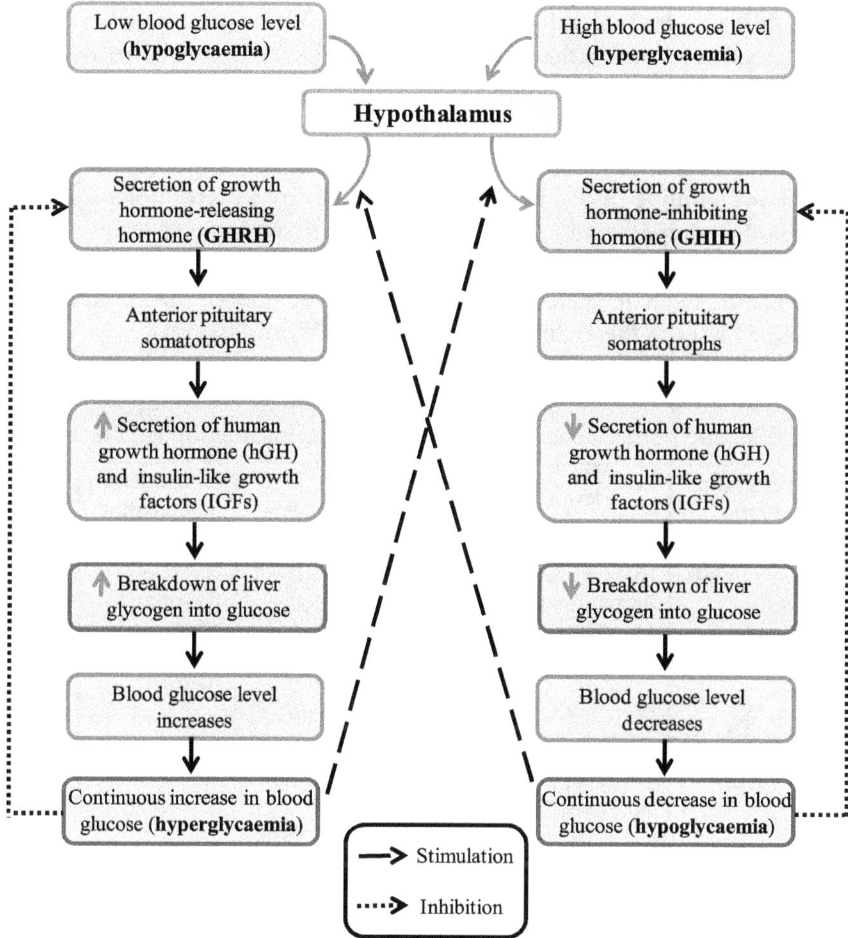

Figure 7-8 Regulation of the release of human growth hormone (hGH) from the anterior pituitary somatotrophs

hormone-releasing hormone (GHRH) and growth hormone-inhibiting hormone (GHIH) (Table 7-5). The secretion of these hormones from the hypothalamus is mainly regulated by blood glucose level. The low level of blood glucose (hypoglycaemia) stimulates the secretion of GHRH, which further promotes the secretion of hGH from somatotrophs. The hGH, in turn, stimulates the secretion of IGFs, which increases the blood glucose level to a normal range by enhancing the breakdown of liver glycogen into glucose (glycogenolysis). An increase in the blood glucose level above the normal value inhibits the release of GHRH from the hypothalamus. On the other hand, the high level of blood glucose (hyperglycaemia) stimulates the secretion of GHIH, which further suppresses the release of hGH. As a result, the breakdown of liver glycogen into glucose is reduced and blood glucose level falls to a normal value. A decease in the blood glucose level below the normal value results in the inhibition of GHIH secretion (Figure 7-8).

II. **Thyrotrophs:** The thyrotrophs of the anterior pituitary releases thyroid-stimulating hormone (TSH), which regulates the secretion of two other hormones from the thyroid gland including triiodothyronine (T_3) and tetraiodothyronine (T_4). The secretion of TSH from thyrotrophs is controlled by another hypothalamic hormone called thyrotropin-releasing hormone (TRH) (Table 7-5). The release of TRH, in turn, depends on the blood levels of T_3 and T_4. The functions, as well as regulation of T3 and T4, are explained later in the chapter under section 'Thyroid gland'.

Table 7-5 The summarization of cells of the anterior pituitary along with hormones released from those cells, their major functions and regulation

Sr. No.	Cells of the anterior pituitary	Hormones released	Major functions	Regulation (stimulating hormone)	Regulation (inhibiting hormone
1	Somatotrophs	Human growth hormone (hGH) or somatotropin	• To synthesize and secrete insulin-like growth factors (IGFs) • Accelerate muscle growth	Growth hormone-releasing hormone (GHRH)	Growth hormone-inhibiting hormone (GHIH)
2	Thyrotrophs	Thyroid-stimulating hormone (TSH)	• Regulation of secretion of T_3 and T_4 from the thyroid gland	Thyrotropin-releasing hormone (TRH)	-
3	Gonadotrophs	Luteinising hormone (LH); Follicle-stimulating hormone (FSH)	• Regulation of secretion of estrogens and progesterone	Gonadotropins-releasing hormone (GnRH)	-
4	Lactotrophs	Prolactin	• Initiation and production of milk in the mammary glands	Prolactin-releasing hormone (PRH)	Prolactin-inhibiting hormone (PIH)
5	Corticotrophs	Adrenocorticotropic hormone (ACTH) or corticotropin	• Stimulation of adrenal cortex to secrete glucocorticoids	Corticotropin-releasing hormone (CRH)	-

III. **Gonadotrophs:** The gonadotrophs of the anterior pituitary secrete two hormones including luteinizing hormone (LH) and follicle-stimulating hormone (FSH), which are collectively known as gonadotropins. The secretion of LH and FSH is regulated by another hypothalamic hormone called gonadotropins-releasing hormone (GnRH) (Table 7-5). The release of

GnRH is further controlled by the blood level of estrogens (in females) and testosterone (in males) via a negative feedback mechanism. The detailed description of functions of LH and FSH and their regulation is explained in the chapter 'Reproductive system'.

IV.   **Lactotrophs:** The lactotrophs of the anterior pituitary release the only hormone called prolactin (PRL) that initiates and maintains the production and release of milk from the mammary glands in females (Table 7-5). The prolactin is also known as the 'maternity hormone'. The exact role of prolactin in males is unknown.

Regulation of the release of prolactin (PRL)

The secretory activity of the anterior pituitary lactotrophs i.e. secretion of prolactin is regulated by two hypothalamic hormones including prolactin-inhibiting hormone (PIH; dopamine) and prolactin-releasing hormone (PRH) (Table 7-5). The secretion of PIH inhibits the prolactin release from the anterior pituitary lactotrophs. The PIH secretion is decreased just before the onset of menstruation that leads to an increase in the blood prolactin level, but this rise in the prolactin level is not enough to cause milk secretion from the mammary glands. However, the secretion of PIH is again increased with the start of a new menstrual cycle and the blood level of prolactin decreases. During pregnancy, the secretion of PRH from the hypothalamus is increased that stimulates the release of prolactin and increases their levels in the blood above the normal range. The increased level of prolactin further results in the initiation of milk production (Figure 7-9).

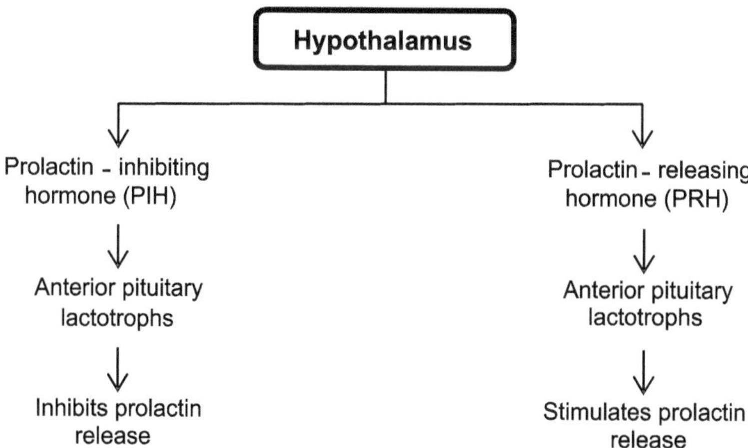

Figure 7-9 Regulation of the prolactin release from the anterior pituitary lactotrophs

V. **Corticotrophs:** The anterior pituitary corticotrophs secrete corticotropin or adrenocorticotropic hormone (ACTH) that stimulates the adrenal gland cortex (the outer portion of the adrenal gland) to secrete glucocorticoids such as cortisol. The release of ACTH from corticotrophs is regulated by a hormone, which is released from the hypothalamus called corticotropin-releasing hormone (CRH) (Table 7-5). The excessive level of glucocorticoids in the blood inhibits the release of both ACTH and CRH via a negative feedback mechanism. The functions and regulation of glucocorticoid secretion are explained later in this chapter under section 'Adrenal gland'.

B. Posterior Pituitary: The posterior pituitary or neurohypophysis is comprised of the remaining portion of the pituitary gland (about 25%). Anatomically, it consists of two portions including the pars nervosa (a larger portion of the posterior pituitary) and the infundibulum (attachment between the hypothalamus and the pituitary gland). Functionally, the posterior pituitary consists of many axons and axon terminals (more than 10,000) of neurosecretory cells of the hypothalamus. The axon terminals are associated with a special kind of cells, present in the posterior pituitary called pituicytes. The cell bodies of the neurosecretory cells are present in the paraventricular nucleus and the supraoptic nucleus of the hypothalamus that produces oxytocin (OT) and antidiuretic hormone (ADH; also called vasopressin), respectively (Table 7-6). These hormones are stored and packaged into the secretory vesicles of the neurosecretory cells. Thereafter, the secretory vesicles move towards the axon terminals in the posterior pituitary, where they secrete their stored hormones into the blood through exocytosis after triggered by some nerve impulses. Unlike the anterior pituitary, the posterior pituitary does not synthesize hormones itself.

I. Oxytocin: The oxytocin is released from the axonal terminals in the posterior pituitary during and after the delivery of a baby. It acts on two major organs in the body including the mother's uterus and the mammary glands. The physiological functions of oxytocin on these target organs include:

1. During delivery, oxytocin increases the smooth muscle contractions of walls of the uterus and helps in the expulsion of a foetus. Therefore, it is also called as the 'Birth hormone'.

2. After delivery, oxytocin causes contraction of myoepithelial cells of the mammary glands and stimulates the ejection of milk from them in response to the stimulus provided by a sucking infant. Therefore, it is also called as the 'milk ejecting hormone' (Table 7-6).

Regulation of the release of oxytocin (OT)

The oxytocin is released from neurosecretory cells of the hypothalamus in response to relaxation of the uterus and activation of nipples in the mammary glands via a positive feedback mechanism (Table 7-6). In other words, uterine relaxation and activation of nipples increase the release of oxytocin to facilitate the delivery of a baby and ejecting the milk from the mammary glands, respectively (Figure 7-10).

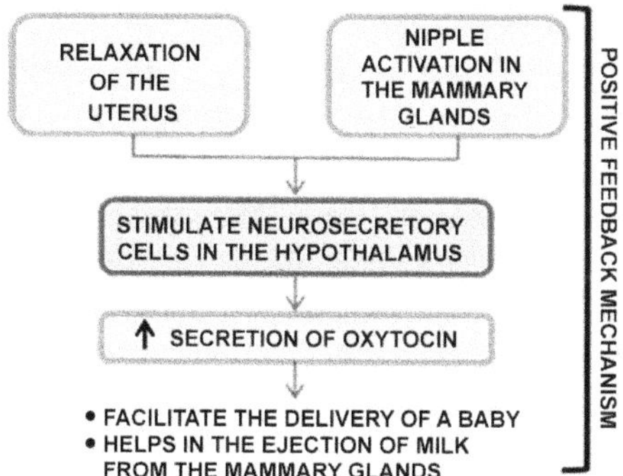

Figure 7-10 Positive-feedback mechanism of regulation of the release of oxytocin

Table 7-6 The summarization of hormones released from the posterior pituitary along with their major functions and regulation

Sr. No.	Hormones	Major functions	Regulation
1	Oxytocin	• Increase uterine contractions and helps in the expulsion of a foetus • Stimulates the ejection of milk from the mammary glands	• In response to the stimuli such as relaxation of the uterus and activation of nipples in the mammary glands via a positive-feedback mechanism
2	Antidiuretic hormone (ADH) or vasopressin	• Decrease the urine output • Decrease water loss by perspiration from the skin • Increase the blood pressure	• Regulated by blood osmotic pressure and blood volume

II. Antidiuretic hormone (ADH or vasopressin): Like oxytocin, the antidiuretic hormone is also released from the axonal terminals, present in the posterior pituitary. The physiological functions of ADH include:

1. The main function of ADH is to decrease the urine output (as its name implies) by acting on the kidneys to reabsorb more water. The urine output increases ten times in the absence of ADH.
2. It acts on the sweat (sudoriferous) glands and causes them to decrease the water loss through perspiration from the skin.
3. It also causes constriction of arterioles, thus increase the blood pressure. Therefore, ADH is also known as vasopressin (Table 7-6).

Regulation of the release of antidiuretic hormone (ADH)

The secretion of ADH from neurosecretory cells of the hypothalamus is controlled by blood osmotic pressure and blood volume (Table 7-6). The conditions such as diarrhoea, hemorrhage, excessive sweating and dehydration cause a decline in the blood volume and consequently increase in the osmotic pressure of blood. This elevated blood osmotic pressure stimulate osmoreceptors (responsible for maintaining the blood osmotic pressure) present in the hypothalamus, which activates the hypothalamic neurosecretory cells to synthesize and store ADH into the axon terminals, present in the posterior pituitary. The excitatory nerve impulses generated from the osmoreceptors triggers the axon terminals to release ADH into the bloodstream. The ADH-containing blood moves to their target tissues such as the kidneys, sweat glands and arterioles to perform various functions. On the other hand, low blood osmotic pressure or increased blood volume inhibits the osmoreceptors that lead to a decline in the release of ADH (Figure 7-11).

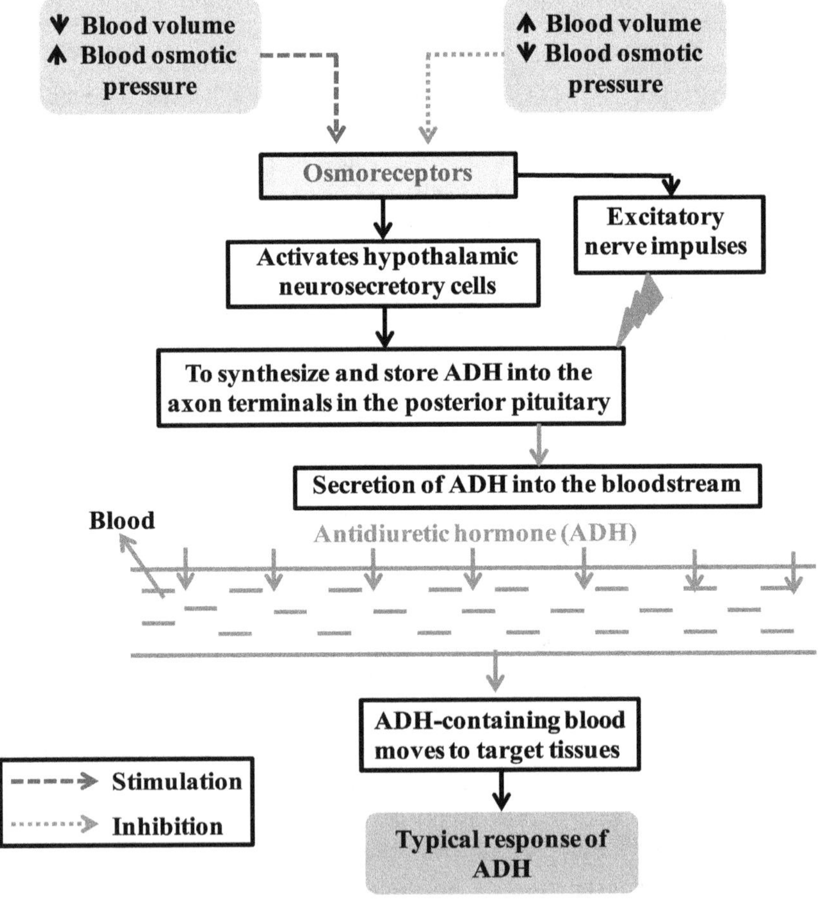

Figure 7-11 Regulation of the release of antidiuretic hormone (ADH)

Disorders of the Pituitary Gland

1. **Dwarfism:** Dwarfism is a condition that is characterized by the hyposecretion of human growth hormone (hGH) from the anterior pituitary somatotrophs during the early growth of a child. This condition is also called pituitary dwarfism. The symptom of dwarfism includes slow growth of bones that further leads to a decline in the body height (short body) (Table 7-7). This decreased patient height is due to the early closure of epiphyseal plates, which occur before a person can achieve their normal height. In dwarfism, the other organs of the body also fail to grow but the body proportions are normal. The person is sexually mature and there is no mental problem associated with this condition.

Table 7-7 Summarization of disorders of the pituitary gland and their characteristic features

Sr. No.	Disorders	Characteristic features
1	Dwarfism	• Hyposecretion of the human growth hormone (hGH) during the early growth of a child • Also called pituitary dwarfism • A major symptom is the slow growth of bones (short body)
2	Gigantism	• Hypersecretion of the human growth hormone (hGH) during childhood • A major symptom is abnormal growth of long bones (large body)
3	Acromegaly	• Hypersecretion of the human growth hormone (hGH) during adulthood • A major symptom includes a disproportionate increase in the size of bones of hands, feet, jaws and cheeks
4	Diabetes insipidus (DI)	• Dysfunctioning of the posterior pituitary • May be due to defects in the release of ADH or defects in the ADH receptors

2. **Gigantism:** Gigantism is a condition that is characterized by the hypersecretion of human growth hormone (hGH) from the anterior pituitary somatotrophs during childhood. The symptom of gigantism includes abnormal growth of long bones that leads to an increase in body height (large body). However, the body proportions are normal in this condition (Table 7-7).
3. **Acromegaly:** Acromegaly is a condition, which is characterized by the hypersecretion of human growth hormone (hGH) during adulthood. The

symptoms of acromegaly include a disproportionate increase in the size of bones of tissues such as hands, feet, jaws and cheeks. In addition, enlargement of the eyelids, lips, tongue and nose is also associated with this condition. Moreover, the thickness of the skin is also increased, and wrinkles are developed on the forehead and soles (Table 7-7).

4. **Diabetes insipidus (DI):** Diabetes insipidus is a disease associated with a dysfunctioning of the posterior pituitary. It may be due to defects in the release of antidiuretic hormone (ADH) from the hypothalamic neurosecretory cells or defects in the ADH receptors (Table 7-8). Diabetes insipidus is of two types including neurogenic diabetes insipidus and nephrogenic diabetes insipidus. In neurogenic diabetes insipidus, there is a decreased release of ADH due to several conditions such as a brain tumor, head trauma or brain surgery that damages the posterior pituitary or the hypothalamus. In nephrogenic diabetes insipidus, the ADH does not produce any actions, which may be due to defects in the ADH receptors or damages in the kidneys. The symptoms of both types of diabetes insipidus are common, which include the increased output of urine (excessive urination), dehydration and excessive thrust. Diabetes insipidus is totally different from diabetes mellitus (DM) and the differences between these both types of diseases are summarized in Table 7-8.

Table 7-8 Key differences between diabetes mellitus (DM) and diabetes insipidus (DI)

Sr. No.	Diabetes mellitus (DM)	Diabetes insipidus (DI)
1	It is a pancreatic disorder	It is a hypothalamic disorder
2	It is due to the deficiency of insulin	It is due to the deficiency of the antidiuretic hormone (ADH)
3	The level of blood glucose is increased	The level of blood glucose is normal
4	Increased glucose in urine (glycosuria)	No glucose in urine (no glycosuria)
5	Frequency of urination is increased but the volume of urine is less	Excessive excretion of urine is the major symptom of diabetes insipidus

Thyroid Gland

The butterfly-shaped thyroid gland is located just inferior to the larynx. Externally, the thyroid gland is composed of two lateral lobes, each one on either side of the trachea called left and right lateral lobe, respectively. These two lobes are connected to each other by an isthmus (a narrow passage), which is present anterior to the trachea (Figure 7-12).

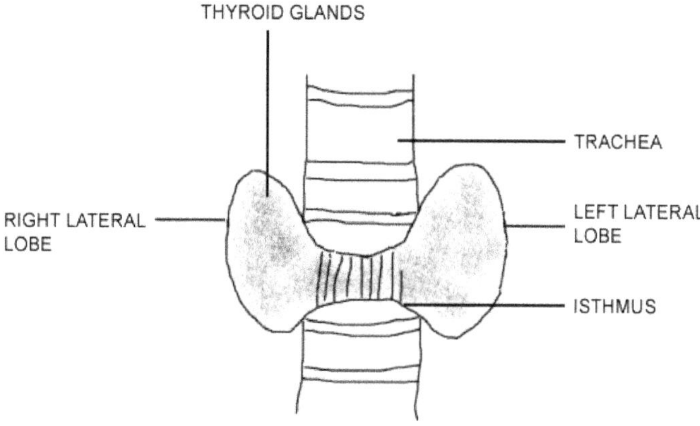

Figure 7-12 The external view of the thyroid glands

The normal mass of the thyroid gland is about 30 g and it receives approximately 80-120 mL of blood per minute. Internally, the thyroid gland is made up of several microscopic spherical sacs, which are known as thyroid follicles (Figure 7-13).

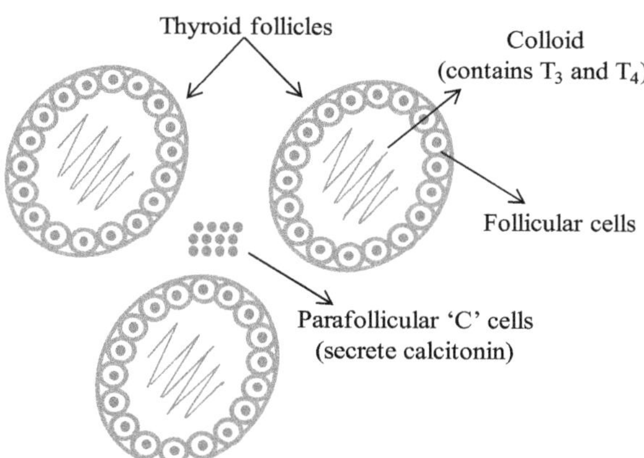

Figure 7-13 Cross-sectional structure of the thyroid gland showing the presence of thyroid follicles and parafollicular cells

The wall of each thyroid follicle consists of follicular cells that produce two hormones including triiodothyronine (T_3) and tetraiodothyronine or thyroxine (T_4), collectively known as thyroid hormones. Moreover, a colloid is present inside each thyroid follicle, which stores these thyroid hormones. In addition, few cells are present in between the thyroid follicles called parafollicular cells or 'C' cells that produce a hormone called calcitonin, which helps in the regulation of calcium homeostasis (Table 7-9).

Table 7-9 Hormones of the thyroid gland, their sources and functions

Sr. No.	Hormones	Source	Functions
1	Triiodothyronine (T$_3$)	Follicular cells	• Regulation of metabolic actions of the body • T$_3$ is the active form and produces action
2	Tetraiodothyronine (thyroxine or T$_4$)	Follicular cells	• Regulation of metabolic actions of the body. • T$_4$ is converted to T$_3$, which produces actions
3	Calcitonin	Parafollicular or 'C' cells	• Regulation of calcium homeostasis

Physiological functions of thyroid hormones

1. Thyroid hormones increase the basal metabolic rate (BMR) and the rate of oxygen consumption of the body.

2. The metabolic action of these hormones results in the production of heat in the body. This phenomenon of an increase in heat production is known as the calorigenic effect. Therefore, thyroid hormones play an important role in the maintenance of normal body temperature. (Table 7-10).

Table 7-10 Summarization of the physiological functions of thyroid hormones, calcitonin and parathormone

Sr. No.	Hormones	Physiological functions
1	Thyroid hormones	• Increase the basal metabolic rate (BMR) and the rate of oxygen consumption • Maintenance of normal body temperature • Enhance the cellular metabolism of proteins, carbohydrates and lipids • Decrease the blood cholesterol level • Increase the utilization of glucose and fatty acids • Stimulate protein synthesis • Increase the synthesis of sodium-potassium pumps • Increase the actions of catecholamines such as epinephrine and norepinephrine • Promote mental development
2	Calcitonin	• Along with parathormone, it helps in the regulation of calcium homeostasis • Inhibits the actions of osteoclasts, thus prevents bone resorption • Decrease the level of Ca^{2+} in the blood

Table 7-10 *Contd...*

Sr. No.	Hormones	Physiological functions
3	Parathyroid hormone (Parathormone)	• Regulation of levels of different ions in the blood such as Ca^{2+}, Mg^{2+} and HPO_4^{2-} • Increase the number and activity of osteoclasts, thus enhance bone resorption • Increase the level of Ca^{2+} in the blood • Along with calcitonin, it helps in the regulation of calcium homeostasis • Promote the formation of an active form of vitamin D (calcitriol)

1. They increase the cellular metabolism of proteins, carbohydrates and lipids.
2. Thyroid hormones increase the lipolysis (the breakdown of lipids) and enhance the cholesterol excretion. Therefore, they help in the reduction of blood cholesterol level.
3. Thyroid hormones increase the utilization of glucose and fatty acids for ATP production.
4. These hormones stimulate protein synthesis.
5. Thyroid hormones also increase the synthesis of sodium-potassium pumps (Na^+-K^+ ATPase), which uses ATP for its functioning.
6. They also increase the actions of catecholamines (epinephrine and norepinephrine) including an increase in the heart rate and blood pressure.
7. Thyroid hormones, together with the human growth hormones (hGH) and insulin, accelerates body growth particularly, the skeletal and nervous systems. They also promote mental development.

Physiological functions of calcitonin

1. Calcitonin functions along with the parathyroid hormone (parathormone), which is released from the parathyroid gland, in the regulation of calcium homeostasis.
2. Calcitonin decreases the level of Ca^{2+} in the blood i.e. it results in hypocalcaemia. Indeed, it decreases the calcium levels by preventing the process of bone resorption by inhibiting the actions of osteoclasts of bones. This action is opposite to that parathormone, which promotes the action of osteoclasts and increases the blood calcium levels (Figure 7-14) (Table 7-10).

Regulation of the release of thyroid hormones

The low levels of thyroid hormones in the blood stimulate the hypothalamus to secrete thyrotropin-releasing hormone (TRH), which further stimulates the thyrotrophs of the anterior pituitary to release thyroid-stimulating hormone (TSH) or thyrotropin. Subsequently, TSH activates the follicular cells of the thyroid gland to synthesis and release T_3 and T_4 in the blood. The excessive release of T_3 and T_4

inhibits the release of TRH from the hypothalamus and TSH from the anterior pituitary thyrotrophs via a negative feedback mechanism (Figure 7-15).

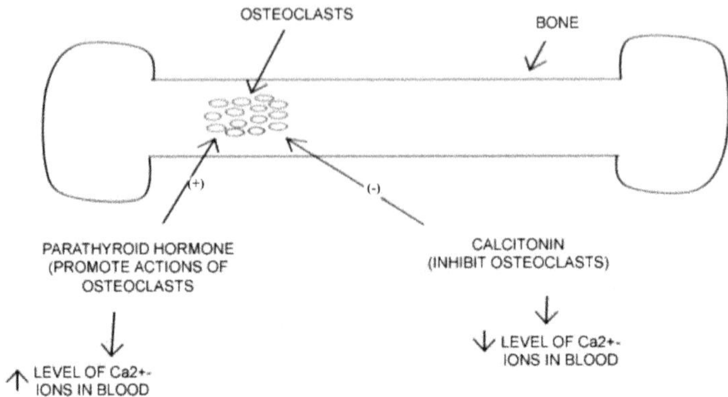

Figure 7-14 Action of parathyroid hormone and calcitonin on the blood calcium levels

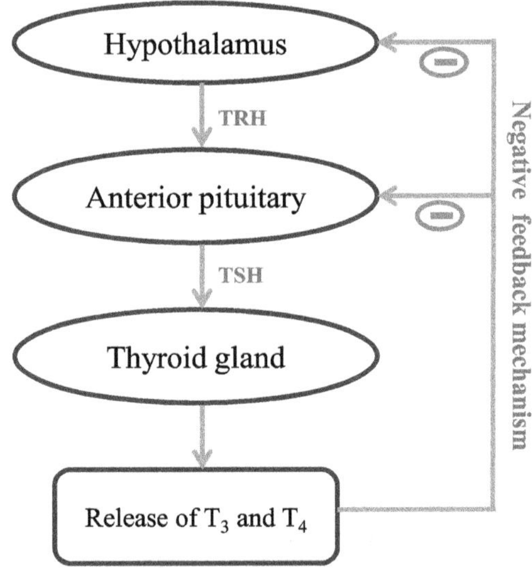

Figure 7-15 Negative feed-back mechanism of regulating the release of thyroid hormones

Disorders of the Thyroid Gland

Thyroid disorders refer to a medical condition in which there is a dysfunction of the thyroid gland and there are abnormalities in the hormonal release. An increase in the release of thyroid hormones (more T_3 and T_4) is termed as hyperthyroidism or thyrotoxicosis. Similarly, a decrease in the secretion of thyroid hormones (lesser T_3 and T_4) is termed as hypothyroidism. In both hyperthyroidism and hypothyroidism, there may be an enlargement/swelling of the thyroid gland, which is termed as goitre.

A. Hyperthyroidism: Hyperthyroidism is a medical condition that is characterized by an increase in the levels of T_3 and T_4 hormones. The disease is diagnosed by an increase in the serum T_3/T_4 levels and low levels of thyroid-stimulating hormone (TSH) in serum. It may occur due to a variety of reasons and accordingly, these have been divided into subcategories. However, in all subtypes, there are common signs and symptoms of hyperthyroidism. These signs and symptoms include increase in heat production leading to heat intolerance, tachycardia (increase in heart rate), nervousness, anxiety, palpitations, irritability, sleeping problems (insomnia), increased appetite but weight loss, increased perspiration, muscle weakness, thinning of the skin, fine brittle hair, diarrhoea and high blood glucose levels (Table 7-11).

Table 7-11 Key differences between the symptoms of hyperthyroidism and hypothyroidism

Sr. No.	Hyperthyroidism	Hypothyroidism
1	More heat production leading to heat intolerance	Less heat production leading to cold intolerance
2	Fast metabolism	Slow metabolism
3	Tachycardia	Bradycardia
4	Nervousness, anxiety	Poor memory (in adults), mental retardation (in children)
5	Diarrhoea	Constipation
6	Loss of weight	Weight gain
7	Insomnia	Excessive sleep

These signs and symptoms are due to the excessive metabolic actions of thyroid hormones. The various types of hyperthyroidism are described in the following sections (Table 7-12).

1. Grave's Disease (Exophthalmic goitre): Grave's disease is the most common type of hyperthyroidism. About 50-80% of the cases of hyperthyroidism are due to the Grave's disease. It is an autoimmune syndrome characterized by an increase in the size of the thyroid gland (goitre). In this disease, there is a production of auto-antibodies called thyroid-stimulating antibodies. These antibodies mimic the actions of TSH and continuously stimulate the thyroid gland to enlarge its size and secrete more amounts of thyroid hormones. The thyroid gland is enlarged in most of the patients and is about 40 to 60 g in weight (two to three times the normal size). The signs and symptoms of Grave's disease are typical of hyperthyroidism as explained above. Additionally, the excessive activity of thyroid hormones is associated with protrusion of the eyes and retraction of the upper lids, a reason for its name i.e. exophthalmic goitre.

Table 7-12 Summarization of different types of hyperthyroidism and their characteristic

Sr. No.	Types of hyperthyroidism	Characteristic features
1	Grave's disease	• Autoimmune disease • Increase in the size of the thyroid gland • Formation of auto-antibodies called thyroid-stimulating antibodies that excessively stimulate the gland to induce hyperthyroidism
2	Multinodular goitre	• The thyroid gland becomes independent of the control of anterior pituitary • Multinodular enlargement of the thyroid gland • It is not a tumour or cancer but may convert to cancer/tumour
3	Toxic adenoma	• Benign tumour of the thyroid gland
4	Pituitary adenoma	• Benign, invasive or carcinoma tumours of the pituitary gland
5	Thyroid storm	• State of severe hyperthyroidism, thyrotoxicosis • Life-threatening medical emergency

2. **Multinodular Goitre:** Multinodular goitre is the second most common cause of hyperthyroidism following Grave's disease. In this type, the thyroid gland becomes autonomous i.e. becomes independent of the control of the anterior pituitary. In other words, the thyroid gland does not require TSH for its stimulation and growth. This disease is characterized by multinodular enlargement of the thyroid gland. Although, multinodular goitre is not a tumour, yet there are increased chances of development of thyroid cancer in these patients. The signs and symptoms of this type are typical of hyperthyroidism.

3. **Toxic Adenoma:** A toxic adenoma is a benign tumour of the thyroid gland in which the thyroid gland becomes autonomous and independent of the pituitary control. There is an excessive release of thyroid hormones and typical symptoms of hyperthyroidism are present.

4. **Pituitary Adenoma:** A pituitary adenoma is a relatively uncommon form of hyperthyroidism and it accounts for less than 1% of the total cases of hyperthyroidism. These are the tumours of the pituitary gland, which may be benign (most of the cases), invasive (about 35% cases) or carcinomas (0.1 to 0.2%). There is an excessive release of TSH from the pituitary adenoma cells that causes persistent stimulation of the thyroid gland to increase the release of thyroid hormones. Along with typical symptoms of hyperthyroidism, the symptoms due to an excessive release of growth hormones (to lead acromegaly) and glucocorticoids (to lead Cushing syndrome) are also present.

5. **Thyroid Storm:** Thyroid storm is not a separate type of thyrotoxicosis; rather it is a state of severe hyperthyroidism and may appear in any type of hyperthyroidism. It is a life-threatening medical emergency, which is characterized by severe thyrotoxicosis, high fever, tachycardia, tachypnea (fast respiration) and diarrhoea that results in dehydration, mental agitation, delirium and coma.

B. **Hypothyroidism:** Hypothyroidism is a state in which the thyroid gland does not produce enough thyroid hormones and there is a significant reduction in the levels of T_3 and T_4 in the serum, along with a rise in the serum TSH levels. It may occur in several different conditions and accordingly, hypothyroidism is of different types. Despite the differences in the aetiology of different types of hypothyroidism, there are common signs and symptoms present in almost all cases. These symptoms are quite opposite to that observed in hyperthyroidism and include a decrease in heat production leading to cold intolerance, bradycardia, growth and mental retardation in children, weight gain, constipation, lethargy, poor memory, slow and hoarse speech and energy loss (Table 7-11). The various types of hypothyroidism are described in the following sections (Table 7-13).

1. **Chronic Autoimmune Thyroiditis (Hashimoto's Disease):** Hashimoto's disease is the most common type of hypothyroidism in adults. There is a specific defect in the functioning of suppressor T cells, which leads to an over-activation of the immune system and some of these cells may attack the thyroid gland. In this type, the activation of both cell-mediated and antibody-mediated immune systems leads to the destruction of the thyroid gland. The patients may have two patterns of disease: either there is an enlargement of the thyroid gland (goitre) with mild hypothyroidism or shrinkage of the thyroid gland (atrophy) with severe hypothyroidism. An increase in the size of the thyroid gland is a compensatory mechanism to overcome the destruction of thyroid follicles. The Hashimoto's disease has general signs and symptoms of hypothyroidism as enlisted above.

2. **Iatrogenic Hypothyroidism:** Iatrogenic hypothyroidism is characterized by the destruction of the thyroid gland either due to

some type of surgery or exposure to the radiations (used to treat hyperthyroidism). It may occur within 3 months to 1 year after the radioactive therapy, used for the treatment of Graves' disease. In other words, during the process of treatment of thyrotoxicosis (hyperthyroidism), the activity of the thyroid glands may be greatly suppressed due to the destruction of the gland, which may result in hypothyroidism.

3. **Iodine (I2) Deficiency Goitre:** Iodine is an essential dietary mineral and thyroid hormones (T_3 and T_4) contain iodine. In some geographical areas such as in mountainous regions, there is a little iodine in the diet, thus more chances of iodine deficiency. Due to iodine deficiency, the synthesis of thyroid hormones is decreased and in order to increase/restore the levels of thyroid hormones, there is an excessive release of TSH from the anterior pituitary. In turn, TSH stimulates the thyroid gland to increase their size, which results in the development of goitre. The symptoms of hypothyroidism are generally mild in this case. This kind of goitre may be prevented by including small amounts of iodine to salt, a product known as iodized salt.

4. **Congenital Hypothyroidism (Cretinism):** Cretinism is the disease of infants and it is a congenital (from birth) hypothyroidism due to maternal hypothyroidism. It may be due to iodine deficiency or enzymatic defects or exposure to goitrogens (goitre-inducing agents) in pregnant mothers. In untreated cases, there may be a mild to severe impairment of both physical and mental growth (mental retardation) in infants. The other symptoms of cretinism are the same as described above.

5. **Pituitary Disease:** Hypothyroidism may be secondary to the dysfunction of the anterior pituitary in which the anterior pituitary gland is unable to secrete enough TSH required to stimulate the thyroid gland. There may be pituitary insufficiency due to the destruction of thyrotrophs (TSH-secreting cells of the pituitary) by pituitary tumours, surgical therapy, or external radiations. In this case, serum TSH levels are low in comparison to other cases of hypothyroidism.

6. **Myxedema Coma:** Myxedema coma is not a separate type of hypothyroidism; rather it may occur in any type of untreated hypothyroidism. It is a life-threatening state of extreme hypothyroidism and is characterized by very low body temperature, confusion, slow heart rate and reduced breathing effort. Indeed, myxedema is a term used synonymously with severe hypothyroidism in adults. It refers to the dermatological change that can occur in hypothyroidism and leads to cutaneous and dermal oedema.

Table 7-13 Summarization of different types of hypothyroidism and their characteristic features

Sr. No.	Types of Hypothyroidism	Characteristic features
1	Hashimoto's disease	• Specific defect in the functioning of suppressor T cells • Over-activation of the immune system • The destruction of the thyroid gland
2	Iatrogenic hypothyroidism	• The destruction of the thyroid gland either due to surgery or exposure to radiations • May occur within 3 months to 1 year after radioactive therapy to treat hyperthyroidism
3	Iodine deficiency goitre	• Due to the deficiency of iodine in diet or other supplements • A mild form of hypothyroidism • Can be prevented by adding a small amount of iodine into edible salt
4	Congenital hypothyroidism (Cretinism)	• A congenital disease of infants • May be due to iodine deficiency, enzymatic defects or exposure to goitrogens in the pregnant mothers • Mental retardation
5	Pituitary disease	• The anterior pituitary is unable to secrete the required amount of TSH to stimulate the thyroid gland • Low TSH levels • May be due to the destruction of thyrotrophs, surgical therapy or external radiations
6	Myxedema coma	• A life-threatening disease of severe hypothyroidism

Parathyroid Gland

Parathyroid glands are small and rounded mass of tissues that are located posterior to the lateral lobes of the thyroid gland. The two parathyroid glands (one superior and one inferior) are attached to each lobe of the thyroid gland. Since there are two lobes of the thyroid gland, therefore, there are four parathyroid glands attached to the surface of the thyroid gland. The normal mass of each parathyroid gland is about 40 mg. Each parathyroid gland contains two types of epithelial cells including the chief (principal) cells and the oxyphil cells. The chief cells are more in number and release parathyroid hormone (PTH), which is also called parathormone. The function of the oxyphil cells is not clearly known (Figure 7-16).

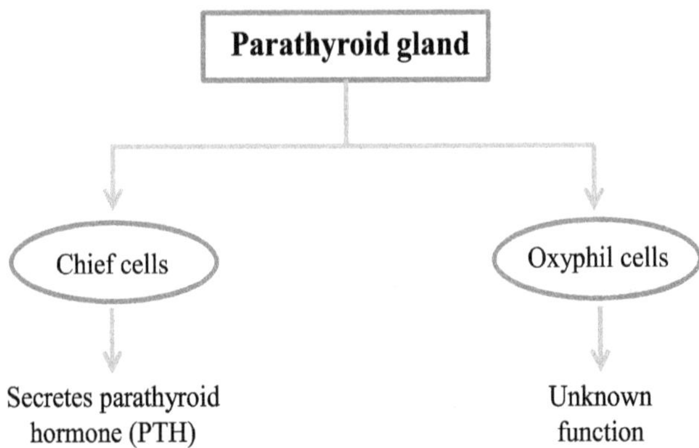

Figure 7-16 The cells of the parathyroid gland

Physiological functions of parathyroid hormone (parathormone, PTH)

1. Parathyroid hormone is the major regulator of different types of ions in the blood including calcium ions (Ca^{2+}), magnesium ions (Mg^{2+}) and phosphate ions (HPO_4^{2-}).
2. The specific physiological function of the parathyroid hormone is to increase the number and activity of osteoclasts (bone dissolving cells) to further enhance the bone resorption.
3. The major action of this hormone is to increase the levels of calcium in the blood.
4. Parathyroid hormone functions along with the calcitonin that is released from the parafollicular cells, in the regulation of calcium homeostasis. The actions of parathormone and calcitonin are opposite to each other (Figure 7-14).
5. Parathyroid hormone also acts on the kidneys to promote the formation of hormone calcitriol, the active form of vitamin D. It further helps in increasing the blood calcium levels (Table 7-10).

Regulation of the release of parathyroid hormone, calcitonin and calcitriol

The low levels of calcium in the blood directly control the secretion of both calcitonin and parathyroid hormone. There is no direct involvement of the hypothalamus and the pituitary gland in regulating their release. In other words, the parathyroid gland is not under the control of the anterior pituitary gland. High levels of calcium in the blood stimulate the parafollicular cells of the thyroid gland to release more calcitonin. Calcitonin inhibits the osteoclasts and decreases the blood calcium level. The low blood calcium level stimulates the chief cells of the parathyroid gland to secrete more parathyroid hormone. The increased level of parathyroid hormone further promotes the release of extracellular calcium into the blood and slows down its secretion into the urine, thus increasing the blood calcium level. Moreover, the parathyroid hormone also stimulates the kidneys to release calcitriol, which further increases the blood calcium level by enhancing its absorption from the foods. Therefore, this increase in the blood calcium level again stimulates the thyroid gland to decrease its level via a negative feedback mechanism (Figure 7-17).

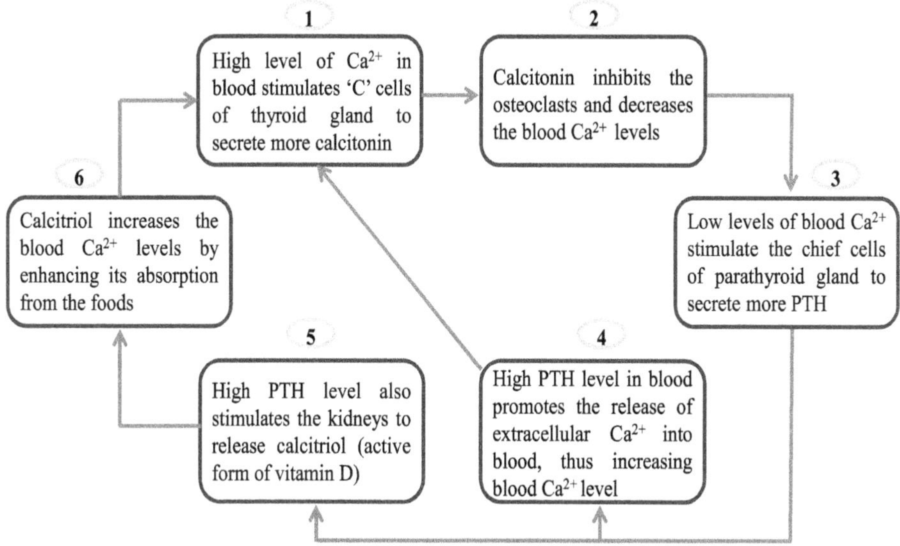

Figure 7-17 Regulation of parathyroid hormone, calcitonin and calcitriol

Disorders of the Parathyroid Gland

1. **Hypoparathyroidism:** Hypoparathyroidism is a condition in which the level of calcium ions are persistently decreased in the blood due to a decrease in the level of parathyroid hormone (PTH). It may be due to accidental damage to the parathyroid glands. This decreased calcium level leads to sustained muscle contractions, which further leads to the development of parathyroid tetany (maintained contraction) of the skeletal muscles (Table 7-14).

2. **Hyperparathyroidism:** The excessive level of calcium ions in the blood due to the high PTH level is called hyperparathyroidism. It may be due to a tumor of one of the parathyroid glands. This excessive calcium is deposited in the body tissues such as the kidneys that results in the formation of kidney stones. Due to the excessive stimulation of osteoclasts in the presence of high PTH, there is excessive bone resorption, which leads to the weakening of bones. The other symptoms of hyperparathyroidism include fatigue, lethargy and personality changes (Table 7-14).

Table 7-14 Key differences between the hypoparathyroidism and hyperparathyroidism

Sr. No.	Hypoparathyroidism	Hyperparathyroidism
1	It is characterised by the decreased release of parathormone (PTH) that leads to a persistent decrease in blood calcium ion level	It is characterised by the excessive release of parathormone (PTH) that leads to increase the blood calcium ion level
2	It may be due to the accidental damage to the parathyroid glands	It may be due to a tumor of one of the parathyroid glands
3	A major symptom is sustainable muscle contractions that may lead to parathyroid tetany	The major symptoms include the formation of kidney stones due to deposition of calcium and weakening of bones

Adrenal Gland

The adrenal glands are flattened pyramidal-shaped glands. They are two in number and are located superior to each kidney (over the kidneys), thus they are also called suprarenal (supra + renal) glands (Figure 7-18).

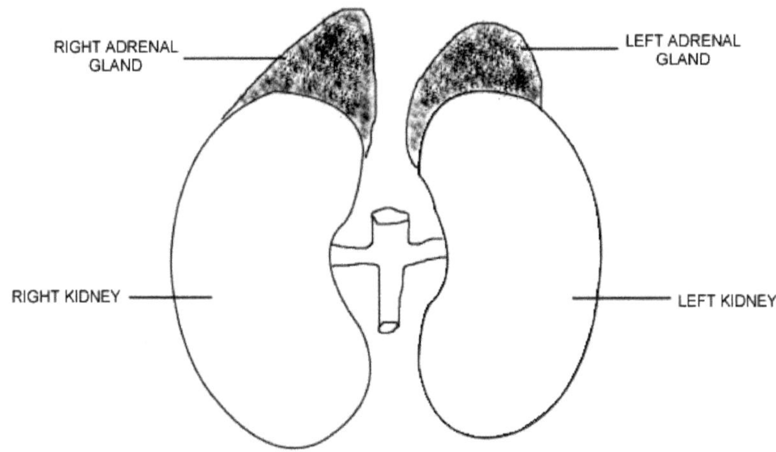

Figure 7-18 The external structure of the adrenal glands

Each adrenal gland measures about 4 cm in height, 2.5 cm in width and 0.75 cm in thickness, with a weight of 4 grams. The size of the adrenal gland is half of its original size during the birth of a child. Anatomically, each adrenal gland is differentiated into two parts including the adrenal cortex and the adrenal medulla (Figure 7-19).

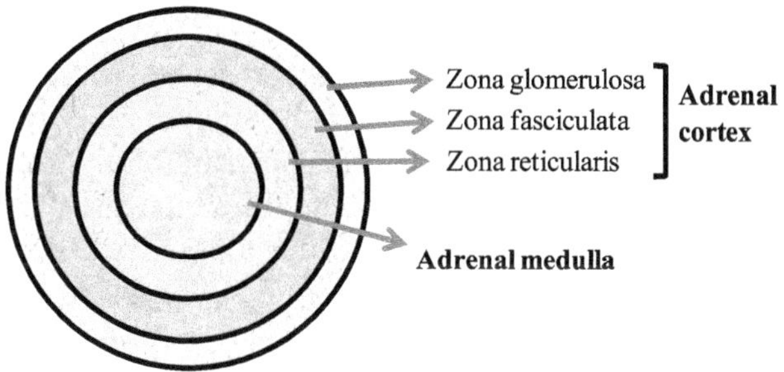

Figure 7-19 The different parts of the adrenal gland

These two parts of the adrenal gland have an entirely different structure and functions. The difference between the adrenal cortex and the adrenal medulla is given in Table 7-15. The whole adrenal gland is covered with the capsule of connective tissues.

Table 7-15 Key differences between the adrenal cortex and the adrenal medulla

Sr. No.	Adrenal Cortex	Adrenal medulla
1	It is the outer part of the adrenal gland	It is the inner part of the adrenal gland
2	It constitutes about 80-85% of the gland	It constitutes about 15-20% of the gland
3	It comprises of three types of cells including zona glomerulosa, zona fasciculata and zona reticularis	It comprises of only chromaffin cells
4	It secretes mineralocorticoids, glucocorticoids and androgens	It secretes hormones, epinephrine and norepinephrine
5	It is essential for life and its destruction leads to death	It is non-essential for life and its death does not lead to death
6	The hormones released from the adrenal cortex has their own physiological functions	The hormones released from the adrenal medulla potentiates the actions of neurotransmitters of the sympathetic nervous system
7	There is no linkage between the adrenal cortex and the sympathetic nervous system	The adrenal medulla acts along with the sympathetic nervous system

A. Adrenal Cortex: The adrenal cortex is a large and peripheral part of the adrenal gland and it constitutes about 80-85% of the total area of the gland. It produces steroidal hormones, which are essential for life. The adrenal cortex is subdivided into three parts including the zona glomerulosa, the zona fasciculata and the zona reticularis (Figure 7-19). These three regions of the cortex secrete different hormones. The zona glomerulosa is an outer part of the cortex that is present beneath the connective tissue capsule. Its cells are closely packed, arranged in the spherical clusters and secrete several hormones known as mineralocorticoids. The zona fasciculata is the middle and widest part of the cortex. It consists of cells arranged in the long and straight columns, which secrete hormones called glucocorticoids. The third and last part of the cortex, zona reticularis, consists of cells arranged in the branching cords. These cells secrete sex hormones called androgens (Figure 7-20) (Table 7-17).

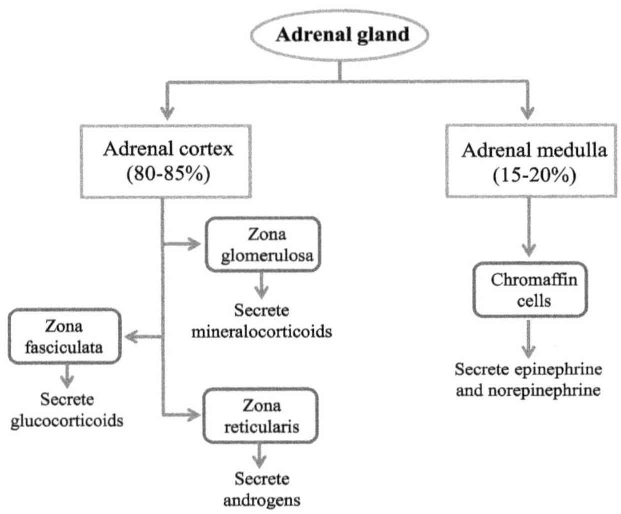

Figure 7-20 The different parts of the adrenal gland and hormones released from those parts

I. **Mineralocorticoids:** The major mineralocorticoid released from the zona glomerulosa is aldosterone. The physiological functions of the aldosterone include: (Table 7-16)

1. It regulates mineral homeostasis of two ions including sodium ions (Na^+) and potassium ions (K^+) in the body.

2. In the kidneys, its major action is on the distal convoluted tubules and collecting ducts of the nephron. It helps in reabsorption of sodium ions from the glomerular filtrate to the blood, and hence, it helps to retain sodium ions in the body. On the other hand, it promotes the excretion of potassium ions in the glomerular filtrate and hence, it decreases the potassium levels in the blood.

3. Due to the retention of sodium ions, it also retains water in the body (due to osmotic action). Accordingly, it helps in the regulation of blood volume and blood pressure.

4. It also helps to prevent acidosis (pH of blood <7) by excreting an excess of H^+ ions in the urine.

Regulation of the secretion of aldosterone

The renin-angiotensin-aldosterone system (RAAS) regulates the secretion of aldosterone from the zona glomerulosa cells of the adrenal cortex. The conditions such as dehydration, Na^+-ions deficiency and hemorrhagic shock lead to a decrease in the blood volume and blood pressure, which stimulates the activation of the RAAS pathway. The decreased blood pressure stimulates the juxtaglomerular cells (JG) of the kidney to secrete renin enzyme, thus the level of renin increases in the blood. Renin converts the plasma protein angiotensinogen (produced by the liver) to the hormone angiotensin I. The angiotensin I is inactive, and it is acted upon by angiotensin-converting enzyme (ACE) to convert it into the hormone angiotensin II. The angiotensin II stimulates the adrenal cortex to secrete aldosterone, which circulates through the blood to reach the kidneys. In the kidneys, aldosterone increases the reabsorption of Na^+-ions and water to reduce their secretion into the urine and leads to an increase in the blood volume. The aldosterone also stimulates the kidneys to increase the excretion of K^+-ions and H^+-ions into the urine. With the restoration of blood volume, blood pressure also returns to normal (Figure 7-21).

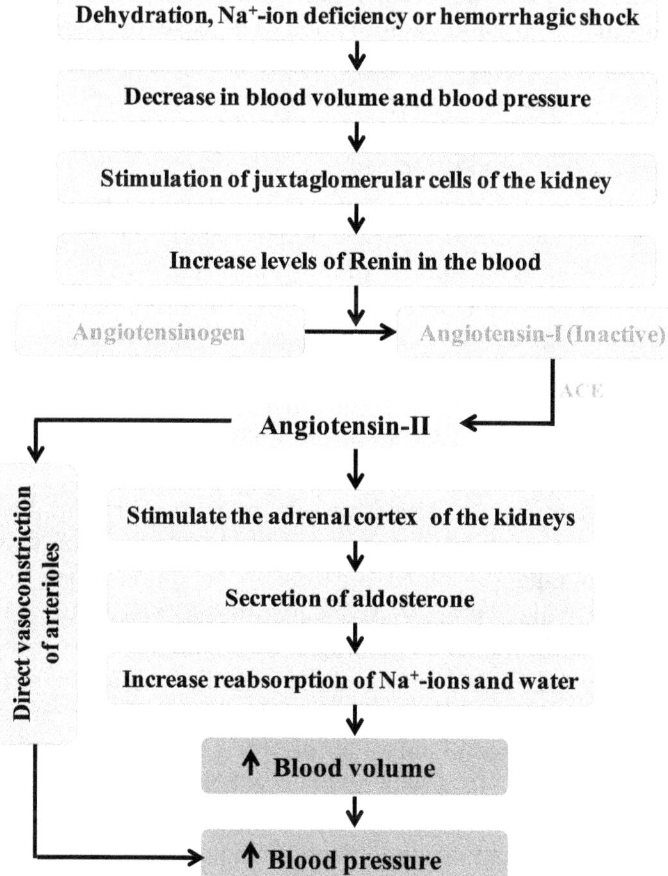

Figure 7-21 Regulation of the secretion of aldosterone

In addition to the above-described pathway of restoring the blood volume and blood pressure, angiotensin II also stimulates the smooth muscles contractions in the walls of arteries. This angiotensin II-mediated vasoconstriction of arterioles leads to increase/restore the blood pressure to a normal range. Moreover, an increase in the K^+-ion concentration in the blood also stimulates the secretion of aldosterone from the adrenal cortex.

II. **Glucocorticoids:** The glucocorticoid hormones are released from the cells of zona fasciculata, which include cortisol (also called hydrocortisone), corticosterone and cortisone. Amongst these hormones, cortisol is the most abundant glucocorticoid (about 95%) present in the body. The physiological functions of the glucocorticoids include: (Table 7-16)

1. The major function of the glucocorticoids is the regulation of metabolism and to provide resistance to stress.

2. They increase the breakdown of proteins in the muscle fibres that leads to accumulation of amino acids in the blood. These amino acids may be used by other body cells for the synthesis of new proteins. Some of these amino acids may be used in the formation of glucose (discussed below).

3. They help in the formation of glucose from the substances other than glycogen by the process called gluconeogenesis. The liver cells under the influence of glucocorticoids convert certain amino acids into glucose that can be used for ATP production.

4. They stimulate the breakdown of triglycerides and other lipids that results in the release of fatty acids from the adipose tissue into the blood. This process of breakdown and release of fatty acids is known as lipolysis.

5. Glucocorticoids provide resistance to a range of stressful condition such as very heavy exercise, fasting, bleeding, high altitude, extreme temperature or cold, infection, surgery and diseases. In these conditions, the body starts to utilize additional glucose formed by the liver cells (through gluconeogenesis) to produce ATPs to counter the stressful conditions.

6. Glucocorticoids make the blood vessels more sensitive to hormones, which cause vasoconstriction and increase blood pressure. This effect helps in maintaining the blood pressure in conditions such as severe blood loss, where blood pressure suddenly drops to a larger extent.

7. They produce anti-inflammatory effects by inhibiting the various steps involved in the inflammatory processes including inhibitory effects on the white blood cells (WBC). Therefore, glucocorticoids are also used in the treatment of chronic inflammatory disorders such as osteoarthritis and bronchial asthma etc, in which excessive activation of inflammation produces pain and discomfort.

8. Glucocorticoids also participate in the inhibition of immune response and act as immunosuppressants. Therefore, these can be used in the treatment of autoimmune diseases (excessive activation of the body's own immune system produces tissue damage) such as rheumatoid arthritis. Moreover,

these may also be very helpful in preventing the immune system-mediated organ/tissue rejection during tissue/organ transplantation.

Regulation of the secretion of glucocorticoids

The secretion of glucocorticoids from the adrenal cortex is controlled via a negative feedback mechanism. The low level of glucocorticoids in the blood stimulate the neurosecretory cells of the hypothalamus to release corticotropin-releasing hormone (CRH), which further stimulates the anterior pituitary to secrete adrenocorticotropic hormone (ACTH). The ACTH then travels toward the adrenal gland via blood circulation, where it stimulates the adrenal cortex to release glucocorticoids to maintain its normal level. In turn, an excessive release of glucocorticoids inhibits the hypothalamus as well as the anterior pituitary to inhibit the release of glucocorticoids via a negative feedback mechanism (Figure 7-22).

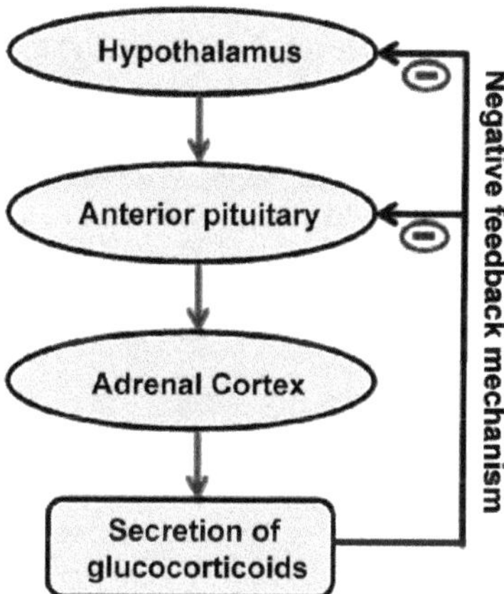

Figure 7-22 Negative feedback mechanism of regulating the release of glucocorticoids

III. **Androgens (Sexocorticoids):** The zona reticularis cells of the adrenal cortex secrete weak androgens in both males and females. The major androgen released from the adrenal cortex is dehydroepiandrosterone (DHEA). In males, the testes release testosterone (an androgen) in larger quantities, during/after the onset of puberty. The adrenal gland secretes a very less quantity of androgens in males and their effects during adulthood in usually insignificant, but they contribute to the onset of puberty and the formation of male organs in the foetus. In females, these hormones play important functions, which include: (Table 7-16)

1. They promote libido (sex drive).
2. They have converted into the female sex steroids i.e. estrogens.
3. After menopause (when the secretion of estrogens from the ovarian follicles stops), all the estrogens in females are formed from the conversion of adrenal androgens.

4. They also stimulate the growth of pubic and axillary hairs in both males and females.

Regulation of the secretion of androgens

The regulation of the secretion of androgens from the adrenal cortex is not fully understood. However, it has been hypothesised that their secretion is stimulated by the hormone ACTH.

Table 7-16 Summarization of physiological functions of different hormones released from the cells of the adrenal cortex

Sr. No.	Hormones	Physiological functions
1	Mineralocorticoids	• Regulation of the mineral homeostasis of Na^+ and K^+ ions • Increase the level of Na^+ ions while decreasing the level of K^+ ions in the blood • Regulation of the blood volume and blood pressure
2	Glucocorticoids	• Regulation of metabolism and provide resistance to stress • Increase the breakdown of proteins • Increase the breakdown of triglycerides • Formation of glucose from amino acids • Produce anti-inflammatory effects • Inhibits the immune response of the body, thus act as an immunosuppressants
3	Androgens	• Promotes libido • Stimulate the growth of pubic and axillary hairs in both males and females

B. Adrenal medulla: The adrenal medulla is centrally located, a very small portion of the adrenal gland, which constitutes about 15-20% of the total area of the gland (Figure 7-20). Indeed, it is a modified form of the ganglion of the sympathetic nervous system. The cells of the adrenal medulla form cluster around the blood vessels and secrete hormones in the blood instead of releasing neurotransmitters in the synaptic cleft (as normal sympathetic ganglion secrete neurotransmitters). The hormone-producing cells of the adrenal medulla are called chromaffin cells, which are directly innervated by the pre-ganglionic fibres of the sympathetic nervous system (Figure 7-23). Due to direct control of the sympathetic nervous system over the chromaffin cells, the latter release hormones very quickly.

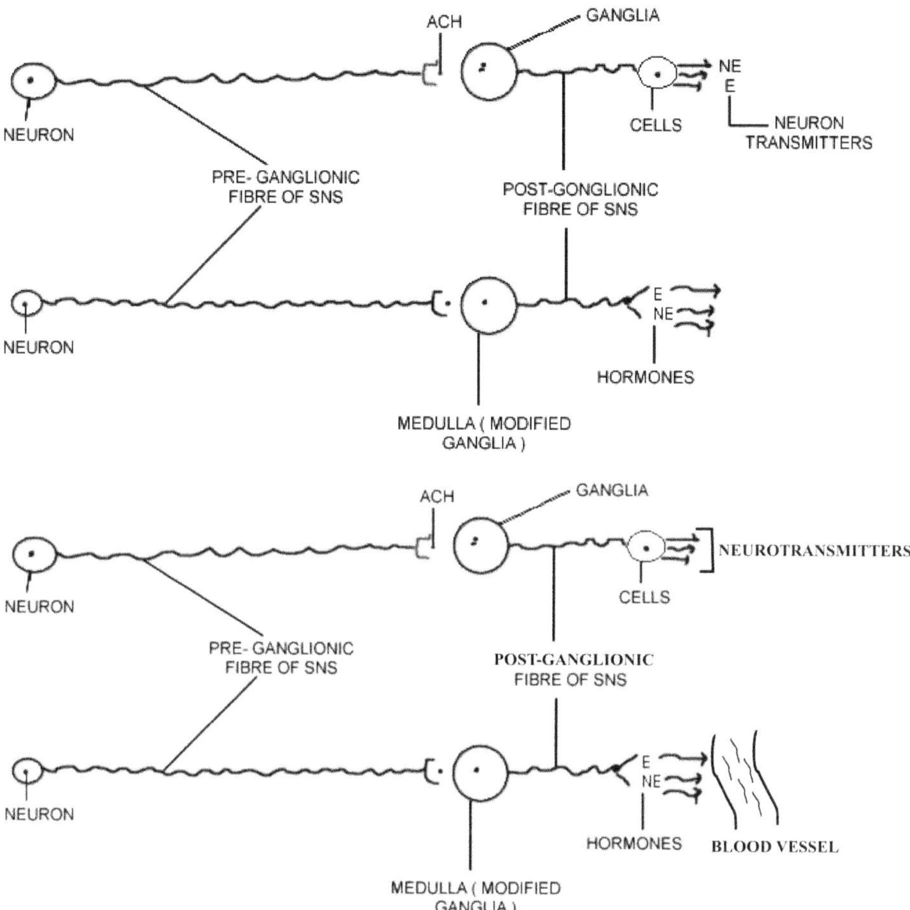

Figure 7-23 Pre-ganglionic innervation of the ganglia and the adrenal medulla (a modified form of ganglia). SNS: Sympathetic nervous system, ACH: Acetylcholine, NE: Norepinephrine, E: Epinephrine.

The chromaffin cells produce two major hormones including epinephrine (also called adrenaline) and norepinephrine (NE; also called noradrenaline). These hormones are released in unequal amount i.e. about 80% of epinephrine and 20% of norepinephrine. In comparison to hormones released from the adrenal cortex, the hormones of the adrenal medulla are not essential for the life because they only work to intensify the sympathetic responses of norepinephrine (neurotransmitter) in other parts of the body (Table 7-17). The physiological responses of epinephrine and norepinephrine are collectively known as fight or flight response, which includes

1. They dilate pupils of the eyes.
2. They increase the heart rate and force of heart contraction.

3. They increase cardiac output, which leads to an increase in blood pressure.
4. In exercise, excitement and emergency-like conditions, they allow greater blood flow towards the tissues involved in them such as cardiac muscles, liver, skeletal muscles and adipose tissues.
5. They dilate bronchi of the lungs, which allow easy movement of air to the lungs.
6. They also increase blood levels of glucose and fatty acids.

Regulation of the secretion of epinephrine and norepinephrine

In stressful conditions and during exercise, signals from the hypothalamus stimulate the sympathetic pre-ganglionic neurons to release acetylcholine, which further stimulates the chromaffin cells of the adrenal medulla to secrete epinephrine and norepinephrine.

Table 7-17 The summarized source, major functions and regulation of different hormones released from the adrenal gland

Sr. No.	Parts	Hormones	Source	Major functions	Regulation
1	Adrenal cortex	Mineralocorticoids e.g. aldosterone	Zona glomerulosa	• Regulation of mineral homeostasis	Activation of the RAAS pathway
		Glucocorticoids e.g. cortisol	Zona fasciculata	• Regulation of metabolism and provide resistance to stress • Anti-inflammatory and immunosuppressant	Release of ACTH and CRH from the anterior pituitary and the hypothalamus, respectively
		Androgens e.g. DHEA	Zona reticularis	• Promotes libido and stimulate the growth of pubic hairs	Not fully understood
2	Adrenal medulla	Epinephrine and Norepinephrine	Chromaffin cells	• Enhancement of the sympathetic responses of norepinephrine	

Disorders of the Adrenal Gland

1. **Cushing's syndrome:** Cushing's syndrome is a group of symptoms in which the adrenal cortex secretes an excessive amount of cortisol. It may be due to the tumor of the adrenal gland or any other tissue, which directly or indirectly (by secreting ACTH) leads to the excessive release of cortisol. The symptoms of this condition include redistribution of body fat, spindly arms and legs, rounded 'moon-like' face, stretch marks on the stomach and 'buffalo hump' on the back (Table 7-18). The elevated level of cortisol also causes an increase in the blood glucose level and blood pressure, which results in the development of hyperglycaemia and hypertension, respectively. Moreover, other common symptoms of Cushing's syndrome include reabsorption of Na^+-ions and water, weakness, delayed wound healing, increased susceptibility to infections, mood swings and osteoporosis.

2. **Addison's disease:** Addison's disease is characterised by the deficiency of both mineralocorticoids and glucocorticoids, therefore, it is also called chronic adrenocortical insufficiency. Most of the cases of Addison's disease are autoimmune in which the antibodies attacks on the adrenal gland and leads to its destruction or block the binding of ACTH to its receptors, which results in the decreased secretion of mineralocorticoids and glucocorticoids from the adrenal cortex. The symptoms of Addison's disease do not appear until 90% of the adrenal cortex has been destroyed. The symptoms due to the deficiency of glucocorticoids include nausea and vomiting, mental lethargy, anorexia, weight loss, muscular weakness and hypoglycaemia. The deficiency of mineralocorticoids in the blood causes a decrease in the reabsorption of Na^+-ions and water, elevation in K^+-ion level, hypotension, decrease in cardiac output and 'bronze-like' pigments on the skin (Table 7-18).

3. **Pheochromocytomas:** A pheochromocytoma is a benign tumor of the chromaffin cells of the adrenal medulla. It is mainly characterised by the hypersecretion of epinephrine (some amount of norepinephrine too) that results in the enhancement of the fight or flight response. The symptoms of pheochromacytomas are typical of the increased actions of epinephrine and norepinephrine, which include an increase in heart rate and very high blood pressure, hyperglycaemia, glycosuria, increase in basal metabolic rate (BMR), nervousness, sweating and decrease in gastrointestinal motility (Table 7-18).

4. **Adrenal virilism:** The adrenal virilism is a syndrome, which is characterised by the excessive release of adrenal androgens. It is more common in females as compared to males. It may be caused due to the tumor of androgen-secreting cells (i.e. zona reticularis cells) or adrenal hyperplasia (increase in size). The symptoms of adrenal virilism include male-like characters in

females, atrophy of the uterus, decrease in breast size, increase in libido and increase in muscularity (Table 7-18).

Table 7-18 The summarized source, major functions and regulation of different hormones released from the adrenal gland

Sr. No.	Disorder	Characteristic features
1	Cushing's syndrome	• Excessive release of cortisol • May be due to the tumor of the adrenal gland • Specific symptoms include redistribution of the body fat, 'moon-like' face and 'buffalo hump' on the back
2	Addison's disease	• Autoimmune disorder • Deficiency of both mineralocorticoids and glucocorticoids • Also called chronic adrenocortical insufficiency • Symptoms include weight loss, hypoglycaemia and 'bronze-like' pigments on the skin
3	Pheochromocyto mas	• Benign tumor of the chromaffin cells of the adrenal medulla • Characterised by the hypersecretion of epinephrine • Symptoms are typical of the increased actions of epinephrine and norepinephrine
4	Adrenal virilism	• Excessive release of adrenal androgens • More common in females • May be due to the tumor of androgen-secreting cells or adrenal hyperplasia • Symptoms include male-like characters in females, atrophy of the uterus, decrease in the breast size and increase in libido

Pancreas

The pancreas is a flattened gland that is present inferior to the stomach, in the curve of the duodenum (first part of the small intestine). It measures about 2.5 cm in thickness and 12.5-15.0 cm in length. It consists of three parts including a head, a body and a tail. The pancreas is a heterocrine gland means it act as both an endocrine gland and an exocrine gland. About 99% cells of the pancreas form the exocrine portion of the organ and they are arranged in a cluster form called acini, which produce digestive enzymes (pancreatic juice) that flow into the gastrointestinal tract through various ducts. The exocrine functions of the pancreas are discussed in the chapter 'Digestive System'. The remaining 1% cells of the pancreas form the endocrine portion of the gland and are known as pancreatic islets or islets of Langerhans.

Each pancreatic islet comprises of four types of hormone-secreting cells including Alpha cells (A cells), Beta cells (B cells), Delta cells (D cells) and F cells. These cells secrete different types of hormones with different functions. Alpha cells constitute about 17% of the cells of the pancreatic islet and secrete glucagon hormone. Similarly, beta cells and delta cells constitute about 70% and about 7% of the pancreatic islet cells and secrete insulin and somatostatin, respectively. The remaining cells of the islet (about 6%) are known as F cells that secrete pancreatic polypeptide (Figure 7-24). The interactions between these four types of pancreatic hormones are very complex and not fully understood. However, some of the physiological functions of these hormones are well known which include:

1. Glucagon increases the level of blood glucose by enhancing the breakdown of glycogen into glucose (glycogenolysis) and increasing the conversion of other nutrients (lactic acid and certain amino acids), present in the liver into glucose (gluconeogenesis).
2. Insulin decreases the blood glucose level by accelerating the transport of glucose into the cells, converting the glucose into glycogen (glycogenesis) and inhibiting the processes of glycogenolysis and gluconeogenesis.
3. Insulin also accelerates the process of lipogenesis (synthesis of fatty acids and triglycerides) and protein synthesis.
4. Somatostatin ac+++ ts in a paracrine manner (local action) and inhibits the release of both glucagon and insulin from the alpha and beta cells, respectively.
5. Somatostatin also slows down the absorption of nutrients from the gastrointestinal tract.
6. Pancreatic polypeptide inhibits the release of somatostatin, contractions of gallbladder and secretion of pancreatic digestive enzymes.

Regulation of the secretion of glucagon and insulin

The principal actions of two major hormones of the pancreas i.e. glucagon and insulin depend on the blood glucose level. The glucagon, released from the alpha cells of the pancreas, increases the blood glucose level when it falls below the normal value. On the other hand, the insulin that is released from the beta cells of the pancreas functions opposite to that of glucagon and lowers the blood glucose level when it is too high. The blood glucose level controls the secretion of glucagon and insulin via a negative feedback mechanism.

The low level of glucose in the blood (hypoglycaemia) stimulates the secretion of glucagon that acts on the liver cells (hepatocytes) to accelerate the processes of glycogenolysis and gluconeogenesis, which leads to a rise in the blood glucose level. The persistent increase in glucose (hyperglycaemia) inhibits the secretion of glucagon via a negative feedback mechanism. Moreover, high blood glucose also stimulates the release of insulin, which acts on the various body cells to speed up the processes of glycogenesis, lipogenesis and protein synthesis and slow down the processes of glycogenolysis and gluconeogenesis. These actions of insulin lead to a decline in the blood glucose level. However, the persistent decline in the level of glucose inhibits the release of insulin via a negative feedback mechanism and again stimulates the secretion of glucagon (Figure 7-25).

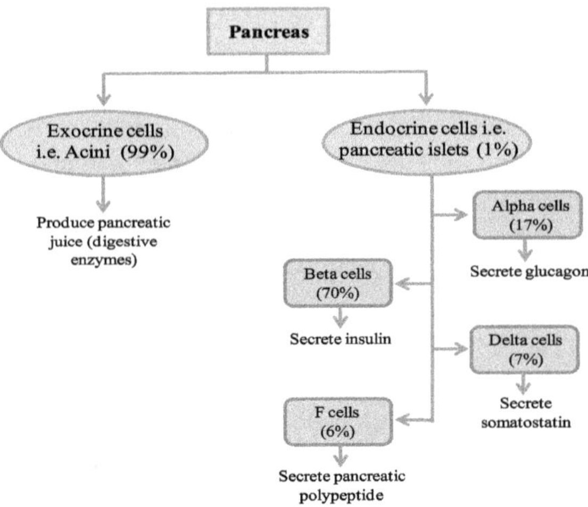

Figure 7-24 The different types of cells of the pancreas and hormones released from those cells

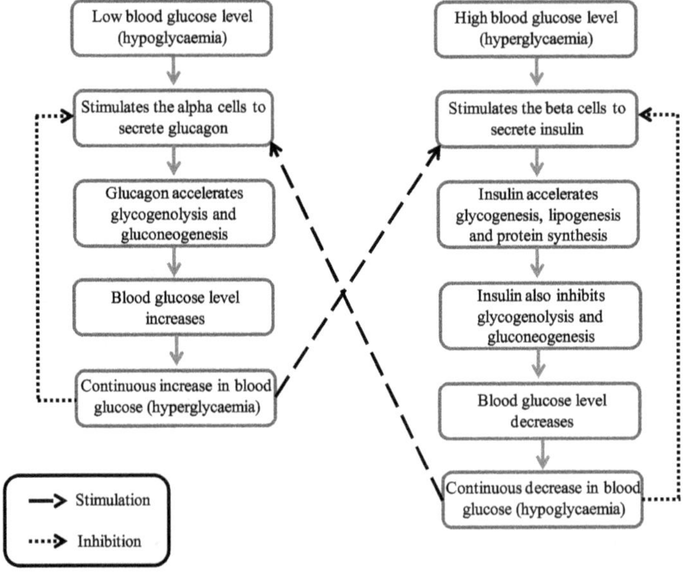

Figure 7-25 Negative feedback mechanism of regulating the release of glucagon and insulin

Disorders of the Pancreas

1. **Diabetes mellitus (DM):** Diabetes mellitus is the most common and chronic metabolic disorder of the endocrine system. It is characterised by the abnormal metabolism of carbohydrates, proteins and fats. Diabetes mellitus may be caused by either a defect in the insulin release from the beta cells of Langerhans or impairment in the functioning of insulin in the body. In short, the disease is characterized by hyperglycaemia (increase in blood glucose level) due to the non-utilization of glucose either due to the absence or loss of functioning of insulin. It is worth mentioning that diabetes mellitus is different from diabetes insipidus, which is caused due to the deficiency of antidiuretic hormone (ADH) and is characterized by an excessive volume of urine.

   Depending on the etiology (pathogenesis) of disease, diabetes mellitus is of two types including primary diabetes mellitus and secondary diabetes mellitus. The primary diabetes mellitus is the most common type of diabetes mellitus and is also called idiopathic because its exact cause of pathogenesis is unknown. It is called primary because the disease itself is primary in nature and it is not secondary to any other disorder. The cause of secondary diabetes mellitus is the presence of some other secondary disorder. The various examples that may cause secondary diabetes mellitus include the usage of drugs such as corticosteroids, post-pancreatectomy (surgical removal of the pancreas), lipodystrophy (loss of body fat) and other disorders such as chronic pancreatitis and pheochromocytoma (tumor of the adrenal medulla).

   Primary diabetes mellitus is further divided into two types that include type I and type II. The type I and type II primary diabetes mellitus are also termed as insulin dependent diabetes mellitus (IDDM) and non-insulin dependent diabetes mellitus (NIDDM), respectively. The key differences between these two types of diabetes mellitus are highlighted in Table 7-19. The clinical symptoms of diabetes mellitus include hyperglycaemia, glycosuria (glucose in the urine), polyuria (increase in urine excretion), polydipsia (increase in water intake), polyphagia (increase in appetite), weight loss and ketoacidosis (in type I diabetes mellitus). Moreover, diabetes mellitus is also associated with various long-term complications such as retinopathy, nephropathy, neuropathy, atherosclerosis and decreased immune response.

Table 7-19 Key differences between type I (IDDM) and type II (NIDDM) primary diabetes mellitus

Sr. No.	Type I (IDDM) diabetes mellitus	Type II (NIDDM) diabetes mellitus
1	About 10-20% of the patients are diagnosed with type I diabetes mellitus	Most of the patients (about 80-90%) are diagnosed with type II diabetes mellitus

Table 7-19 *Contd...*

Sr. No.	Type I (IDDM) diabetes mellitus	Type II (NIDDM) diabetes mellitus
2	Early onset of disease, approximately at about 20 years of age, also termed as juvenile diabetes mellitus	Late onset of disease, approximately at about 35-40 years of age
3	Mainly due to an 'autoimmune disorder' that causes destruction of islet beta cells	Development of 'insulin resistance' is mainly responsible for the development of type II diabetes
4	Characterized by ketoacidosis (decrease in pH) due to the accumulation of ketone bodies in the blood	Ketone bodies are not accumulated in the blood i.e. there is no ketoacidosis
5	Absolute lack of insulin	The level of insulin may be lower or higher than normal
6	Mainly occur in lean people	Mainly occur in obese people.
7	50% concordance in twins (genetic linkage)	60 to 80% concordance in twins (genetic linkage)
8	Severe loss of beta cells of the pancreas	A modest loss of beta cells of the pancreas
9	Drug therapy involves the use of insulin	Drug therapy involves the use of oral hypoglycaemic agents

Pineal Gland

The pineal gland is a small gland that is a part of the epithalamus (a part of the forebrain) and is located in between the two superior colliculi. It is attached to the roof of the third ventricle of the brain. The weight of the pineal gland is about 0.1-0.2 g and it consists of two types of cells including neuroglia cells and secretory cells, which are collectively known as pinealocytes. The whole pineal gland is covered by a capsule that is made up of pia mater (innermost layer of the meninges). The cells of the pineal gland secrete an amine hormone called melatonin that is derived from the serotonin (a neurotransmitter in the brain). Melatonin has several physiological functions in the body, which include:

1. Melatonin contributes to the maintenance of the biological clock (produce circadian rhythms) of the body that is controlled by the suprachiasmatic nucleus (SCN) of the hypothalamus.

2. The secretion of melatonin from the pineal gland is higher in the darkness as compared to the daylight thus it may be involved in the onset of sleep. Therefore, it can be used to induce sleep and reset the circadian pattern in people who work in the alternate shifts of day and night.

3. Melatonin is a potent antioxidant that provides protection against the reactive oxygen species (ROS) or oxygen free radical associated neuronal or any other damages.
4. Melatonin inhibits reproductive functions in the animals, which breed during the specific seasons. The effect of melatonin on human reproductive functions is still unknown.

Regulation of the secretion of melatonin

The secretion of melatonin from the cells of the pineal gland is controlled by the visual inputs from the eyes (retina). In response to these visual inputs, the suprachiasmatic nucleus (SCN) of the hypothalamus stimulates the postganglionic neurons of the sympathetic superior cervical ganglion. The stimulation of these postganglionic neurons further activates the cells of the pineal gland i.e. pinealocytes to secrete melatonin, which is released in a rhythmic pattern with lower level during the day and higher level during the night. The plasma level of melatonin is ten times higher than that of the normal values during sleep (Figure 7-26).

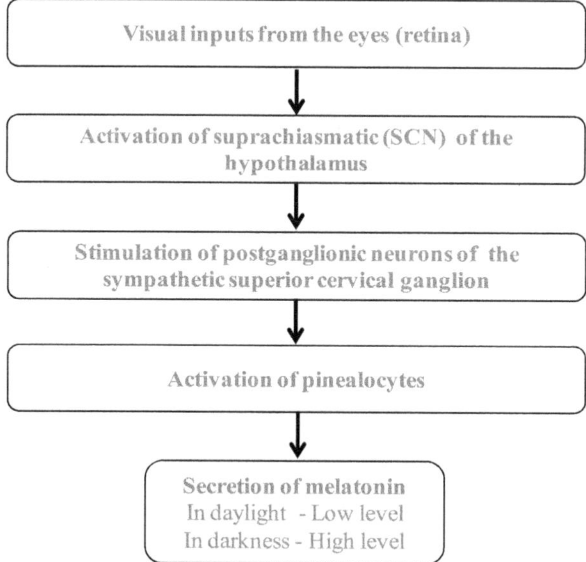

Figure 7-26 Various steps involved in the release of melatonin from pinealocytes

Thymus

The thymus is a soft and bilobed gland that is made up of lymphoid tissues. It is located behind the sternum, in between the lungs. It is covered with a capsule of connective tissues. The size of the thymus is large in children with a weight of about 70 g. However, the size of the thymus starts decreasing after the onset of puberty and weighs only about 3 g in the old age. The thymus secretes four different hormones including thymosin, thymic humoral factor (THF), thymic factor (TF) and thymopoietin. The physiological functions of these hormones are to promote the maturation of T cells (a type of WBCs) and retard the aging process (Table 7-20).

Table 7-20 The different hormones released from the thymus and their functions

Sr. No.	Hormones	Functions
1	Thymosin	• To promote the maturation of T cells
2	Thymic humoral factor (THF)	• To retard the aging process
3	Thymic factor (TF)	
4	Thymopoietin	

7.2 Chapter at a Glance

Term	Description
Endocrine system	Combination of hormone-secreting tissues and endocrine glands
Endocrinology	Branch of science that deals with structure and function of endocrine glands along with diagnosis and treatment of disorders associated with them
Endocrine glands	Ductless glands that release hormones in the blood
Exocrine glands	Glands with ducts that release enzymes in body cavities
Heterocrine glands	Glands that act like both endocrine and exocrine glands
Holocrine glands	Glands that act only as endocrine glands
Hormones	Mediators of endocrine system that regulate the activities of various cells of the body
Circulating hormones	Circulates in the blood and act on various cells
Local hormones	Released from some types of cells and act locally
IL-2	Interleukin-2
Neurotransmitters	Mediators of nervous system
NO	Nitric oxide
Catecholamines	Epinephrine, Norepinephrine and Dopamine
PGs	Prostaglandins
LTs	Leukotrienes
cAMP	Cyclic Adenosine Mono-Phosphates
ATPs	Adenosine Tri-Phosphates

Contd...

Term	Description
Pituitary gland/Hypophysis	Master endocrine glands
Anterior pituitary/adenohypophysis	75% part of the pituitary gland that secrete various hormones
Posterior pituitary/neurohypophysis	About 25% part of the pituitary gland that contain axons and axon terminals
MSH	Melanocyte-stimulating hormone
OT	Oxytocin/Birth hormone/Milk-ejecting hormone
ADH	Antidiuretic hormone
hGH	Human growth hormone
LH	Luteinizing hormone
FSH	Follicle-stimulating hormone
ACTH	Adrenocorticotropic hormone
CRH	Corticotropin-releasing hormone
IGFs	Insulin-like growth factors
GHRH	Growth hormone-releasing hormone
GHIH	Growth hormone-inhibiting hormone
Hypoglycemia	Low level of glucose in blood
Hyperglycemia	High level of glucose in blood
Glycogenolysis	Breakdown of liver glycogen into glucose
Gluconeogenesis	Formation of glucose from substances other than glycogen
Glycogenesis	Conversion of glucose into glycogen
TRH	Thyrotropin-releasing hormone
TSH	Thyroid-stimulating hormone
PRL	Prolactin/Maternity hormone
PRH	Prolactin-releasing hormone
PIH	Prolactin-inhibiting hormone
Osmoreceptors	Maintain osmotic pressure in blood
Dwarfism	Short body height due to slow growth of bones
Gigantism	Large body height due to abnormal growth of long bones
Acromegaly	Inappropriate increase in the size of bones of hands, feet, jaws and cheeks
DI	Diabetes insipidus
DM	Diabetes mellitus

Contd...

Term	Description
IDDM	Insulin-dependent diabetes mellitus
NIDDM	Non-insulin dependent diabetes mellitus
Thyroid hormones	T_3 and T_4 released from thyroid gland
T_3	Triiodothyronine
T_4	Tetraiodothyronine or Thyroxine
Lipolysis	Breakdown of lipids
PTH	Parathyroid hormone/Parathormone released from parathyroid gland
BMR	Basal metabolic rate
Hyperthyroidism/Thyrotoxicosis	Increase in release of T_3 and T_4
Hypothyroidism	Decrease in secretion of T_3 and T_4
Goiter	Enlargement of thyroid gland
Toxic adenoma	Benign tumor of thyroid gland
Pituitary adenoma	Tumors of pituitary gland
Thyroid storm	Severe form of hyperthyroidism
Cretinism	Hypothyroidism from birth/congenital
Hypoparathyroidism	Persistent decrease of calcium ions in blood due to decreased blood PTH level
Hyperparathyroidism	Excessive level of calcium ions due to high blood PTH level
Suprarenal	Located over the kidneys
Adrenal cortex	Outer portion of adrenal gland
Adrenal medulla	Inner portion of adrenal gland
Chromaffin cells	Hormone-producing cells of adrenal medulla
RAAS	Renin-angiotensin-aldosterone system
JG	Juxtaglomerular cells
ACE	Angiotensin-converting enzyme
WBC	White blood cells
DHEA	Dehydroepiandrosterone
Libido	Sex drive
NE	Norepinephrine
Cushing's syndrome	Excessive release of cortisol due to tumor of adrenal gland or any other issue
Addison's disease	Autoimmune disease due to deficiency of mineralocorticoids and glucocorticoids
Pheochromocytomas	Benign tumor of chromaffin cells of adrenal medulla

Contd...

Term	Description
Adrenal virilism	Syndrome due to excessive release of adrenal androgens
Hepatocytes	Liver cells
Glycosuria	Increase of glucose in urine
Polyuria	Increase in urine excretion
Polydipsia	Increase water intake
Polyphagia	Increase appetite
SCN	Suprachiasmatic nucleus
ROS	Reactive oxygen species
THF	Thymic humoral factor
TF	Thymic factor

Exercises

Multiple Choice Questions

1. The example of a heterocrine gland is?
   - (a) Pituitary gland
   - (b) Pancreas
   - (c) Ovaries
   - (d) Sweat glands

2. What are autocrines?
   - (a) Hormones that act on the neighbouring cells
   - (b) Hormones that act on the same cells from which they are released
   - (c) Hormones that enters the bloodstream
   - (d) None of the above

3. Which are lipid-soluble hormones?
   - (a) Steroid hormones
   - (b) Thyroid hormones
   - (c) Nitric oxide
   - (d) All of the above

4. Eicosanoid hormones are
   - (a) Lipid-soluble hormones
   - (b) Water-soluble hormones
   - (c) Both a and b
   - (d) None of the above

5. The pituitary gland is also known as
   - (a) Adenohypophysis
   - (b) Neurohypophysis
   - (c) Hypophysis
   - (d) None of the above

6. Which hormone is released from the remnants of pars intermedia?
   - (a) Prolactin
   - (b) Vasopressin
   - (c) Melanocyte-stimulating hormone
   - (d) Human growth hormone

7. Anterior pituitary gonadotrophs release
   (a) Adrenocorticotropic hormone (ACTH)
   (b) Luteinising hormone (LH)
   (c) Follicle-stimulating hormone (FSH)
   (d) Both b and c

8. Gigantism is characterised by
   (a) Hypersecretion of human growth hormone during childhood
   (b) Hypersecretion of human growth hormone during adulthood
   (c) Hyposecretion of human growth hormone
   (d) None of the above

9. Prolactin-inhibiting hormone (PIH) is also known as
   (a) Serotonin   (b) Acetylcholine
   (c) Dopamine   (d) Epinephrine

10. Oxytocin is also known as
    (a) Milk-ejecting hormone (b) Birth hormone
    (c) Both a and b   (d) None of the above

11. Hashimoto's disease is characterised by
    (a) Destruction of the thyroid gland
    (b) Over-activation of an immune response
    (c) Iodine deficiency
    (d) Congenital abnormalities

12. What are the different layers of the adrenal cortex
    (a) Zona glomerulosa   (b) Zona fasciculata
    (c) Zona reticularis   (d) All of the above

13. Chromaffin cells of the adrenal medulla secrete
    (a) Epinephrine   (b) Glucocorticoids
    (c) Androgens   (d) Mineralocorticoids

14. 'Moon-like face' and 'Buffalo hump' are the characteristic features of
    (a) Adrenal virilism   (b) Pheochromocytoma
    (c) Cushing's syndrome   (d) Addison's disease

15. Insulin is released from
    (a) Alpha cells of the pancreas   (b) F cells of the pancreas
    (c) Delta cells of the pancreas   (d) Beta cells of the pancreas

Short Answer Questions

1. What are the types of glands? Give their examples.
2. What are the differences between hormones and enzymes?
3. What are the characteristic features of circulating hormones and local hormones?

4. What are the two major differences between hormones and neurotransmitters?

5. What is hormone? Mention its types along with their examples.

6. Why pituitary gland is also called 'master endocrine gland'? Give the composition of the pituitary gland.

7. Describe the hormones secreted by different parts of the pituitary gland.

8. Classify different types of cells of the anterior pituitary along with their hormones.

9. What is the antidiuretic hormone (ADH)? Give its two physiological functions.

10. What are the differences between dwarfism and gigantism?

11. What are the common symptoms of hyperthyroidism?

12. Write a brief note on Grave's disease.

13. What are the major differences between diabetes mellitus and diabetes insipidus?

14. What is Hashimoto's disease?

15. Give two major functions of parathormone?

16. Write the differences between hyperparathyroidism and hypoparathyroidism.

17. What are the major differences between the adrenal cortex and adrenal medulla?

18. What is Cushing's syndrome?

19. What is Addison's disease?

20. What is thymus? Mention the hormones released from it.

Long Answer Questions

1. Write a note on the mechanism of hormone action.

2. Write a note on posterior pituitary. Give functions of oxytocin and vasopressin.

3. Write about different types of disorders of the pituitary gland.

4. Explain the structure of the thyroid gland. What are the physiological functions of thyroid hormones?

5. Write a note on different types of hypothyroidism-related disorders?

6. Write a note on mineralocorticoids along with their regulation.

7. Explain the physiological functions of glucocorticoids.

8. Write a brief note on different types of adrenal gland disorders.

9. How the secretion of insulin and glucagon is regulated?

10. What is diabetes mellitus? Describe the differences between type I and type II diabetes mellitus.

Bibliography

Costanzo LS. Physiology. 4th Edition. Lippincott Williams & Wilkins.

Guyton AC, Hall JE. Textbook of Medical Physiology. 11th Edition. Elsevier Saunders. 2006.

Jaggi AS, Bali A, Singh N. Pathophysiology. 1st Edition. Vallabh Prakashan. 2019.

Jain AK. Human Anatomy and Physiology for Pharmacy. 3rd Edition. Arya publications. 2017.

Lodish H, Berk A, Kaiser CA. Molecular Cell Biology. 6th Edition. W. H. Freeman & Co Ltd. 2007.

Tortora GJ, Derrickson B. Principles of Anatomy and Physiology. 15th Edition. John Wiley and Sons, Inc. 2017.

Waugh A, Grant A. Ross and Wilson Anatomy and Physiology in Health and Illness. 12th Edition. Churchill Livingstone. 2014.

Answer Key MCQs

1. (b)	2. (b)	3. (d)	4. (b)	5. (c)
6. (c)	7. (d)	8. (a)	9. (c)	10. (c)
11. (b)	12. (d)	13. (a)	14. (c)	15. (d)

Reproduction System

After completing this lesson, the Reader should be able to understand:

- *Introduction*
- *Male reproductive system*
- *Reproduction in Humans*
- *Anatomy of the Male reproductive system*
- *Semen*
- *Gametogenesis*
- *Spermatogenesis*
- *Structure of sperm*
- *Anatomy of the Female reproductive system*
- *Composition of human milk*
- *Oogenesis*
- *Structure of ovum*
- *Menstrual cycle*
- *Fertilisation*
- *Parturition*

8.1 Introduction

Reproductive system is defined as the collection of both internal and external organs that are used for the purpose of sexual reproduction in humans. Humans are unisexual, which means that male and female sex organs are present in the different individuals. There are two types of sex organs present in the humans i.e. primary sex organs and secondary sex organs. Both primary and secondary sex organs are different in males and females.

Primary sex organs

These are the organs that produce male and female gametes along with sex hormones. The testes are male primary sex organs and they produce sperms (male gametes) and testosterone (male sex hormone). On the other hand, the ovaries are female primary sex organs and they produce eggs (female gametes) and female sex hormones including estrogens and progesterone. The functioning of these primary sex organs is controlled by the gonadotropic hormones such as follicle follicle-stimulating hormone (FSH) and luteinizing hormone (LH), which are released from the anterior pituitary gland (Table 8-1 and 8-2) (Figure 8-1).

Table 8-1 Characteristic features of primary sex organs

Sr. No.		Male	Female
1	Organs	Testes	Ovaries
2	Gametes	Sperms	Eggs
3	Hormones	Testosterone	Estrogens, Progesterone
4	Regulation	FSH and LH	FSH and LH

Secondary sex organs

These are the organs, which neither produce gametes nor produce hormones, but they play an important role in the reproduction of humans. The examples of male secondary sex organs include the prostate gland, the seminal vesicles, the vas deferens, and the penis. On the other hand, the fallopian tubes, the uterus, the vagina, and the mammary glands are female secondary sex organs (Table 8-2) (Figure 8-1).

Table 8-2 Summarized differences between the primary and secondary sex organs

Sr. No.	Primary sex organs	Secondary sex organs
1	Primary sex organs produce male and female gametes	Secondary sex organs do not produce male and female gametes
2	These organs also produce sex hormones including testosterone, estrogens, and progesterone, which are required for the reproduction in humans	These organs do not produce sex hormones, but these organs play an important role in the reproduction of humans
3	The examples include the testes (in males) and the ovaries (in females)	The examples include the prostate gland and the penis (in males) and the uterus and the vagina (in females)

External (accessory) sex characters

The external sex characters are the characters that distinguish males and females externally. The examples of these characters include beard, moustache, body build up, and voice.

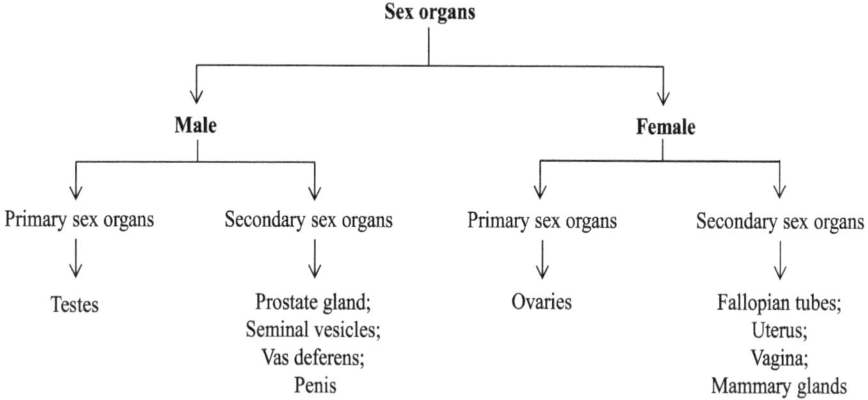

Figure 8-1 Summary of different types of Human Sex Organs

Male Reproductive System

The male reproductive system comprised of several parts (Figure 8.2) including (1) Scrotum; (2) Testes; (3) Epididymis; (4) Vas deferens; (5) Ejaculatory ducts; (6) Urethra; (7) Penis; and (8) Accessory sex glands (Table 8-3).

Table 8-3 Functions of different parts of the male reproductive system

S. No.	Organ/Part	Functions
1	Scrotum	It helps in the regulation of the temperature of the testes
2	Testes	The formation of the sperms takes place in the seminiferous tubules of the testes Interstitial cells present between the seminiferous tubules of the testes secrete testosterone, which is the most prevalent male sex hormone
3	Epididymis	Epididymis store the sperms for several months The final maturation of the sperms also takes place in the epididymis
4	Vas deferens	Vas deferens carry the sperms from the epididymis to the ejaculatory duct It also helps in the storage of sperms
5	Ejaculatory duct	It ejects the sperms and secretions of the seminal vesicles into the urethra
6	Urethra	The urethra is the passageway for both the semen and the urine
7	Penis	Penis transfer the sperms into the female vagina It also helps in the excretion of urine

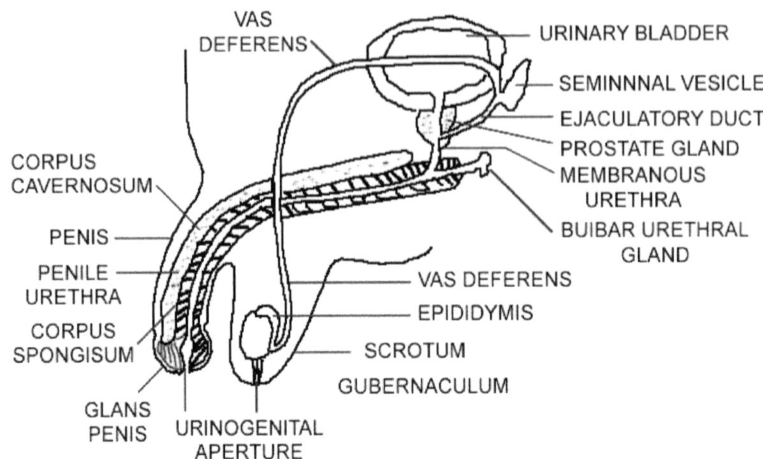

Figure 8-2 Structure of the male reproductive system

1. **Scrotum:** The scrotum is a pouch-like supporting structure of the testes and it is present outside the pelvic cavity. Externally, the scrotum is separated into two lateral parts by a middle ridge, called raphe. Internally, the scrotal septum divides the scrotum into two portions, which are known as scrotal sacs and each sac contains one testis (Figure 8-3). The scrotum is connected to the abdomen by an inguinal canal. The dartos muscle tissue and the cremaster muscle tissue are two muscle tissues present in the scrotum, which plays an important role in the regulation of the temperature of the testes. The production of sperm requires lower temperature, about 2-3°C less in comparison to the normal body temperature. The low temperature is essential for the formation of sperms because they are killed at a higher temperature. This lower temperature of the testes is maintained by the location of the scrotum i.e. outside the pelvic cavity.

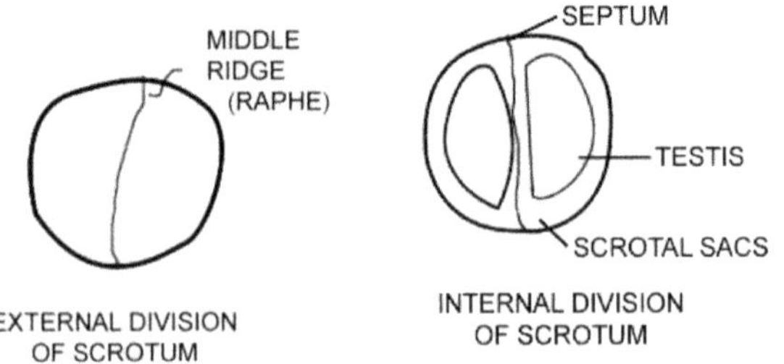

Figure 8-3 External and internal divisions of the scrotum

Moreover, the dartos and the cremaster muscle tissues also help in protecting the sperms from a very low temperature. In winters, the cremaster muscles contract and bring the testes closer to the pelvic cavity, where they absorb the body heat and protect the sperms from the cold environment. The contraction of the dartos muscle causes the scrotum to become tight (wrinkled in appearance) in the cold environment, which reduces the heat loss from the body.

2. **Testes (Testicles):** The testes are the primary sex organs in males and a pair of the testis is present in the scrotum. Each testis is about 5 cm long and about 2.5 cm in diameter, with a weight of about 10-15 grams. They develop near the kidneys, in the posterior part of the abdomen and start their descent from the abdomen into the scrotum through inguinal canals during the seventh month of fetal development. The testes are suspended in the scrotum with the help of spermatic cords and a white fibrous cord, known as gubernaculum.

The testes are covered with three types of layers including the tunica vaginalis, the tunica albuginea, and the tunica vasculosa. The tunica vaginalis is the outer covering of the testes and it forms during the descent of them. The tunica albuginea is a white fibrous layer that is located internal to the tunica vaginalis. It is folded inward and form septa, which divides each testis into 200-300 internal compartments called testicular lobules. The tunica vasculosa consists of a network of capillaries that lines with the tunica albuginea (Figure 8-4).

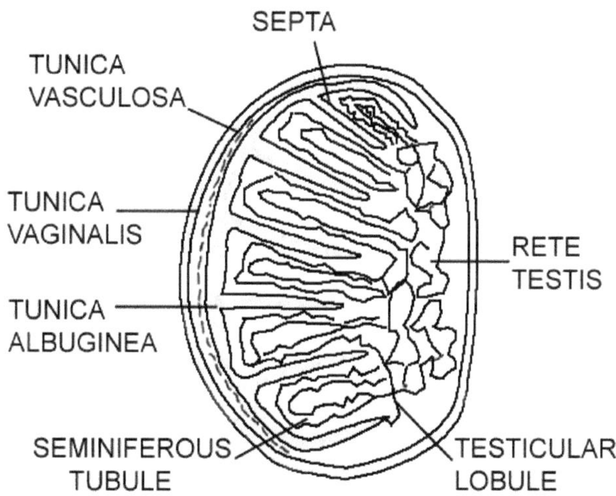

Figure 8-4 Diagram of the longitudinal section of the testis

Each testicular lobule contains 2-3 tightly coiled tubules, which are known as the seminiferous tubules. The production of the sperms take place in these tubules by the process of spermatogenesis. The seminiferous tubules are lined with a single layer of cells called germinal epithelium and it contains two types of cells i.e. cuboidal cells and sertoli cells. Cuboidal cells are large in number and smaller in size and they help in the production of sperms, therefore, cuboidal cells are also known as spermatogenic cells. However, sertoli cells are large and less in number and they provide nourishment to the developing sperms, therefore, sertoli cells are also known as nurse cells. Sertoli cells secrete a fluid, which control the movements of spermatogonia and sperms in the lumen of the seminiferous tubules. In between the seminiferous tubules, a small group of cells are present called interstitial or Leydig's cells. These cells secrete testosterone, the most prevalent male sex hormone (Figure 8-5). The seminiferous tubules are closed at one end and at other end, they join with one another to form a network of tubules called rete testis (Figure 8-4). Rete testis further join to form small ductules (lined inside by cilia), which are known as vasa efferentia. Vasa efferentia then end to the epididymis.

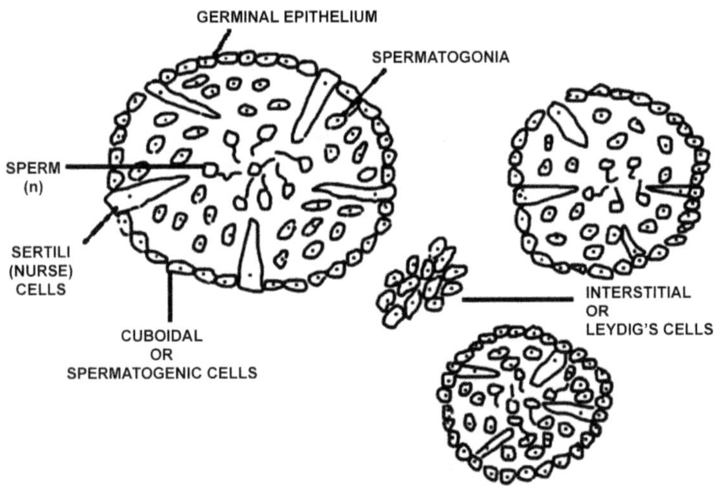

Figure 8-5 Transverse section of the seminiferous tubules

3. **Epididymis:** The epididymis is a long (about 4 cm) and a comma-shaped organ that lies along the inner side of each testis. Each epididymis is comprised of three portions including the caput epididymis, the corpus epididymis, and the cauda epididymis. The caput epididymis is the anterior end of the epididymis and it is attached to the vasa efferentia. The corpus epididymis and the cauda epididymis are the middle and posterior parts of the epididymis, respectively. The cauda epididymis is continuous with the next part of the male reproductive system i.e. vas deferens (Figure 8-6). The major function of the epididymis is to store the sperms where they remain viable for several months. The final maturation of the sperms also take place in the epididymis.

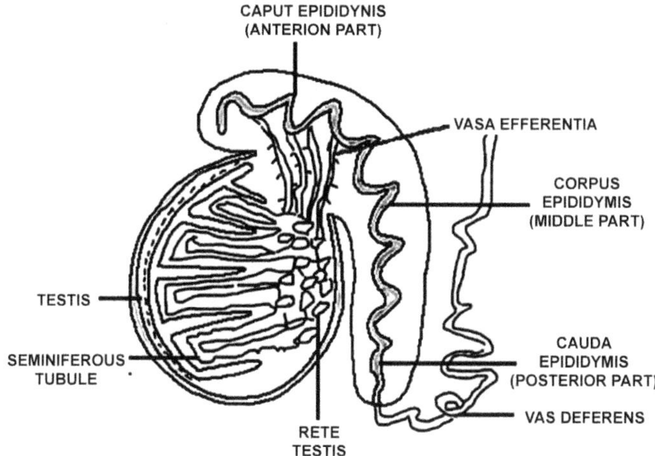

Figure 8-6 Diagram showing a section of the testis, the epididymis and the vas deferens

4. **Vas deferens:** The vas deferens is the pair of long tubules (about 45 cm) that arises from the cauda epididymis. These tubules move upwards and ascend towards the urinary bladder. Each vas deferens joins with the duct of seminal vesicles to form the ejaculatory ducts (Figure 8-5 and 8-6). The major function of the vas deferens is to carry the sperms from the epididymis to the ejaculatory duct during sexual arousal. Like the epididymis, the vas deferens can also store the sperms for several months.

5. **Ejaculatory ducts:** The ejaculatory ducts are the pair of short tubules (about 2 cm), which are formed by the union of the duct from the seminal vesicles and the vas deferens. They further terminate in the prostatic urethra, where they eject the sperms and secretions of the seminal vesicles (Figure 8-7).

6. **Urethra:** The urethra is a tubular structure and it is the major part of the male reproductive system, which carries both semen and urine. It is about 20 cm long and is subdivided into three parts including the prostate (prostatic) urethra, the membranous urethra, and the penile or spongy urethra. The prostate urethra is the first part (about 2-3 cm long) of the urethra and it passes through the prostate gland. The membranous urethra is a very short (about 1 cm) and middle part of the urethra (Figure 8-6). The penile urethra is the last and longest (about 15-20 cm) part of the urethra and it passes through the penis. The penile urethra ends at the external urethral orifice. The prostate urethra carries only urine, while the membranous and the penile urethra carry both semen and urine.

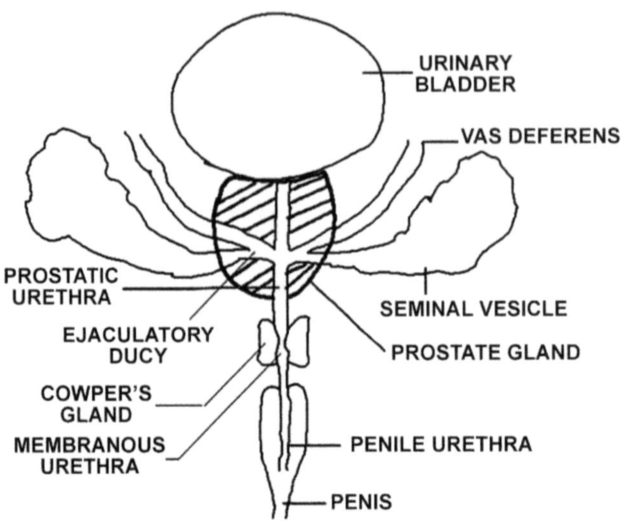

Figure 8-7 Diagram showing the ejaculatory duct, the urethra and accessory sex glands

7. **Penis:** The penis is a male copulatory organ and is cylindrical in shape that transfer the male gametes into the female reproductive tract. The penis also helps in the excretion of urine from the body. It is composed of three cylindrical tissues including two corpora cavernosa (dorsolateral tissues) and one corpus spongiosum (mid-ventral tissue). The corpus spongiosum tissue contains the penile urethra and keep it open during the ejaculation. The terminal end of this tissue is slightly enlarged and swollen called the glans penis. This glans penis is covered with a loose skin called the prepuce.

8. **Accessory sex glands**

   (i) **Seminal vesicles:** The seminal vesicles (two in number) are convoluted pouch-like structures, measuring about 5 cm in length and located posterior to the urinary bladder and anterior to the rectum. The ducts arise from these seminal vesicles and join with the vas deferens to form the ejaculatory duct (Figure 8-7). The seminal vesicles secrete a fluid that forms the bulk part (about 60%) of semen. This fluid is alkaline in nature and contain fructose, amino acids, clotting proteins, prostaglandins, and ascorbic acid. The alkaline nature of the seminal fluid helps to neutralize the acidic environment of the male urethra and the female reproductive tract to prevent the killing of sperms in the acidic environment. The fructose is the source of energy for the movement of sperms and prostaglandins stimulates the uterine contractions that helps in the motility of sperms towards the fallopian tubes. The clotting proteins present in the seminal fluid helps in the coagulation of semen after ejaculation (Table 8-4)

Table 8-4 Components and functions of the secretion of seminal vesicles

S. No.	Components/nature of fluid	Functions
1	Alkaline nature of a fluid	Neutralize the acidic environment of the male urethra and the female reproductive tract
2	Fructose	Source of energy for the movement of sperms
3	Prostaglandins	Causes uterine contractions to make easy passage of sperms towards the fallopian tubes
4	Clotting proteins	Helps in the coagulation of semen after their ejaculation

(ii) **Prostate gland:** The prostate gland is a single largest and doughnut-shaped gland, which measures about 4 cm from side to side, 3 cm from top to bottom and 2 cm from front to back. It lies inferior to the urinary bladder and surrounds the urethra (Figure 8-6). The secretions of this gland are slightly acidic and include prostaglandins, citric acid, lipids, enzymes and bicarbonate ions (HCO_3^-). The citric acid is used for the ATP production and bicarbonate ions make the semen alkaline, so that acidic pH of the vagina can be neutralised. These secretions also give milky colour to the semen and make up about 25% volume of semen (Table 8-5).

(iii) **Cowper's glands (Bulbourethral glands):** The Cowper's glands (two in number) are very small in size. They are present inferior to the prostate gland on either side of the membranous urethra (Figure 8-6). The Cowper's glands secrete alkaline fluid and contain a large amount of mucus that helps in the lubrication of the penis and lining of the urethra. The secretions of Cowper's glands make up the remaining volume (about 15%) of semen (Table 8-5).

Table 8-5 Components and functions of the secretions of prostate gland and Cowper's glands

S. No.	Components/nature of fluid	Functions
1	**Prostatic fluid**	
2	Slightly acidic nature of fluid	Helps in the motility of sperms
3	Citric acid	Used for ATP production
4	Bicarbonate ions	Neutralize the acidic pH of the vagina
	Cowper's fluid	
5	Mucus	Helps in the lubrication of the penis and lining of the urethra

Semen

Semen is a fluid that is ejected from the penis during ejaculation. It is a mixture of the secretions of seminiferous tubules (sperms) and accessory sex glands. In other words, it has sperms and secretions of the seminal vesicles, prostate gland, and Cowper's glands. Apart from the sperms, other components of the semen include prostaglandins, fructose, amino acids, enzymes, and mucus. The volume of the semen in a typical ejaculation is about 2.5-5 ml. The number of sperms in the semen is very large i.e. about 200-300 million sperms per ejaculation. The semen has a slightly alkaline pH of around 7.3-7.5 that helps in the neutralisation of the acidic pH of the vagina.

Gametogenesis

Gametogenesis is the process of the formation of male and female gametes i.e. sperms and ovum. It comprises of the spermatogenesis (formation of sperms) and the oogenesis (formation of ovum).

Spermatogenesis

Spermatogenesis is the process of the formation of sperms and it takes place in the seminiferous tubules of the testes. It starts with the beginning of puberty. Sperms are formed by the cuboidal cells of the germinal epithelium of the seminiferous tubules. Spermatogenesis takes about 65-75 days for the complete production of sperms. The process of spermatogenesis is divided into two parts: (1) Formation of spermatids, and (2) Formation of sperms from spermatids (Spermiogenesis).

1. **Formation of spermatids:** The process of the formation of spermatids is divided into three phases: (i) Multiplication phase; (ii) Growth phase, and (iii) Maturation phase.

    (i) **Multiplication phase:** The multiplication phase begins with the spermatogonia cells. Spermatogonia are the types of stem cells, which are diploid (2n) in nature (Table 8-6). In this phase, spermatogonia cells undergo mitosis to increase their number. During mitosis, some of the spermatogonia remain near the basement membrane of the seminiferous tubules in the undifferentiated state. These undifferentiated cells are known as spermatogonia type A cells. They serve as a reservoir of stem cells for future cell division and subsequent, sperm formation. The rest of the spermatogonia loses contact with the basement membrane of the seminiferous tubules and squeezes through the tight junctions of the blood-testis barrier. These cells are known as spermatogonia type B cells (Table 8-6, 8-7 and 8-8) (Figure 8-8).

    (ii) **Growth phase:** In the growth phase, type B spermatogonia cells grow by obtaining nourishment from the sertoli cells (nurse cells). Thereafter, these are differentiated into the primary spermatocytes after some developmental changes. Like spermatogonia, the primary spermatocytes contain a diploid number (2n) of chromosomes (Table 8-7 and 8-8) (Figure 8-8).

Table 8-6 Differentiation between the types of spermatogonia cells

S. No.	Spermatogonia type A cells	Spermatogonia type B cells
1	The type A cells are undifferentiated spermatogonia cells	The type B cells are differentiated spermatogonia cells
2	These cells remain attached to the basement membrane of the seminiferous tubules during mitosis	These cells lose contact with the basement membrane of the seminiferous tubules during mitosis and squeeze through the tight junctions of the blood-testis barrier
3	Type A spermatogonia cells serve as a reservoir of stem cells for future cell division and subsequently helps in the formation of sperms	Type B spermatogonia cells obtain nourishment from the sertoli cells and differentiated into the primary spermatocytes, which further leads to the formation of sperms

Table 8-7 Characteristic features of different phases of the formation of spermatids

S. No.	Phase	Characteristic features
1	Multiplication phase	Spermatogonia undergo mitosis to increase their number Spermatogonia type A and spermatogonia type B cells are formed
2	Growth phase	Differentiation of spermatogonia type B cells into the primary spermatocytes
3	Maturation phase	Meiosis I and meiosis II takes place in this phase In meiosis I, the primary spermatocytes divide into the secondary spermatocytes by reductional division In meiosis II, the secondary spermatocytes further divide into the spermatids by equatorial division

(iii) Maturation phase: The primary spermatocytes undergo meiosis during this phase, which is called the maturation phase. Two types of meiotic divisions take place in this maturation phase that include meiosis I and meiosis II. In meiosis I, each diploid primary spermatocyte (2n) divides to form two haploid secondary spermatocytes (n) and this division of diploid primary spermatocytes into haploid secondary spermatocytes is called reductional division. In meiosis II, each haploid secondary spermatocyte (n) divides to form two haploid spermatids (n) and this division of haploid secondary spermatocytes into haploid spermatids is known equatorial division. Therefore, a single diploid primary spermatocyte divides into four haploid spermatids through two types of cell division i.e. meiosis I and meiosis II (Tables 8-7 and 8-8) (Figure 8-8).

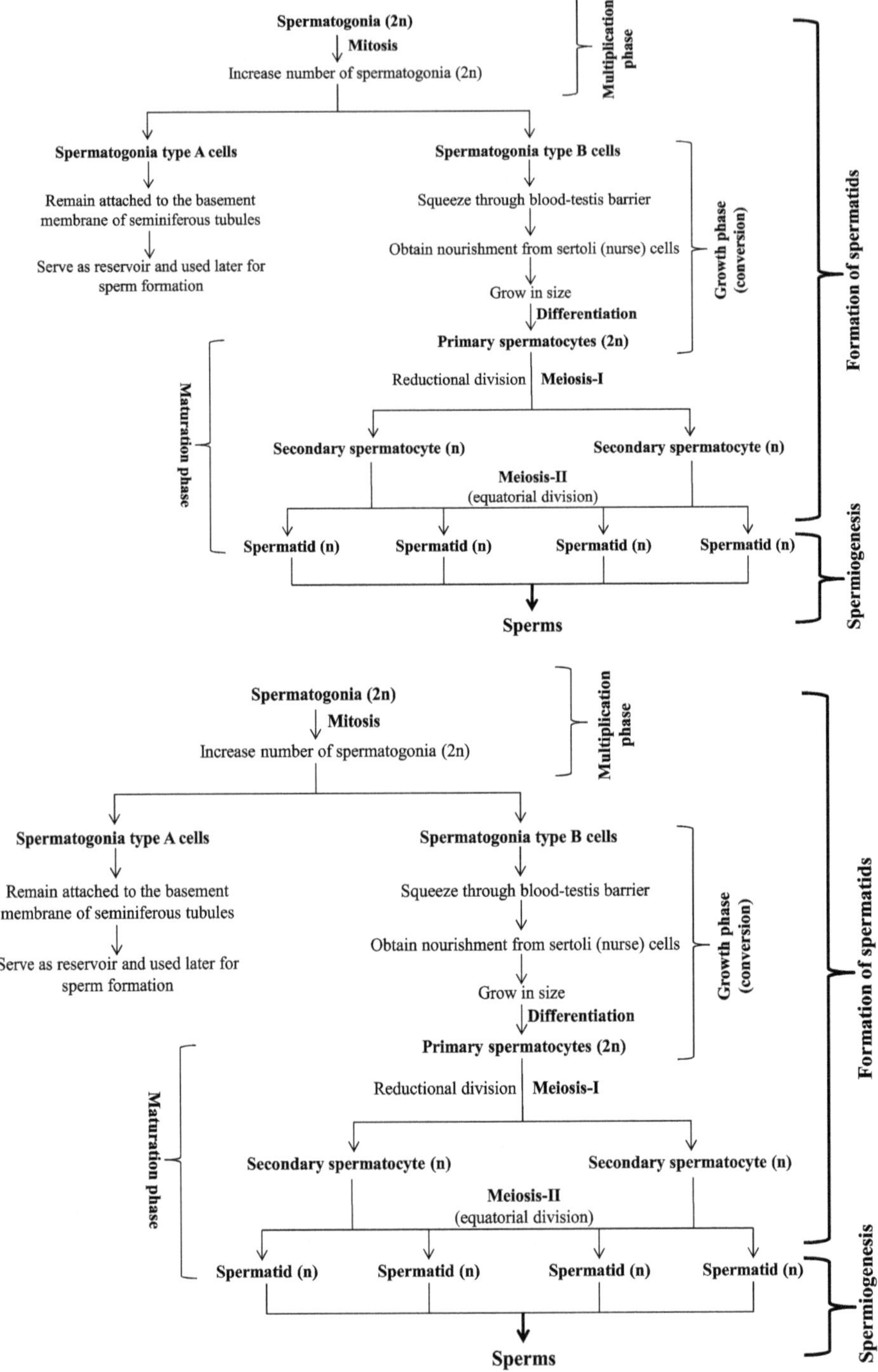

Figure 8-8 Flow chart of the process of spermatogenesis

2. **Formation of sperms from spermatids (Spermiogenesis):** Spermiogenesis is the process of the transformation of spermatids into sperms (spermatozoa) (Table 8-8). Each haploid spermatid (n) transforms into an elongated sperm cell and no cell division takes place in this process. Finally, sperms are released into the lumen of the seminiferous tubules (Figure 8-8).

Table 8-8 Haploid/diploid number of chromosomes in the process of spermatogenesis

S. No.	Stages of Spermatogenesis	Sub-stages of spermatogenesis	Haploid/diploid
1	Formation of spermatids	Multiplication phase	Diploid (2n)
		Growth phase	Diploid (2n)
		Maturation phase	Haploid (n)
2	Spermiogenesis	Transformation of spermatids into sperms	Haploid (n)

Role of hormones in spermatogenesis

Luteinizing hormone (LH) and follicle-stimulating hormone (FSH) control the process of spermatogenesis. These hormones are released from the gonadotrophs of

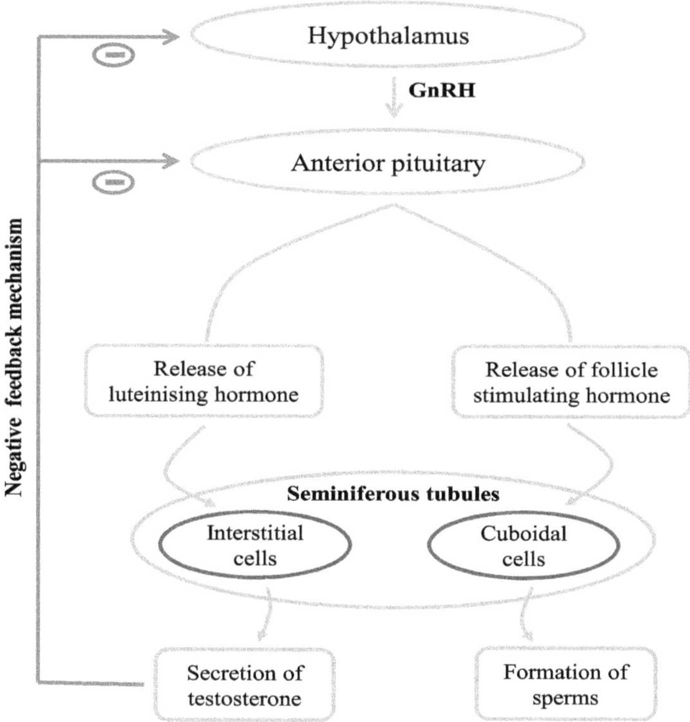

Figure 8-9 Role of hormones in the process of spermatogenesis

the anterior pituitary under the influence of gonadotropin-releasing hormone (GnRH). Collectively, LH and FSH are called gonadotropins. The luteinizing hormone stimulates the interstitial cells, present between the seminiferous tubules of the testes, to secrete the hormone testosterone, which is the principal androgenic hormone in males and stimulates the formation of sperms. Testosterone suppresses the release of gonadotropins from the anterior pituitary gonadotrophs and gonadotropin-releasing hormone from the hypothalamic neurosecretory cells via a negative feedback mechanism (Figure 8-9).

Follicle-stimulating hormone directly stimulates the cuboidal cells of the seminiferous tubules to form sperms. Follicle-stimulating hormone also stimulates the sertoli cells to release androgen binding protein (ABP) into the lumen of the seminiferous tubules. Androgen binding protein binds to the testosterone and concentrates it in the seminiferous tubules, which further stimulates the final step of spermatogenesis i.e. spermiogenesis. After achieving the required degree of spermatogenesis for male reproductive functions, the sertoli cells release a protein known as inhibin, which inhibits the secretion of follicle-stimulating hormone from the anterior pituitary (Table 8-9).

Table 8-9 Role of different hormones in spermatogenesis

Sr. No.	Hormones	Sources	Functions
1	Luteinizing hormone (LH)	Anterior pituitary	Stimulates the interstitial cells to secrete testosterone
2	Follicle-stimulating hormone (FSH)	Anterior pituitary	Directly stimulates the cuboidal cells to form sperms Stimulates the sertoli cells to release androgen binding protein, which concentrates testosterone into the seminiferous tubules
3	Testosterone	Seminiferous tubules	The principal androgenic hormone in males Stimulates the formation of sperms Controls the secretion of luteinizing hormone and gonadotropin-releasing hormone via negative feedback mechanism
4	Inhibin	Sertoli cells	Inhibits the release of follicle-stimulating hormone

Significance of spermatogenesis

1. Sperms are produced during spermatogenesis, which is required for fertilization.

2. Sperms are haploid (n) in nature and after fertilisation with haploid egg (n), a diploid zygote (2n) is formed. Thus, the chromosome number is maintained in the process of fertilization.

3. Crossing over takes place during meiosis I, so that variations are introduced in the gametes (sperm) and then in to the individual.

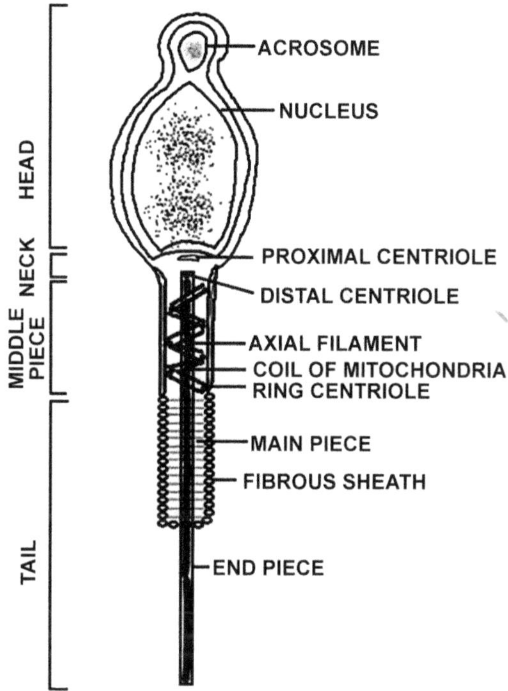

Figure 8-10 The transverse section of sperm

Structure of sperm (spermatozoa)

Sperms are the male gametes and are motile in nature. About 300 million sperms complete the process of spermatogenesis every day. The size of sperm is microscopic (about 60 μm long). The structure of sperm consists of four parts: (1) Head, (2) Neck, (3) Middle piece, and (4) Tail (Table 8-10) (Figure 8-10).

1. **Head:** Head is the upper and major part of sperm. The size of the head is about 4-5 μm long. Almost all the space in the head is occupied by a highly condensed nucleus. The acrosome is present at the tip of the head, which covers almost two-third part of the nucleus. The acrosome is a cap-like vesicle, which contains two hydrolytic enzymes i.e. protease and hyaluronidase, that helps the sperm to penetrate the egg to start the process of fertilization.

2. **Neck:** It is a small part present between the head and the middle piece. It contains two centrioles i.e. proximal centriole and distal centriole. The

proximal centriole is present towards the nucleus and it helps in the first division of zygote. The distal centriole is present towards the middle piece and it helps in forming the axial filament.

3. **Middle piece:** The middle piece consists of a coil of mitochondria, which provides energy for the locomotion of sperms to the site of fertilization. Mitochondria are coiled around the axial filament and ring centriole is present at the end of the middle piece.

4. **Tail:** It is the last and longest portion of sperm. It is very long in length and much larger than the head. The motility of the sperm is due to its tail. It consists of two parts including the main piece and the end piece. The main piece consists of an axial filament surrounded by a thin layer of cytoplasm and fibrous sheath. The end-piece is a terminal portion of the tail and it contains only naked axial filaments.

Table 8-10 Summary of characteristic features and functions of the different parts of sperm

Sr. No.	Part	Characteristic features	Functions
1	Head	Upper and major part of sperm Almost all space is occupied by a nucleus The acrosome is present at the tip of the head, which contains two hydrolytic enzymes i.e. protease and hyaluronidase	Hydrolytic enzymes help the sperm to penetrate the egg during fertilization
2	Neck	A mall part present between the head and the middle piece It contains two centrioles i.e. proximal and distal	Proximal and distal centrioles help in the division of zygote and formation of axial filament, respectively.
3	Middle piece	It consists of a coil of mitochondria Ring centriole is present	It provides energy for the locomotion of sperms
4	Tail	Last and longest portion of sperm It consists of the main piece and the end piece Axial filaments are present	The motility of the sperm is due to its tail

Functions of the Male Reproductive System

1. The testes produce the sperms and the male sex hormone i.e. testosterone.
2. The various ducts of the male reproductive system help in the transport, storage, and maturation of sperms.
3. The accessory sex glands including the seminal vesicles, the prostate gland, and the Cowper's glands secrete most of the liquid portion of semen.

4. The penis contains the penile urethra, which is a passage-way for the ejaculation of both semen and excretion of urine.

Female Reproductive System

The female reproductive system comprises of several parts including (1) Ovaries, (2) Fallopian (uterine) tubes, (3) Uterus, (4) Vagina, (5) External genitalia, and (6) Mammary glands (Table 8-13) (Figure 8-14).

1. **Ovaries:** The ovaries (female gonads) are the female primary sex organs. These are almond-sized glands and two in number. These produce secondary oocytes, which transforms into mature eggs after fertilization, and two major female sex hormones including estrogens and progesterone. The ovaries are present inside the pelvic cavity on the sides of the uterus. These are attached to the pelvic cavity by suspensory ligaments and the uterus by ovarian ligaments. The broad ligament of the uterus (a part of parietal peritoneum) connects to the ovaries by a double-layered membrane of peritoneum called the mesovarium.

   The ovaries are surrounded by two outermost coverings called the visceral peritoneum and the germinal epithelium. The germinal epithelium is present inner to the visceral peritoneum. Below the germinal epithelium, three types of tissues including the tunica albuginea, the ovarian cortex, and the ovarian medulla are present. The tunica albuginea is a whitish capsule of dense and irregular connective tissues. The ovarian cortex is present just below the tunica albuginea and it consists of ovarian or graafian follicles surrounded by irregular connective tissues, which contain fibroblast-like cells called the stromal cells. The ovarian medulla lies deep to the ovarian cortex and the border between the cortex and the medulla is indistinct. The medulla part of the ovaries consists of loosely arranged connective tissues, nerves, blood vessels and lymphatic vessels (Figure 8-11).

   The characteristaic feature of the ovaries is the presence of many follicles in the different stages of development. A follicle containing one primary oocyte and surrounded by a single layer of follicular cells is called the primordial follicle. The primordial follicle grows and converts into the primary follicle. In this stage, the primary oocyte is surrounded by several layers of cuboidal cells called the granulosa cells. The granulosa cells are also called the membranous granulosa and these surrounding cells provide nourishment to the developing oocyte. As the growth of primary follicle continues, a layer of glycoproteins is formed between the primary oocyte and the granulosa cells called the zona pellucida. Afterwards, the primary follicle develops into the secondary follicle with continuing growth. In this secondary follicle, the basement membrane of the follicle is differentiated into two membranes, which are known as theca interna and theca externa. In addition, the granulosa cells start to secrete follicular fluid, which forms a cavity in the center of the secondary follicle called the antrum or the follicular cavity. The inner most granulosa cells remain attached to the zona pellucida of oocyte and these are known as corona radiata. Thereafter, the secondary follicle becomes larger and converts into the mature graafian follicle (Table 8-11) (Figure 8-12).

Table 8-11 Stages of follicles in the ovary based on their developmental state

Sr. No.	Follicle	Characteristic feature	Shape
1	Primordial follicle	The primary oocyte is surrounded by a single layer of follicular cells	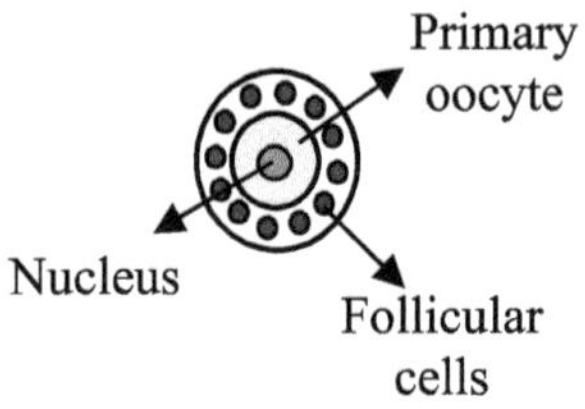
2	Primary follicle	The primary oocyte is surrounded by several layers of granulosa cells	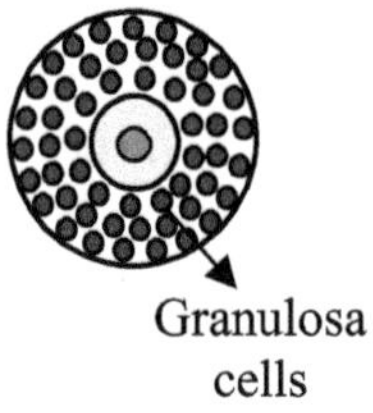
3	Secondary follicle	The basement membrane of the follicle is differentiated into theca interna and theca externa The follicular cavity is formed	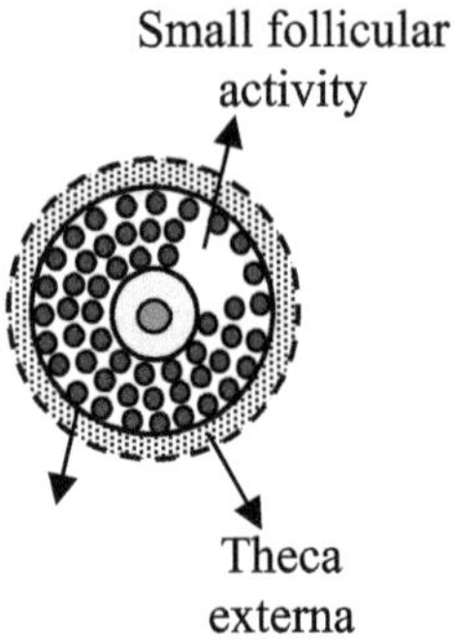
4	Mature graafian follicle	Large and fluid-filled follicle Release secondary oocytes after their rupturing by the process of ovulation	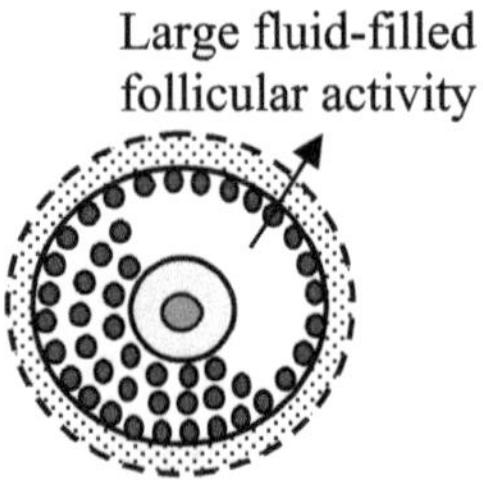

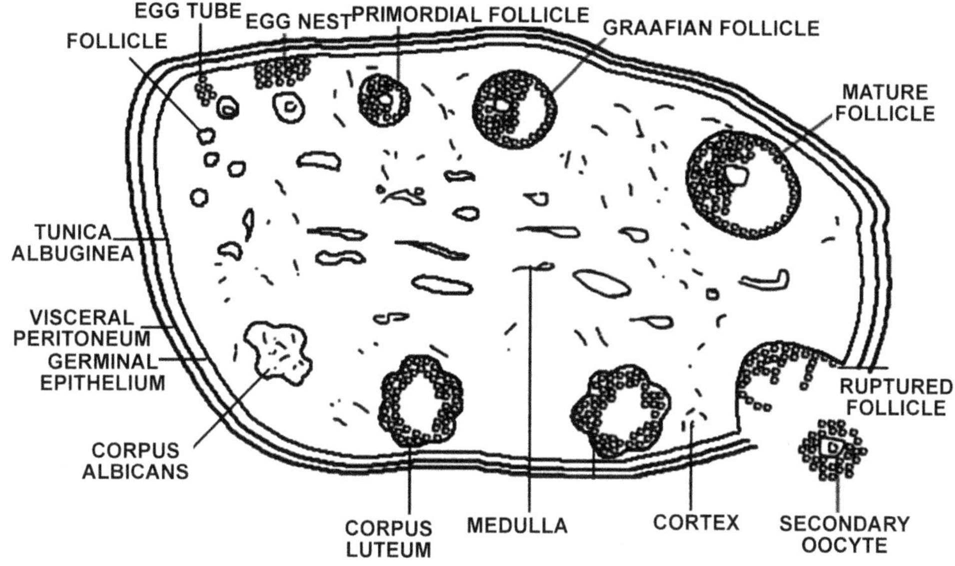

Figure 8-11 The structure of mammalian ovary

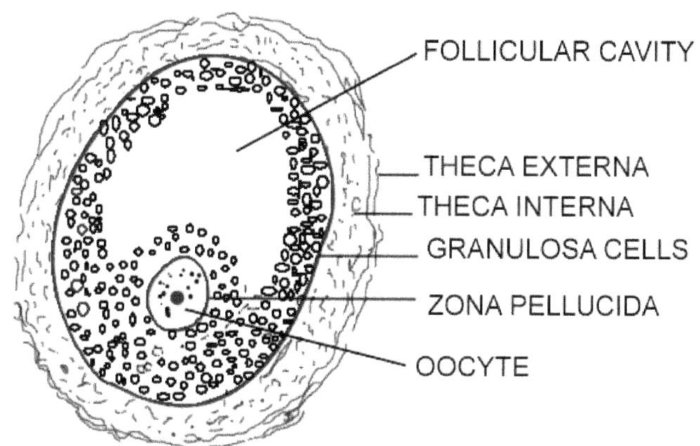

Figure 8-12 The transverse section of mature graafian follicle

There are about 4 lakh graafian follicles present in both the ovaries and most of them undergo degeneration by the process known as follicular atresia. The mature follicles are larger and fluid-filled, which release secondary oocytes after their rupturing. The process of release of secondary oocytes from the mature follicles is known as ovulation. After ovulation, the remaining follicular cells are rearranged, become enlarged and get filled with the yellow pigment called lutein and such a follicle is known as corpus luteum (yellow body). The major function of corpus luteum is to secrete female sex hormones including progesterone, estrogens, inhibin, and relaxin. Thereafter, the corpus luteum gets degenerated and changes into the corpus albicans (whitish body), which is much smaller in size than corpus luteum (Figure 8-13).

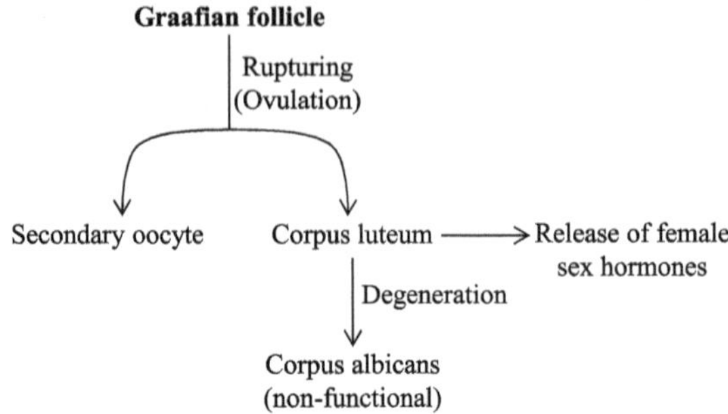

Figure 8-13 Depiction of a series of events after ovulation

2. **Uterine tubes (fallopian tubes or oviducts):** The fallopian tubes are pair of tubes that lies between the ovaries and the uterus. Each fallopian tube measures about 10 cm in length, and it consists of three parts including the infundibulum, the ampulla and the isthmus. The infundibulum is the funnel-shaped dilated portion of the tube and it's one end has finger-like projections called fimbriae. These fimbriae make a connection with the ovaries. The ampulla is the widest and longest portion (about 2/3rd part) of the fallopian tube. The fertilization between the sperm and the egg take place in this ampulla. The isthmus is the short and narrow portion of the tube, which is connected to the uterus. The major function of the fallopian tubes is that they provide a route for the sperm transport to reach an ovum. The transport of the fertilized egg to the uterus also takes place through the fallopian tubes.

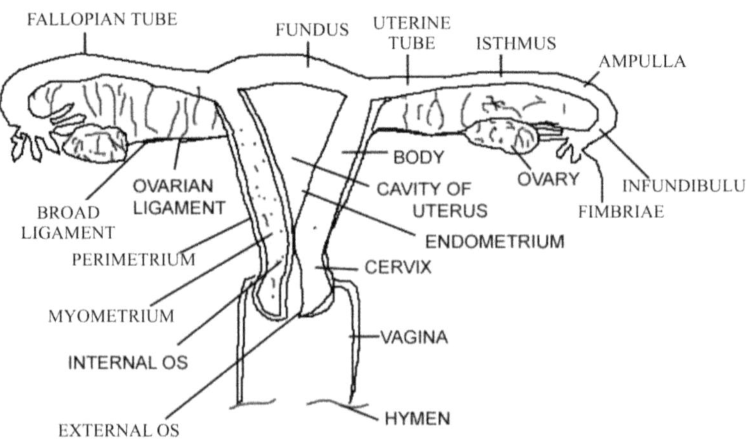

Figure 8-14 Structure of the female reproductive system

3. **Uterus (Womb):** The uterus is a hollow muscular structure, which is present between the urinary bladder and the rectum. The size of the uterus varies according to the pregnancy condition of the female. In non-pregnant females, the uterus is measuring about 7.5 cm long, 5 cm wide, and 2.5 cm thick, whereas in pregnant females, the size of the uterus becomes larger. After menopause, when the level of sex hormones is low, the uterus becomes smaller. Anatomically, the uterus consists of three parts including the fundus, the body, and the cervix. The fundus is an upper dome-shaped structure of the uterus and the body is a central and main portion of the uterus. The narrow portion of the uterus is known as the cervix, which further opens into the vagina. The opening between the middle part of the uterus and the cervix is known as internal OS and the opening between the cervix and the vagina is known as external OS (OS = mouth-like opening).

Histologically, the wall of the uterus is composed of three layers of tissues called the perimetrium, the myometrium and the endometrium. The perimetrium or serosa is the outermost covering of the uterus and it is composed of simple squamous epithelial cells. The myometrium is the middle layer of the uterus and it is made up of smooth muscle fibers. It is the thickest layer of the uterus. The uterine contractions during childbirth are due to the response of myometrium in the presence of oxytocin. The endometrium is the innermost and highly vascularised layer of the uterus. It is composed of simple columnar epithelium and endometrial stromal cells. The endometrium layer undergoes various changes during the menstrual cycle (Table 8-12).

Table 8-12 Characteristic features of the parts and layers of the uterus

Sr. No.	Name	Characteristic features or functions
Parts of uterus		
1	Fundus	Upper dome-shaped part of the uterus
2	Body	Central and main part of the uterus
3	Cervix	Narrow and last part of the uterus
Layers of uterus		
1	Perimetrium	Outermost covering of the uterus and composed of simple squamous epithelial cells
2	Myometrium	Middle and thickest layer of the uterus and composed of smooth muscle fibres Myometrium produce uterine contractions during childbirth
3	Endometrium	Innermost and highly vascularised layer of the uterus Composed of simple columnar epithelium and endometrial stromal cells

The major function of the uterus is to serve as the site of implantation of fertilized egg. During pregnancy, the development of embryo also occurs inside the uterus. The uterus also provides the passage for sperms, deposited in the vagina to reach the fallopian tubes.

4. **Vagina:** The vagina is a small tube, measuring about 10 cm long and it extends from the cervix to outside of the body. It consists of three types of layers including the mucosa, the muscularis and the adventitia. The innermost layer i.e. mucosa of the vagina consists of nonkeratinized stratified epithelial cells and it is continuous with the uterus. It contains large stores of glycogen, which produce organic acids. The acidic environment of the vagina resulting from the production of organic acids prevents the growth of microbes in it. The muscularis is the middle layer of the vagina and it is composed of smooth muscles, which helps in the accommodation of the penis in the vagina during sexual intercourse. The stretching smooth muscles of the muscularis also helps in the expulsion of child during their birth. The last and outermost layer of the vagina is called the adventitia and it consists of areolar connective tissues. The adventitia attaches the vagina to the adjacent organs including the urethra, the urinary bladder, the rectum and the anal canal.

The opening of the vagina to the exterior is called the vaginal orifice. It is partially covered by a thin fold of vascularised mucous membrane called the hymen. The hymen usually ruptures after the first sexual intercourse, but it is not a marker of the virginity. The main functions of the vagina include the receptacle for the penis during sexual intercourse and a passageway for the menstrual flow. It also acts as birth canal for the expulsion of chid during its birth.

5. **External genitalia (Vulva):** The vulva or the pudendum is the external genitalia of the female. It consists of six parts including the mons pubis, the labia majora, the labia minora, the clitoris, the vestibule and the perineum. The mons pubis is a fatty area covered by the skin and coarse pubic hairs. It lies anterior to the vaginal orifice. The labia majora are two thick folds of the skin, which are covered by the pubic hairs and they form boundary of the vulva. It contains large amounts of adipose tissues, sebaceous (oil) glands and sweat glands. Moreover, the labia majora are homologous to the scrotum in males. The labia minora are two smaller folds of the skin, which lies in between the labia majora. They do not contain the pubic hairs and adipose tissues, but it consists of few sebaceous glands and sweat glands. The labia minora are homologous to the penile urethra in males.

The clitoris is a small and cylindrical mass composed of two erectile tissues, called the corpora cavernosa. A layer of the skin is formed at the point, where the labia minora joins and this point is known as prepuce of the clitoris. It covers the body of the clitoris. The exposed portion of the clitoris is called glans clitoris and it is homologous to the glans penis in males, but it has no opening for the passage of substances. The clitoris has a role in the initiation of sexual excitement in the females. The vestibule is the next part of the external genitalia and it is present between the labia minora. It comprises of the hymen, the vaginal orifice, the external urethral orifice and the openings of several glands. The vestibule is homologous to the membranous urethra of males. The perineum is the last and diamond-shaped area of the external genitalia, which is present between the thighs and the buttocks. It contains both the parts of external genitalia and the anus.

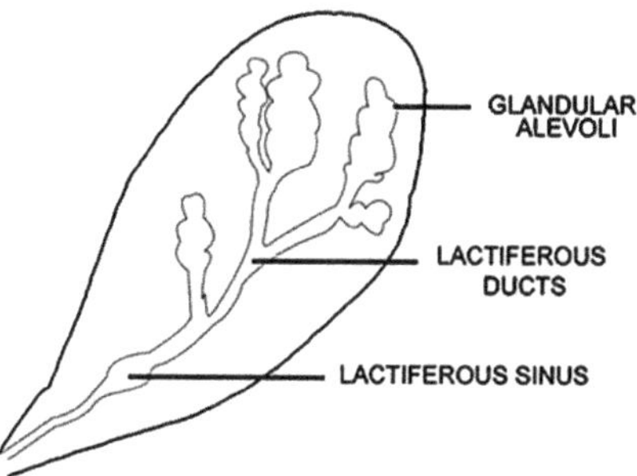

Figure 8-15 The structure of lobule

6. **Mammary glands (Breasts):** The mammary glands are modified sweat glands, which produces milk. Each mammary gland consists of the glandular tissues, the fibrous tissues, and the fatty tissues. The glandular tissue comprises of around 20 lobes or compartments, which are separated by the varying amount of adipose tissue. Each lobe is in-turn made up of several smaller compartments called lobules. These lobules are composed of grape-like clusters of the milk-secreting glands called the alveoli. The alveolis further open into the ducts, which are known as the lactiferous ducts (Figure 8-15). The milk produced in the alveoli travels to the exterior through these lactiferous ducts. The lactiferous ducts join and form an expanded structure called the lactiferous sinus, where the milk is stored before its ejection. The fibrous tissue of the mammary glands provides support to the glandular tissue. Moreover, the fatty tissue of the mammary glands is present between the lobes. The size of the mammary glands depends on the amount of fatty tissue present in them. After the onset of puberty, the mammary glands begin to develop under the influence of estrogens and progesterone. They are also present in males but the size of them is very small in males.

Externally, the breast is a hemispheric projection of variable size, which is present anterior to the pectoralis major and serratus muscles. Each breast has one pigmented projection called the nipple. The nipple has a series of closely spaced openings, through which the milk is oozing out called the lactiferous ducts. The circulated pigmented area of the skin surrounding the nipple is known as the areola, which contains the modified oil glands. The strands of connective tissue called the Cooper's ligaments or suspensory ligaments, support the breast. The major functions of the mammary glands include the synthesis, secretion and ejection of milk. These functions are collectively known as lactation. After child birth, the milk production occurs under the influence of hormone prolactin, which is released from the anterior pituitary and the ejection of milk is stimulated by the hormone oxytocin, which is secreted from the posterior pituitary in response to the sucking of an infant on the mother's nipple.

Table 8-13 Functions of the different parts of the female reproductive system

Sr. No.	Organ/Part	Functions
1	Ovaries	The ovaries produce secondary oocytes, which transforms into the mature eggs after fertilization The corpus luteum secretes different female sex hormones including progesterone, estrogens, inhibin, and relaxin
2	Fallopian tubes	Fertilisation takes place in the fallopian tubes The fallopian tubes provide a route for the transport of sperms to reach an ovum and for the transport of fertilized egg to reach the uterus
3	Uterus	It serves as the site of implantation of the fertilized egg It also serves as the site of development of embryo during pregnancy
4	Vagina	It is the receptacle for the penis during sexual intercourse It serves as a passageway for the menstrual flow It acts as birth canal for the expulsion of chid during its birth
5	External genitalia (vulva)	The clitoris of the external genitalia has a role in the initiation of sexual excitement in the females.
6	Mammary glands (Breasts)	The synthesis, secretion and ejection of the milk occur in the mammary glands. These functions are collectively known as lactation.

Composition of human milk

Human milk is the mixture of water, organic substances and inorganic substances. It contains 3-5% fat, 0.8-0.9% casein (milk protein), 6.9-7.2% carbohydrates (lactose or milk sugar), 0.2% minerals (calcium, sodium, potassium and magnesium) and vitamins. The energy content of human milk is 60-75 kcal/100 ml.

Oogenesis

Oogenesis is the process of the formation of ovum and it takes place in the ovaries. Oogenesis begins in the ovaries even before they are born. The process of oogenesis consists of three phases: (1) Multiplication phase, (2) Growth phase, and (3) Maturation phase.

1. **Multiplication phase:** The primitive germ cells migrate from the yolk sac into the ovaries during early fetal development. These primitive germ cells present in the ovaries then differentiate into the oogonia. The oogonia are the types of stem cells, which are diploid (2n) in nature. In this multiplication phase, the oogonia cells undergo mitosis very rapidly and produce many germ cells, which are also called egg mother cells. Most of these egg mother cells undergo degeneration before the birth of a female child by the process known as atresia. The remaining group of cells are present in the form of egg tube of pfluger. The egg tube of pfluger then changes into the rounded mass called the egg nest (Table 8-14) (Figure 8-16).

2. **Growth phase:** The growth phase of the oogenesis is very prolonged, and it may take 12-13 years for its completion. It continues till the onset of puberty in females. In this phase, the oogonia (cells of the egg nest) transforms into the primary oocytes, which are also diploid (2n) in nature. These primary oocytes enter the prophase of the meiosis I during fetal development, but do not complete this phase before the onset of puberty. During this arrested stage of development, each primary oocyte gets surrounded with a single layer of the follicular cells and this entire structure is called the primordial follicle (Table 8-14) (Figure 8-16).

Table 8-14 Characteristic features of the different phases of oogenesis

Sr. No.	Phase	Characteristic features
1	Multiplication phase	Oogonia cells undergo mitosis very rapidly to produce large number of egg mother cells Egg mother cells are present in the form of egg tube of pfluger The egg tube of pfluger is changes into the rounded mass called the egg nest
2	Growth phase	It is very prolonged phase of the oogenesis Oogonia cells of the egg nest transforms into the primary oocytes Primordial follicles are formed in this phase
3	Maturation phase	Primordial follicles convert into the mature graafian follicles Meiosis I and meiosis II take place in this phase In meiosis I, the primary oocyte divides into the secondary oocyte and the first polar body by reductional division In meiosis II, the secondary oocyte further splits into the ovum and the second polar body by equatorial division

3. **Maturation phase:** In maturation phase, the primordial follicles convert into the mature graafian follicles after a series of developments (described in section 'ovaries') (Figure 8-11). This phase is characterised by two types of meiotic divisions including meiosis I and meiosis II. Just before the ovulation, the diploid primary oocyte present in the mature graafian follicle completes meiosis I (reductional division) and forms two haploid (n) cells of

unequal size. The larger haploid cell is called the secondary oocyte (n) and the smaller haploid cell is called the first polar body (n). The secondary oocyte contains most of the cytoplasm and first polar body is the packet of discarded nuclear material.

The meiosis II (equatorial division) begins after the formation of haploid secondary oocyte, but it then stops in the metaphase. During ovulation, the mature graafian follicle ruptures and release its secondary oocyte into the pelvic cavity, specifically into the fallopian tube. If the sperms are not present in the fallopian tube, then fertilization does not occur and the secondary oocyte degenerates. On the other side, the meiosis II resumes if the sperms are present in the fallopian tube and one sperm get penetrate the secondary oocyte. In meiosis II, the secondary oocyte (n) again splits into the two unequal sized haploid cells. The larger cell is called the ovum (n) or the mature egg and the smaller cell is known as second polar body. Thereafter, the nuclei of both the sperm and the ovum unite to form a diploid zygote (2n) (Table 8-14) (Figure 8-16).

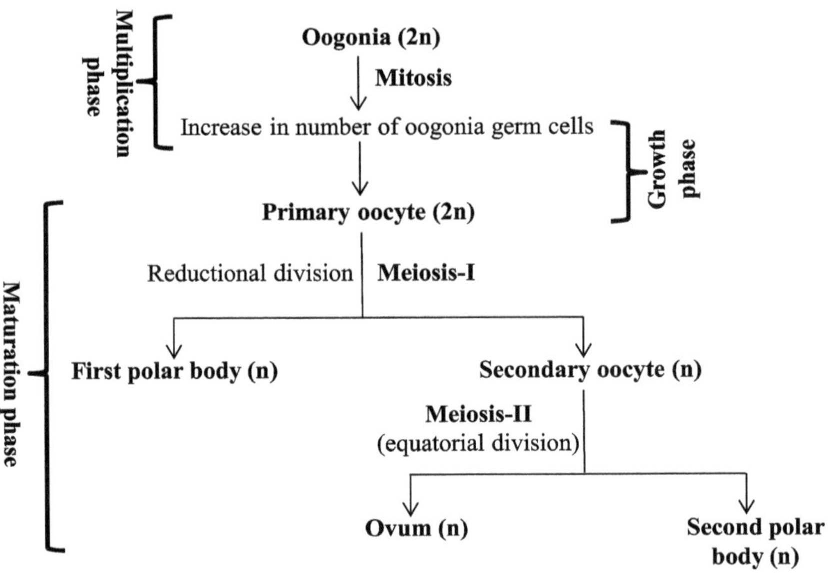

Figure 8-16 Flow chart of the process of oogenesis

Role of hormones in oogenesis

Luteinizing hormone (LH) and follicle-stimulating hormone (FSH) control the process of oogenesis. These hormones are released from the gonadotrophs of the anterior pituitary under the influence of gonadotropin-releasing hormone (GnRH), therefore, they are also called gonadotropins. Follicle-stimulating hormone initiates the growth of follicles, while luteinizing hormone stimulates the further development of the graafian follicles to trigger the process of ovulation. The luteinizing hormone also stimulates the formation of corpus luteum, which helps in the production and secretion of estrogens, progesterone, relaxin, and inhibin. Follicle-stimulating hormone also stimulates the development of primary oocytes present in the graafian follicles and the follicles to secrete estrogens.

Table 8-15 Sources and functions of the different hormones used in oogenesis

Sr. No.	Hormones	Sources	Functions
1	Luteinizing hormone (LH)	Anterior pituitary	Stimulates the development of graafian follicles Stimulates the formation of corpus luteum, which helps in the secretion of estrogens, progesterone, relaxin, and inhibin
2	Follicle-stimulating hormone (FSH)	Anterior pituitary	Initiates the growth of graafian follicles Stimulates the development of primary oocytes present in the graafian follicles Stimulates the follicles to secrete estrogens
3	Estrogens	Graafian follicles	Helps in the development and maintenance of the female reproductive structures, secondary sex characters and the breasts Controls the release of LH, FSH, and GnRH via a negative feedback mechanism
4	Progesterone	Corpus luteum	Along with estrogens, it helps in the preparation of endometrium for implantation of the ovum Prepare the mammary glands for the secretion of milk
5	Relaxin	Corpus luteum	Inhibit the contractions of the myometrium, thus helps in the relaxation of the uterus
6	Inhibin	Corpus luteum	Inhibits the release of follicle-stimulating hormone

Estrogens released from the graafian follicles have several important functions including the development and maintenance of the female reproductive structures, secondary sex characters, and the breasts. The high level of estrogens in the blood inhibits the release of GnRH from the hypothalamus along with the secretion of LH and FSH from the anterior pituitary via a negative feedback mechanism (Figure 8-17). Progesterone secreted from the corpus luteum unites with the estrogens to prepare and maintain the endometrium for implantation of a fertilized ovum and to prepare the mammary glands for the secretion of milk. A high level of progesterone also inhibits the secretion of GnRH and LH. The secretion of relaxin from the corpus luteum inhibit the contractions of the myometrium, thus helps in the relaxation of the uterus. Inhibin, released from the cells of corpus luteum, inhibits the release of FSH from the anterior pituitary (Table 8-15).

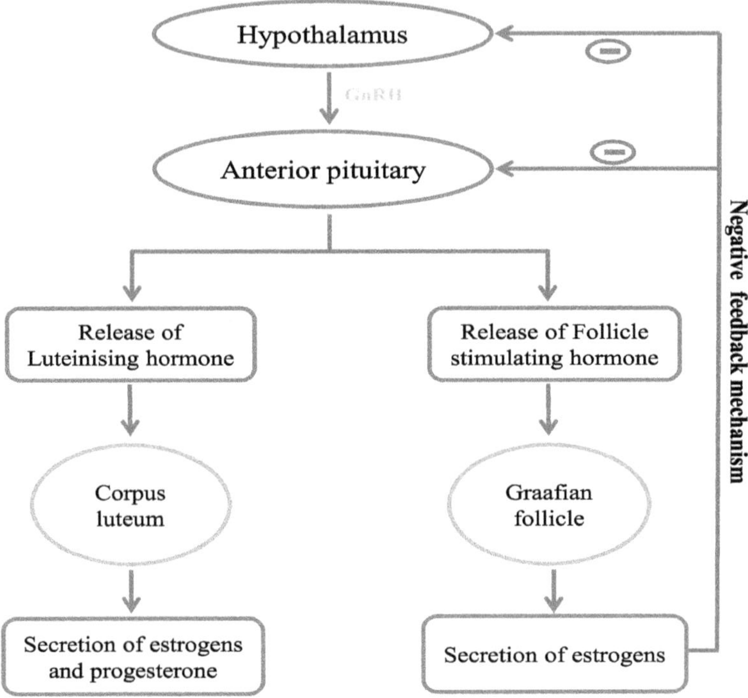

Figure 8-17 Role of hormones in the oogenesis

Significance of oogenesis

1. Ovum is produced during the process of oogenesis, which can fuse with the sperm during fertilisation.
2. Ovum is haploid (n) in nature and after fertilisation with haploid sperm (n), a diploid zygote (2n) is formed. It is essential to maintain the chromosomal number constant (2n) in an individual.
3. Crossing over takes place during meiosis I, so that the variations are introduced into an individual.
4. Formation of two unequal sized cells means that most of the cytoplasm is retained in the ovum. This large amount of cytoplasm in the ovum is essential for the early growth of an embryo.

Table 8-16 Differences between the spermatogenesis and the oogenesis

Sr. No.	Spermatogenesis	Oogenesis
1	It is the process of the formation of sperms in males	It is the process of the formation of ovum (eggs) in females
2	It occurs in the seminiferous tubules of the testes	It occurs inside the ovaries
3	In this process, one spermatogonium leads to the production of four sperms	In this process, one oogonium leads to only one ovum
4	Growth phase of the spermatogenesis is shorter	Growth phase of the oogenesis is very longer
5	The primary spermatocyte divides to form two secondary spermatocytes	The primary oocyte divides to form one secondary oocyte and one polar body
6	No polar bodies are formed	Polar bodies are formed
7	Sperm formed is much smaller than spermatogonium	Ovum formed is much larger than oogonium
8	Spermatogenesis is completed inside the testes	Oogenesis is completed inside the fallopian tubes

Structure of ovum

Ovum is a haploid female gamete and is generally spherical in shape. It receives the sperms in the fallopian tube and then develops into the zygote by the process of fertilization. The size of the ovum varies in different animals and it depends on the amount of yolk present in it. The mature ovum is free of yolk and is known as alecithal, but it contains large amount of cytoplasm. The cytoplasm of the ovum is differentiated into the outer part called egg cortex and the inner part called ooplasm or endoplasm.

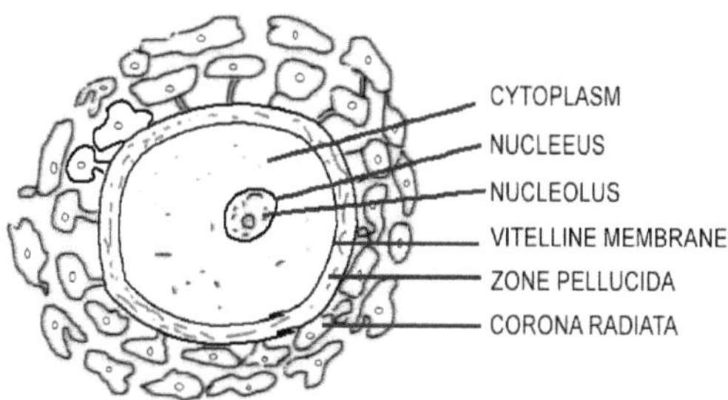

Figure 8-18 The structure of Mature Ovum

The cytoplasm is surrounded by a thinner and transparent layer, which is called a plasma membrane or vitelline membrane. Outside the vitelline membrane, there is a thick, transparent and non-cellular membrane, which is known as zona pellucida. Zona pellucida is further surrounded with by a thick layer of the follicular cells called corona radiata. There is a small space present between the zona pellucida, and the vitelline membrane called the perivitelline space. Moreover, there is a large nucleus present in the ovum. It is excentric in position and has a polarity. The side of the ovum with the nucleus and the polar body is called the animal pole, while the opposite side is called the vegetal pole (Figure 8-18).

Table 8-17 Differences between the sperm and the ovum

Sr. No.	Sperm	Ovum
1	The nucleus is very large in size	The nucleus is comparatively smaller in size
2	A small amount of cytoplasm is present	A large amount of cytoplasm is present
3	Sperm has a tail and it is motile in nature	Ovum does not have its tail and it is not-motile in nature
4	It is elongated in shape	It is spherical in shape
5	It is surrounded by only one plasma membrane	It is surrounded with three layers including the vitelline membrane, the zona pellucida and the corona radiata
6	Centrioles are present in the sperm	Centrioles are absent in the ovum

Menstrual Cycle

The reproductive period in the female extends from the puberty to the menopause. During this reproductive period, a series of cyclical changes occur in the ovaries and the uterus. These changes are meant for the fertilization and the pregnancy. These changes are collectively known as the menstrual cycle. In other words, the rhythmical cycle in females during which one or more mature ova are released is known as the menstrual cycle. The average length of the menstrual cycle is about 28 days. The most important characteristic feature of the menstrual cycle is the periodic vaginal bleeding called menstruation (lasting for about 4-5 days). The menstrual cycle is divided into three phases: (1) Post-menstrual phase, (2) Secretory phase, and (3) Menstrual phase. Since it is a cyclical process, therefore, different scientists have given the counting of these phases from different starting points. However, in this book, the counting has been done starting from the menstrual phase (bleeding). For a better understanding, the menstrual phase is discussed at the last.

1. **Post-menstrual phase:** The post-menstrual phase lasts for 14 days, from 5th day to 18th day of the menstrual cycle. This phase further divides into two phases: (i) Proliferative phase, and (ii) Ovulatory phase (Figure 8-19 and 8-20).

(i) Proliferative phase (Pre-ovulatory phase): In this phase, the secretion of follicle-stimulating hormone increases from the anterior pituitary. Under the influence of follicle-stimulating hormone, the graafian follicles grow and enlarge in size. The enlarged graafian follicles start releasing estrogens. After the menstrual phase (bleeding), only a thin layer of the endometrium is left. Estrogens act on this thin layer of the endometrium of the uterus to increase its thickness, therefore, this phase is also called proliferative phase. The epithelial cells divide and proliferate rapidly to increase the thickness of the endometrium. The uterine glands and blood vessels also proliferate in this phase. However, this growth of glands and blood vessels is more prominent in the secretory phase.

(ii) Ovulatory phase: Graafian follicle changes into a mature follicle in the ovulatory phase. Luteinizing hormone is released from the anterior pituitary around the 17th-18th days of the menstrual cycle. The luteinizing hormone acts on the enlarged mature follicles and lead to its rupturing. It causes the release of the secondary oocyte (ovum) from the mature follicle into the fallopian tubes and this process of release of ovum is known as ovulation.

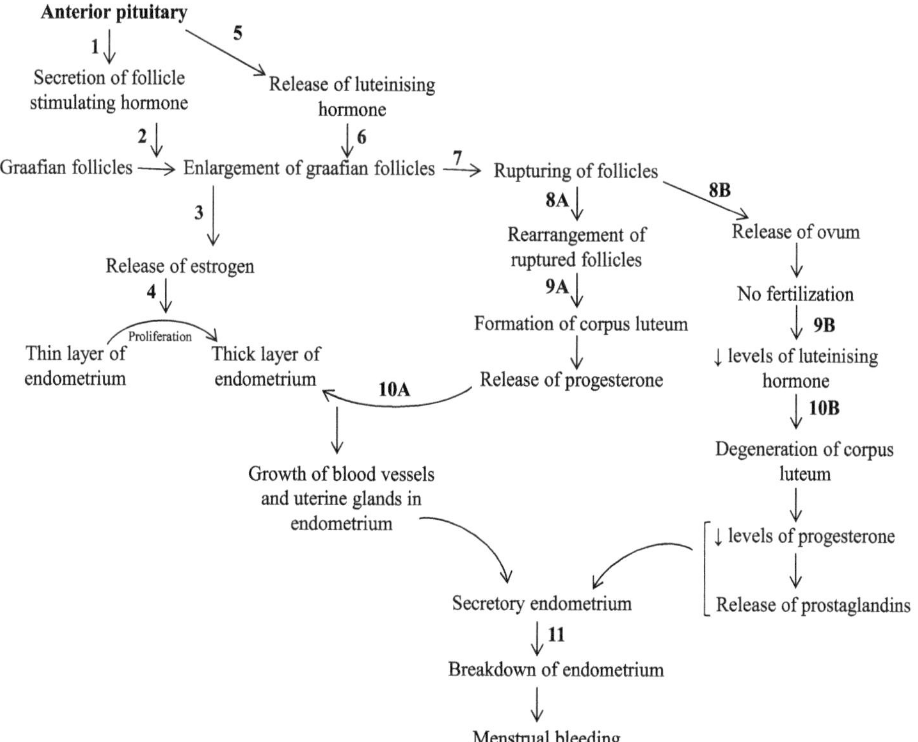

Figure 8-19 Cyclic events of the female menstrual cycle

2. **Secretory phase (Post-ovulatory phase):** The secretory phase is the time between the ovulation and the onset of menstrual phase, and it lasts for about 10 days. The levels of luteinizing hormone are high in this phase. After ovulation, the ruptured follicle rearranges into the corpus luteum and start releasing both estrogens and progesterone. However, the release of progesterone is more as compared to estrogens. Therefore, this phase is also called progestational phase. Estrogens cause a slight increase in the proliferation of the endometrium and progesterone acts on this proliferated endometrium and converts it to the secretory endometrium. The uterine glands increase in number and excess of the secretory substances accumulate in the epithelial cells. Moreover, blood supply to the endometrium increases in proportion to its development. The purpose of these changes is to produce secretory endometrium that can provide conditions for implantation of fertilised ovum (Figure 8-19 and 8-20).

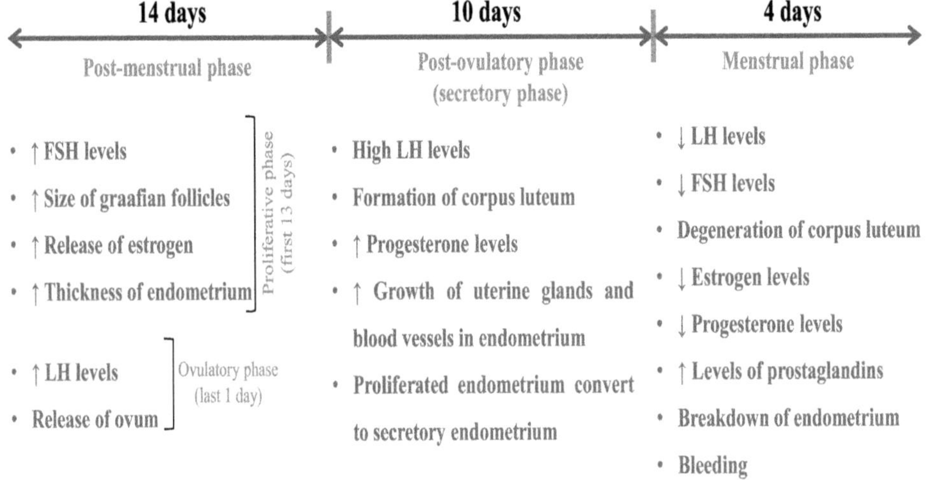

Figure 8-20 Characteristic features of the different phases of the female menstrual cycle

3. **Menstrual phase (Bleeding):** The first 4 days of the menstrual cycle comprises of the menstrual phase and it is characterised by decreased levels of both luteinizing hormone and follicle-stimulating hormone. In the absence of luteinizing hormone, the corpus luteum degenerates and the release of estrogens and progesterone decreases. The decrease in the level of progesterone stimulates the release of prostaglandins that causes the uterine arteries to constrict, thus, causes the breakdown of the endometrium. The mixture of proliferated cells, blood, tissue fluid, mucus and unfertilized ovum is discharged from the uterus through the cervix and the vagina to the exterior in the form of menstrual flow (Figure 8-19 and 8-20).

Functions of the Female Reproductive System

The ovaries produce secondary oocytes (ovum) and female sex hormones including progesterone and estrogens.

The uterine (fallopian) tubes transport the secondary oocyte to the uterus and they provide the site for the fertilization to occur.

The uterus is the site of implantation of a fertilized ovum and development of the foetus during pregnancy.

The vagina receives the penis during sexual intercourse, and it is a passageway for childbirth.

The mammary glands synthesize, secrete and eject milk for the nourishment of the new-born.

Fertilization

Fertilization is the process of the fusion of a haploid sperm and a haploid egg to form the diploid zygote (Figure 8-21). It occurs in the ampulla portion of the fallopian tube of the female reproductive tract. The process of the fertilization is divided into three parts: (1) Movement of sperms, (2) Capacitation of sperms, and (3) Arrival of the secondary oocyte.

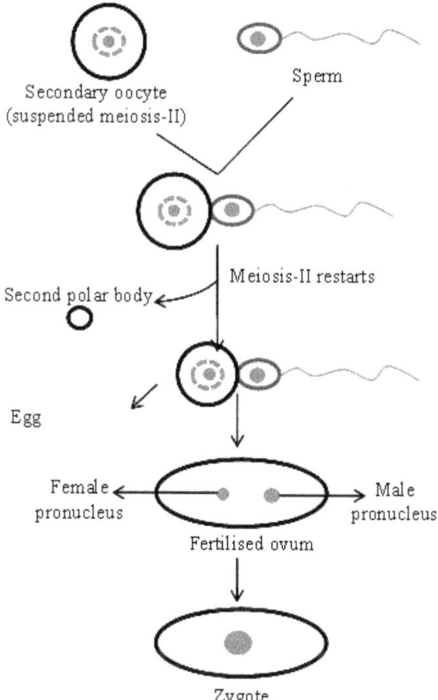

Figure 8-21 The process of fertilization

1. **Movement of sperms:** The male discharge the sperms into the vagina of the female reproductive tract during copulation. Thereafter, the sperms move upward from the vagina to the uterus and then, to the ampulla portion of the fallopian tube. This movement of sperms is due to its tail; thus, they are motile in nature. Moreover, the prostaglandins present in the semen produce contractions of the walls of the uterus and the fallopian tubes, which help in the upward movement of sperms from the vagina to the uterus. The sperms travel into the female reproductive tract at a speed of 1.5-3.0 mm/minute.

2. **Capacitation of sperms:** It is the phenomenon of the activation of sperms, which occurs inside the female reproductive tract. The various functional changes activate the sperms and make them ready for the fertilization. These changes occur when sperms encounter fluids of the female reproductive tract. The various functional changes that help in the activation of sperms include:

   (i)   The secretions of the seminal vesicles and the prostate gland provide the nutrients, which helps in the activation of sperms.

   (ii) The secretions of the prostate gland present in the semen neutralize the acidic pH of the vagina. Hence, sperms are activated at the neutral pH of the vagina.

   (iii) The coating substances are removed from the acrosome part of the sperm in the female reproductive tract. Thus, the acrosomal enzymes are released, which help the sperms to penetrate the secondary oocyte.

   (iv) The head portion of the sperm is much thicker because it is covered with the layer of cholesterol. This cholesterol layer is washed off inside the female reproductive tract, which leads to the weakening of the cell membrane that covering the head of sperm.

   (v)   The permeability of the cell membrane also increases. It leads to a more influx of Ca^{2+}- ions in the sperm through a cell membrane, which results in the more release of enzymes from the acrosome.

3. **Arrival of secondary oocyte:** The secondary oocyte is released from the mature graafian follicle during the ovulation and then enter the ampulla part of the fallopian tube. The male sperms encounter the secondary oocyte present in the fallopian tube and one sperm penetrates the secondary oocyte. The entry of sperm stimulates meiosis II in the secondary oocyte, which causes the formation of egg or the ovum.

Physical and chemical events of fertilization

1. **Acrosomal reactions:** After the capacitation of sperms, the acrosome releases various enzymes including hyaluronidase, corona penetrating enzyme and zona lysine. These enzymes help in the penetration of sperm into the secondary oocyte. Hyaluronidase digests the ground substances while corona penetrating enzyme and zona lysine (acrosin) helps in the digestion of corona radiata and the zona pellucida, respectively. These all the events are known as acrosomal reactions.

2. **Monospermy:** Monospermy is defined as the process in which only one sperm gains the entry into the secondary oocyte for the fertilization. It occurs because the fusion of the sperm's membrane with the membrane of secondary oocyte causes depolarisation, which prevents the polyspermy (entry of many sperms into the secondary oocyte) to take place. After the fusion of two membranes, cortical granules fuse with the membrane of the secondary oocyte. The fusion of cortical granules thickens the zona pellucida, which further prevents the polyspermy to take place.

3. **Karyogamy (Amphimixis):** The entry of the sperm into the secondary oocyte stimulates meiosis II, which results in a division of the latter into the larger ovum and the smaller second polar body. The nuclei's present in the head of the sperm and the ovum is termed as the male pronucleus and the female pronucleus, respectively. Thereafter, the male and female pronuclei fuse together and form the diploid nucleus called zygote. This process of formation of the zygote from the male and female pronuclei's is called karyogamy.

Significance of fertilization

1. Fertilization restores the diploid number of the chromosomes in humans.
2. Fertilization helps in the determination of sex i.e. male or female
3. It initiates the cleavage of the zygote, which is required for further embryonic development and to form new individuals.

Parturition

Parturition is the process of the expulsion of baby from the uterus through the vagina with the help of uterine contractions. During pregnancy, the uterus undergoes weak and rhythmic contractions that becomes much stronger at the end of pregnancy. These strong contractions result in the expulsion of baby are called labor contractions and this process is known as labor. The labor lasts for about 14 hours during first pregnancy, but this time duration of labor decreases during any subsequent pregnancy, typically about 8 hours. The followings are the various factors, which helps in the process of parturition are:

1. **Hormonal factors:** Progesterone inhibits the uterine contractions during pregnancy, while estrogens cause the uterine contractions. The ratio of estrogens to progesterone increases during the end of pregnancy. Thus, the relative excess of estrogens at the end of pregnancy overcomes the inhibitory effects of progesterone on the uterine contractions, which leads to the initiation of the parturition process.

   The high level of estrogens during the end of pregnancy also increases the number of oxytocin receptors on the uterine muscle fibers. Oxytocin released from the posterior pituitary act on these receptors and lead to the stimulation of uterine contractions. The control of these uterine or labor contractions during the parturition occurs via a positive feedback mechanism.

2. **Stretching of cervix:** Stretching of the cervix also plays an important role in increasing the frequency of uterine contractions. Stretch receptors present on the cervix send nerve impulses to the neurosecretory cells of the hypothalamus in the brain and cause them to release oxytocin from the posterior pituitary gland. Thereafter, the released oxytocin moves towards the uterus through blood, where it stimulates the myometrium of the uterus to contract more frequently and forcefully. As the uterine contractions intensify, the expulsion of the baby's body stretches the cervix to a great extent and the resulting nerve impulses stimulate the secretion of more oxytocin from the posterior pituitary gland. This positive feedback mechanism of the uterine contractions is broken at the birth of a child, which leads to a decrease in the cervical distensions.

8.2 Chapter at a Glance

Term	Description
Reproductive system	Collection of organs required for sexual reproduction
Male gametes	Sperms
Male sex hormone	Testosterone
Female gametes	Eggs (Ovum)
Female sex hormone	Estrogens and Progesterone
FSH	Follicle stimulating hormone
LH	Luteinizing hormone
Scrotum	Supporting pouches for the testes
Testes	Primary male sex organs
Seminiferous tubules	Sperm production factories
Interstitial/Leydig's cells	Secrete testosterone
Rete testis	Network of seminiferous tubules
Epididymis	Sperm storage house
Vas deferens	Responsible for the transportation of sperms
Ejaculatory duct	Union of vas deferens and duct of seminal vesicles
Urethra	Responsible for the transportation of semen and urine
Penis	Male copulatory organ
Semen	Fluid containing sperms
Gametogenesis	Spermatogenesis and Oogenesis

Contd...

Term	Description
Spermatogenesis	Formation of sperms
Oogenesis	Formation of ovum
Spermiogenesis	Conversion of spermatids into sperms
GnRH	Gonadotropins-releasing hormone
Gonadotropins	LH and FSH
Acrosome	Upper part of sperm that penetrates the egg to start fertilization
Ovaries	Primary female sex organs
Corpus luteum	Yellow body that secrete female sex hormones
Uterine/Fallopian tubes	Passage of sperm transport to reach ovum
Ampulla	Part of fallopian tubes where fertilization take place
Fertilization	Fusion of sperm and egg
Uterus/Womb	Site of implantation of fertilized egg and development of embryo
Vagina	Receptacle for penis, passageway for menstrual flow and act as a birth canal for expulsion of child
Clitoris	Produce sexual excitement in females
Mammary glands/Breasts	Responsible for synthesis, secretion and ejection of milk (lactation) in females
Alveoli	Milk-secreting glands
Prolactin	Milk-producing hormone/Maternity hormone
Oxytocin	Milk-ejecting hormone/Birth hormone
Human milk	Mixture of water, organic and inorganic substances
Menstrual cycle	Reproductive period of cyclical changes in the uterus and ovaries in females
Menstruation	Periodic vaginal bleeding
Capacitation of sperms	Activation of sperms
Karyogamy/Amphimixis	Formation of zygote from male and female pronuclei's
Parturition	Process of expulsion of child from the uterus

Exercises

Multiple Choice Questions

1. The major hormone released by the corpus luteum is?
   (a) Estrogens   (b) Progesterone
   (c) Relaxin   (d) Inhibin

2. Testosterone is produced by which type of cells?
   (a) Cuboidal cells   (b) Sertoli cells
   (c) Interstitial cells   (d) None of the above

3. The function of the inhibin is?
   (a) To stimulate the formation of sperms
   (b) To control the release of LH
   (c) To inhibit the release of FSH
   (d) All of the above

4. The bleeding phase of the menstrual cycle is characterised by?
   (a) Decrease in LH levels   (b) Decrease in progesterone levels
   (c) Degeneration of corpus luteum   (d)   All of the above

5. The major function of the epididymis is?
   (a) To store the sperms   (b) To carry the sperms
   (c) To eject the sperms into the urethra (d)   None of the above

6. The main function of the scrotum is?
   (a) To provide a support to the testes
   (b) Regulation of temperature of the testes
   (c) Both a and b
   (d) None of the above

7. What is the function of fructose in the composition of seminal vesicle's fluid?
   (a) Helps in the coagulation of semen
   (b) Source of energy for the movement of sperms
   (c) Helps in the motility of sperms
   (d) To neutralise neutralize the acidic pH

8. Presence The presence of acrosome is the characteristic feature of which part of the sperm?
   (a) Head   (b) Neck
   (c) Middle piece   (d) Tail

9. What is the characteristic feature of secondary follicles?
   (a) Presence of zona pellucida
   (b) Presence of follicular cavity or antrum
   (c) Surrounded by a single layer of cells
   (d) None of the above

10. The opening between the cervix and the vagina is called?
    - (a) Internal OS
    - (b) External OS
    - (c) External urethral orifice
    - (d) None of the above

Short Answer Questions

1. What are the differences between primary sex organs and secondary sex organs?
2. What are the different parts of the male urethra?
3. What is the composition of the secretion of seminal vesicles?
4. Write one function of each component of the secretions of the prostate gland and Cowper's gland.
5. What is semen? Describe its composition.
6. Write about the role of luteinizing hormone (LH) and follicle stimulation hormone (FSH) in spermatogenesis.
7. Give one characteristic feature of each part of the structure of sperm.
8. What is graafian follicle?
9. Write the functions of the uterus.
10. What are labia majora and labia minora? Give its characteristic features.
11. What is the composition of human milk?
12. What is corpus luteum? Write its function.
13. What do you mean by the capacitation of sperms?
14. What is fertilization? What types of events occur in this process?
15. What is parturition?

Long Answer Questions

1. Explain the structure of testes with special emphasis on seminiferous tubules.
2. What is spermatogenesis? Explain the different steps involved in it.
3. Explain the structure of sperm with a suitable diagram.
4. Explain the structure of the uterus with a suitable diagram.
5. Write the functions of different parts of the female reproductive system.
6. Explain the role and regulation of different hormones in oogenesis.
7. Write the differences between spermatogenesis and oogenesis.
8. Write the differences between the sperm and ovum.
9. What is the menstrual cycle? Give a detailed description of its pre-menstrual phase.
10. Explain the process of fertilization.

Bibliography

Costanzo LS. Physiology. 4th Edition. Lippincott Williams & Wilkins.

Guyton AC, Hall JE. Textbook of Medical Physiology. 11th Edition. Elsevier Saunders. 2006.

Jaggi AS, Bali A, Singh N. Pathophysiology. 1st Edition. Vallabh Prakashan. 2019.

Jain AK. Human Anatomy and Physiology for Pharmacy. 3rd Edition. Arya publications. 2017.

Lodish H, Berk A, Kaiser CA. Molecular Cell Biology. 6th Edition. W. H. Freeman & Co Ltd. 2007.

Tortora GJ, Derrickson B. Principles of Anatomy and Physiology. 15th Edition. John Wiley and Sons, Inc. 2017.

Waugh A, Grant A. Ross and Wilson Anatomy and Physiology in Health and Illness. 12th Edition. Churchill Livingstone. 2014.

Answer Key MCQs

1. (b)	2. (c)	3. (c)	4. (d)	5. (a)
6. (c)	7. (b)	8. (a)	9. (b)	10. (b)

Introduction to Genetics

After completing this lesson, the Reader should be able to understand:

- *Chromosomes (Introduction)*
- *Gene*
- *Deoxyribonucleic acid (DNA)*
- *Protein synthesis*
- *Genetic pattern of Inheritance*

9.1 Introduction

Chromosomes are defined as the tightly coiled DNA molecules that are packaged into thread-like structures and contain genetic information. In humans, chromosomes are present in the nucleus of each cell. The word 'chromosome' comes from two Greek words i.e. chroma (colour) and soma (body). In other words, they are so called chromosomes because they are cell bodies, which can get strongly stained with different types of basic dyes and produce colours. This colour producing feature of the chromosomes is a characteristic feature of them.

Chromosomes are made up of two major components including DNA (about 40%) and histone proteins (about 50%). The DNA molecules (negatively charged)

Table 9-1 Different components of the chromosomes and their percentage

Sr. No.	Components	Percentage
1	DNA	40 %
2	Histone proteins	50 %
3	Non-histone proteins	8.5 %
4	RNA	1.5 %
5	Lipids	Trace amount
6	Ions (Ca^{2+}, Mg^{2+})	Trace amount

are coiled around the histone proteins (positively charged basic proteins) that support the structure of chromosomes. In addition, the other components of chromosomes include non-histone proteins (acidic proteins, constitute about 8.5%), RNA (about 1.5%), lipids (trace amounts) and trace quantity of ions (Ca^{2+}, Mg^{2+}) (Table 9-1).

Basic features and shapes of chromosomes

The basic structural feature of the chromosomes is the presence of a constriction point called centromere that divides the latter into two arms including a short arm (also called p arm) and a long arm (also called q arm). The position of the centromere gives a characteristic shape to each chromosome. Depending on the position of the centromere, different shapes of chromosomes can be categorised into the following types (Figure 9-1) (Table 9-2).

Metacentric chromosomes: In metacentric chromosomes, the centromere is present in the centre of each chromosome. Therefore, these chromosomes have two equal sized arms i.e. the size of both p and q arms are same (isobrachial chromosomes).

Submetacentric chromosomes: In this type, the centromere is located near the centre of each chromosome. As a result, these chromosomes have two unequal sized arms i.e. the size of p arm and q arm is different (heterobrachial chromosomes).

Acrocentric chromosomes: In acrocentric chromosomes, the centromere is present near the ends of each chromosome i.e. at subterminal positions. These chromosomes have also two unequal sized arms.

Telocentric chromosomes: In this type, the centromere is located at the terminal position of each chromosome. Thus, these types of chromosomes have only one arm.

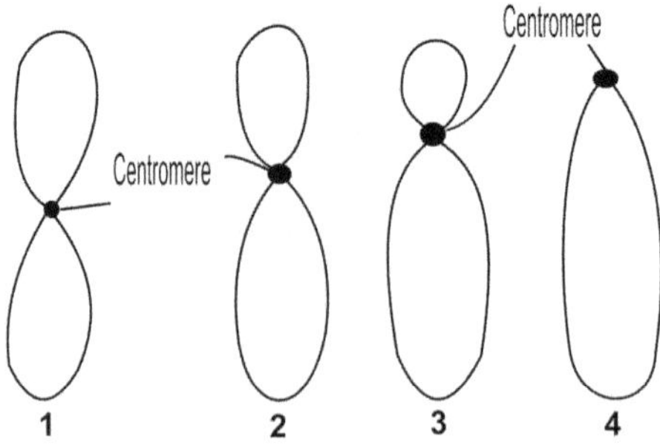

Figure 9-1 Different types of chromosomes depending on the position of the centromere. (1) Metacentric, (2) Submetacentric, (3) Acrocentric, (4) Telocentric.

Table 9-2 Different types of chromosomes depending on the position of the centromere

Sr. No.	Types of chromosomes	Position of centromere
1	Metacentric chromosomes	Centre of each chromosome
2	Submetacentric chromosomes	Near the centre of each chromosome
3	Acrocentric chromosomes	Near the ends of each chromosome i.e. at subterminal position
4	Telocentric chromosomes	Terminal position of each chromosome

Depending on the number of centromeres present on each chromosome, they are divided into four types (Table 9-3).

Holocentric: The centromere is absent in this type of chromosomes. Holocentric chromosomes can be found in the plants.

Monocentric: As the name implies, one centromere is present on each monocentric chromosome. This is the most common type of chromosomes present in humans.

Dicentric: In this type, two centromeres are present on each chromosome. Dicentric chromosomes are not present in humans.

Polycentric: In polycentric chromosomes, multiple centromeres are located at the different positions on each chromosome.

Table 9-3 Different types of chromosomes depending on the number of centromeres

Sr. No.	Types of chromosomes	Number of centromeres
1	Holocentric chromosomes	No centromere is present
2	Monocentric chromosomes	One
3	Dicentric chromosomes	Two
4	Polycentric chromosomes	Multiple

Types of Chromosomes

In humans, 46 chromosomes are present in the form of pairs i.e. 23 pairs of chromosomes. Out of these, the first 22 pairs of chromosomes are called autosomes. Each pair of chromosomes consists of two homologous chromosomes (chromosomes having similar size, shape and arrangement of genes) that include one chromosome inherited from the mother and one chromosome inherited from the father.

In addition to autosomes, 23rd or last pair of the chromosomes is called sex chromosomes (also called allosomes). Allosomes determine the sex of an individual. Sex chromosomes are labelled with letters such as XX or XY. In females, XX pair of sex chromosomes are present. Out of which, one X chromosome comes from the mother and one X chromosome comes from the father. In males, XY pair of chromosomes are present in which X chromosomes come from the mother and Y chromosome comes from the father (Figure 9-2).

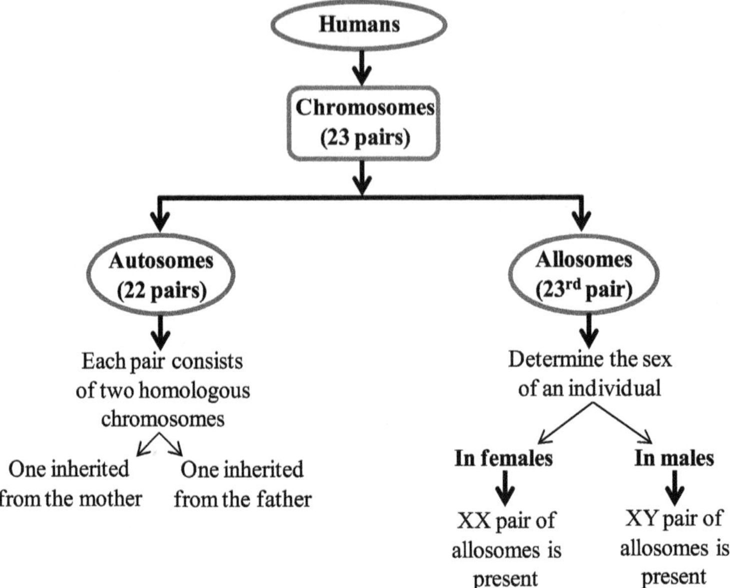

Figure 9-2 Chart of number and different types of Chromosomes present in Humans

Chromatin and Chromosomes

As already discussed, the DNA in the chromosomes does not exist by itself but are coiled around specialized proteins called histone proteins. These proteins help in the organisation of the DNA in the chromosomes and support the structure of the

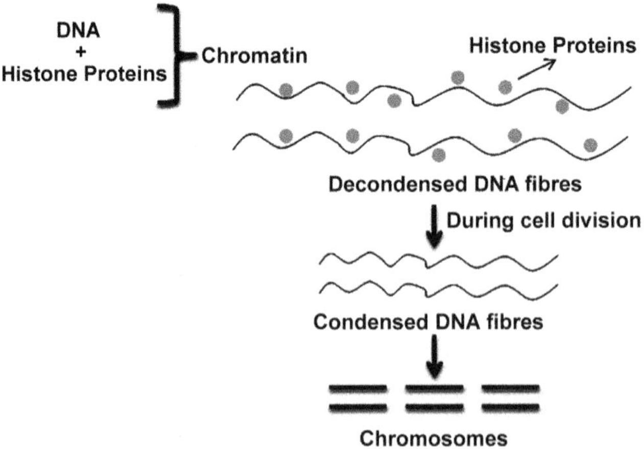

Figure 9-3 Diagram of the representation of chromatin and chromosomes

latter. The resultant complex of the DNA and histone proteins is known as chromatin. In other words, chromatin exists in very long and thin strings of fibres (decondensed form) of the DNA coiled around histone proteins. In most of the life of a cell and during the non-dividing state of a cell (resting state or interphase), chromatin is present in the decondensed form. Due to this decondensed form, the DNA molecules are not visible in the nucleus of a cell even under the microscope.

However, during cell division, the DNA molecules in the chromatin fibres get condensed and break into small linear units. These linear pieces of chromatin fibres are known as chromosomes. In this condensed form of chromosomes, the DNA molecules are visible under the microscope. Chromosomes are best visualised in the metaphase followed by the prophase of cell division (Table 9-4) (Figure 9-3).

Table 9-4 Differences between chromatin and chromosomes

Sr. No.	Chromatin	Chromosomes
1	It is a complex of the DNA and histone proteins	Chromosomes are tightly coiled DNA molecules packaged into thread-like structures
2	Chromatin exists in very long and thin strings of coiled fibres i.e. in decondensed form	Chromosomes are condensed forms of chromatin
3	In the non-dividing state of the cell (resting state or interphase), chromosomes exist in the form of chromatin	In the dividing state of the cell, the DNA molecules in chromatin get condensed and form chromosomes
4	The DNA molecules in chromatin structure are not visible even under the microscope	Chromosomes are visualised under the microscope especially in the metaphase and prophase of the cell division

Functions of Chromosomes

Chromosomes store, replicate (copying of the DNA) and transcribe (Convert the DNA into mRNA) the hereditary material. Thus, they function as hereditary vehicles.

The centromeres (constriction points on the chromosomes) help in the separation of the chromosome during cell division.

Chromosomes are essential for the process of cell division, replication, division, and creation of daughter cells.

Gene

The term 'gene' was coined by Wilhelm Johanssen in 1909. It is defined as the unit of inheritance that is made up of the DNA sections. Genes encoding for the synthesis of either RNA or proteins, which have specific inheritable functions.

They are located at the specific positions (called locus) on the structure of the DNA molecules. Genes can also replicate themselves. In humans, the size of the genes varies from few DNA base pairs to a million base pairs. The term 'genome' refers to the total genetic information contained in a single cell. The human genome is very complex in which approximately 20,000-25,000 genes express only a fraction of the genome.

There are various historical hypotheses related to the evolution of genes or gene concept. 'One gene-one enzyme' hypothesis was given by Beadle and Tatum, which explained that one gene specifies or codes for one enzyme. Another hypothesis called 'one gene-one polypeptide' was given by Yanofsky and this theory explained that one enzyme may consist of several polypeptides, therefore, one gene code for a single polypeptide rather than a whole enzyme.

Most of the genes code for the proteins means they contain the information regarding the sequence of amino acid residues in a protein as every protein has its specific amino acid sequence and function. However, some of the genes do not code for proteins but codes for the RNA. Nowadays, a term 'cistron' is used in the place of 'gene', which is defined as a segment of the DNA that may encode for one polypeptide, one ribosomal RNA (rRNA) or one transfer RNA (tRNA).

Types of Genes

The genes are categorised into various types that include (Table 9-5):

Constitutive genes: Constitutive genes are expressed continuously in almost all types of cells. The products of these genes i.e. proteins are required all the time for the growth of a cell. Therefore, constitutive genes are also known as housekeeping genes.

Non-constitutive genes: Non-constitutive genes are not expressed continuously in a cell. They are switched on or off depending upon the requirement. These are of two types including the inducible genes and the repressible genes. Inducible genes are those genes whose expression is increased or those are switched on in the presence of a chemical called an inducer. Similarly, repressible genes are those genes whose expression is decreased (switched off) in the presence of a chemical called repressor. Repressor genes are expressed constantly in a cell until a repressor comes and stops the expression of these genes (Figure 9-4).

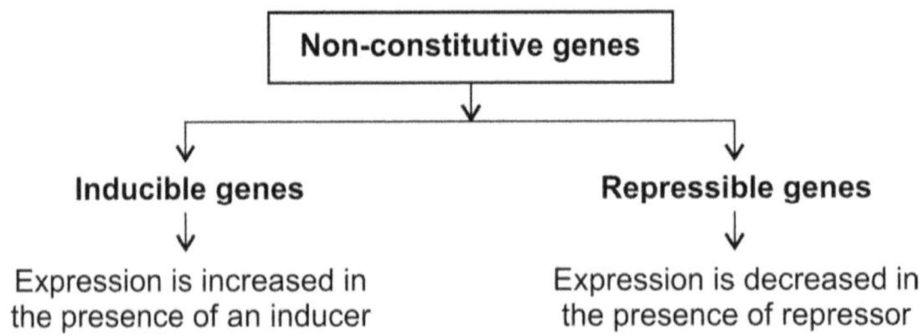

Figure 9-4 Types of non-constitutive genes

Multiple genes: Multiple genes are defined as multiple copies of a single gene that are present in a cell. Example of multiple genes includes histone genes.

Single copy genes: Single copy genes are present in a cell in the form of a single copy, as their name implies.

Functional genes: Functional genes are the genes that perform specific functions in a cell.

Pseudo genes: Pseudo genes are like the functional genes, but they do not produce any specific functions in a cell.

Transposons: Transposons are the genes that can move from one part of the DNA to another part of the DNA, therefore, these are also called jumping genes.

Split genes: Split genes contain two types of regions including the coding region and the non-coding region. The coding region is the essential part of a split gene, which is also known as exons. This region codes for the formation of proteins. The non-coding region does not code for any proteins and it is also known as introns. Introns are present in between the exons (Figure 9-5).

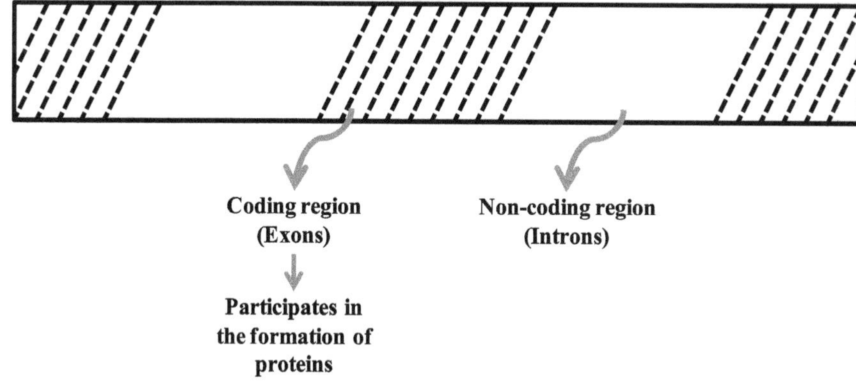

Figure 9-5 Diagram showing the pattern of spilt genes

Processed genes: Processed genes are split genes, which are formed after their processing. These genes contain only exons (coding region) as all the introns (non-coding region) have been removed from the split genes during their processing.

Structural genes: Structural genes are the genes that have information related to the synthesis of proteins.

Regulatory genes: Regulatory genes are the genes that do not code for either the RNA or the proteins, but they control the functioning of other structural genes.

Table 9-5 Various types of genes and their characteristic features

Sr. No.	Types of genes	Characteristic features
1	Constitutive genes	They express continuously in cells Also called housekeeping genes
2	Non-constitutive genes	They do not express continuously in cells They are of two types including inducible genes and repressible genes
3	Multiple genes	They are present in multiple copies in a cell An example includes histone proteins
4	Single copy genes	They are present in a single copy in a cell
5	Functional genes	Functional genes perform specific functions in a cell
6	Pseudo genes	Pseudo genes are like functional genes, but they do not perform any specific function in a cell
7	Transposons	They can move from one part of the DNA to another part of the DNA Also called jumping genes
8	Split genes	They contain two types of regions including the coding region and the non-coding region The coding region and the non-coding region is also called as exons and introns, respectively.
9	Processed genes	They are the processed form of split genes They contain only the coding region (exons)
10	Structural genes	They have the information related to the synthesis of proteins
11	Regulatory genes	Regulatory genes control the functioning of other structural genes

Functions of Genes

The major function of the genes is to store genetic information.

Genes are the unit of inheritance means genetic traits or information from the parents to the child is passed through genes.

The genes direct the formation of proteins from the DNA to perform a specific function in the body.

Genes determine the outer appearance of an individual such as the colour of eyes.

Genes control the structure and metabolism of the body.

Deoxyribonucleic Acid (DNA)

DNA is a deoxyribonucleic acid and it contains the hereditary information of almost every type of organisms. In humans, most of the DNA is present in the nucleus of a cell, thus, called nuclear DNA. It is made up of four types of chemical (nitrogenous) bases, which includes adenine (A), guanine (G), cytosine (C) and thymine (T). Adenine (A) and guanine (G) are collectively known as purines and cytosine (C) and thymine (T) are collectively known as pyrimidines. The genetic information in the DNA is stored in the form of codes that are made up of these chemical bases. The human DNA is comprised of approximately 3 billion bases and out of them, more than 99% is the same in all the people. The remaining less than 1% of the total bases make people different from each other.

Table 9-6 Differences between chromatin and chromosomes

Sr. No.	Nitrogenous bases	Paired with
1	Adenine (A)	Thymine (T)
2	Guanine (G)	Cytosine (C)
3	Cytosine (C)	Guanine (G)
4	Thymine (T)	Adenine (A)

The chemical bases join with each other to form base pairs. For example, adenine (A) pairs up with thymine (T) and cytosine (C) pairs up with guanine (G) (Table 9-6). These base pairs in the DNA structure are also attached with a sugar molecule and a phosphate group. The complex of base pairs with sugar moieties and phosphate groups is known as a nucleotide. The nucleotides are arranged in two long spiral strands that help in the formation of a double helix structure of the DNA, which is discussed in the following section:

Structure of the DNA

The double helix structure of the DNA was discovered by James Watson and Francis Crick along with their co-workers in 1953. Therefore, the model of the DNA is also known as 'Watson and Crick' model. As discussed earlier, the DNA structure consists of two long identical strands of nucleotides. Each of the nucleotide strands has two ends i.e. 5' end and 3' end. These two strands run in the opposite direction from one other i.e. one strand run towards 5' end to 3' end and the second strand run towards 3' end to 5' end. This anti-parallel configuration of the nucleotide strands makes the DNA structure like a twisted ladder in which both the strands are intertwining around an axis and form a right-handed helix.

The nucleotides present in the one strand are joined together by phosphate-sugar linking in which the phosphate group of one nucleotide is linked with the sugar molecule of the next nucleotide through covalent bonds. Similarly, the two nucleotide strands are joined together by hydrogen bonds between the bases of two adjacent strands (Figure 9-6). This hydrogen bonding between the chemical bases is very specific like adenine (A) bonds only with thymine (T) and cytosine (C) bonds only with guanine (G). The resultant A-T and C-G base pairs are known as complementary base pairs.

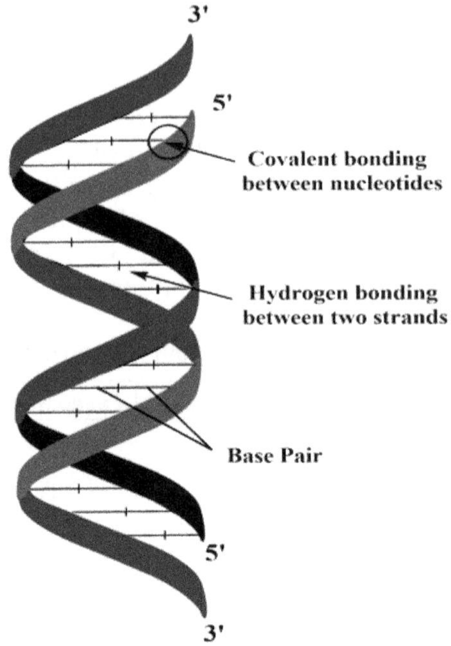

Figure 9-6 Double-helix structure of the DNA

Packaging of DNA

In humans, the DNA is present in the nucleus of a cell in the form of two long strands of nucleotides. To make the DNA fit into the nucleus, it is packaged by specialized proteins called histone proteins. The resultant structure of the DNA and histone proteins is known as chromatin (Figure 9-3). Histone proteins are a family of positively charged basic proteins, which are of five types including H_1, H_{2A}, H_{2B}, H_3 and H_4. On the other hand, the DNA is negatively charged due to the presence of phosphate (PO_4^{2-}) group in its phosphate-sugar backbone. Therefore, the positively charged histone proteins bind tightly with the negatively charged DNA molecules.

The nucleosome is the basic structural and functional unit of chromatin. Each nucleosome consists of 8 histone proteins and 146 DNA base pairs. These 8 histone proteins (two each of H_{2A}, H_{2B}, H_3, and H_4) combine to form a protein octamer. Over this histone octamer, 1.7 turns of the DNA (consists of 146 base pairs) are wrapped to form one nucleosome (Figure 9-7). In one chromosome, hundreds to thousands of nucleosomes are present. Moreover, about 20 base pairs of linker DNA (that links the two nucleosomes) are wrapped around H_1 histone proteins. Thus, a single nucleosome along with the 20 base pairs of linker DNA and H_1

histone proteins form a 166 base pairs long structure called chromatosome (Figure 9-8).

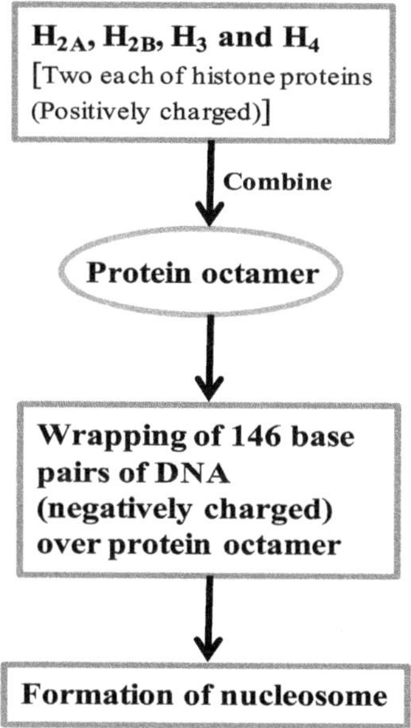

Figure 9-7 Flow chart of the formation of nucleosome

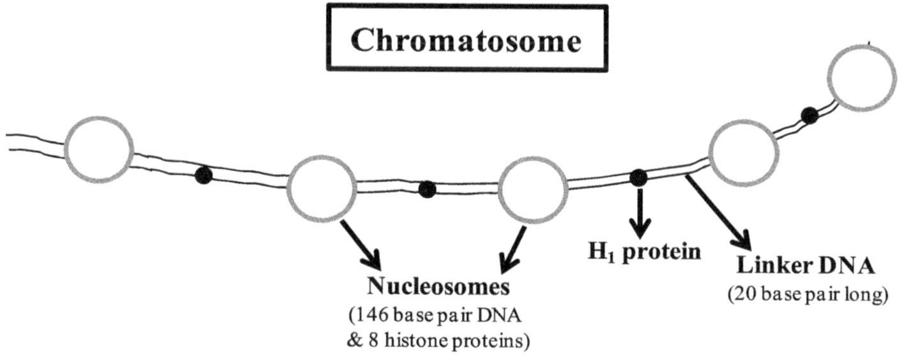

Figure 9-8 Structure of chromatosome

In the nucleus, chromatin may exist in two forms i.e. euchromatin and heterochromatin. Euchromatin is a loosely packed form of the DNA that appears lighter on staining. Euchromatin regions can undergo transcription due to their loose packaging. On the other hand, heterochromatin is a tightly packed form of the DNA that appears darker on staining. The regions of heterochromatin do not undergo transcription due to their tight packaging (Table 9-7).

Table 9-7 Differences between chromatin and chromosomes

Sr. No.	Euchromatin	Heterochromatin
1	Euchromatin represents the loose packed form of the DNA	Heterochromatin represents the tightly packed form of the DNA
2	These regions appear light on staining	These regions appear dark on staining
3	These regions of the DNA undergo transcription	These regions of the DNA do not undergo transcription

DNA Replication

DNA replication is one of the most important characteristic features of the DNA. It is semi-conservative in nature because the DNA can replicate its own or make identical copies of himself. Replication of the DNA is necessary to transfer the genetic information from one cell to other cells during cell division. One of the two strands of the DNA double helix model serve as a template to duplicate their genetic information on the new strand in the form of a complementary sequence of bases. The resultant copies of the DNA duplex consist of one strand derived from the parent DNA (template strand) and the other strand is a newly synthesized strand. The process of the DNA replication requires many enzymes such as DNA polymerase etc. The procedure of the DNA replication is out of the scope of this book.

Functions of the DNA

The DNA contains genetic information that is transferred from one cell to another by DNA replication.

The DNA store genetic information of an individual for a lifetime.

The important function of the DNA is to encode the amino acid sequences to direct the synthesis of proteins.

The DNA gives instructions to a cell for the synthesis of proteins and RNA molecules.

Protein Synthesis

Protein synthesis is the process of formation of new proteins that perform specific functions in the body. In this process, some part of the DNA i.e. gene is used as a template for the synthesis of a specific protein. The process of protein synthesis is divided into two parts including transcription and translation. Transcription is defined as the process in which the genetic information encoded in a gene is transcribed (copied) to produce specific molecules of the RNAs. On the other hand, translation is defined as the process in which the genetic information is translated from the RNAs into a corresponding set of amino acids that leads to the formation of new proteins.

Transcription

Transcription is the process of copying the genetic information from a sequence of base triplets in the DNA (double stranded) into a complementary sequence of codons (a group of three nucleotides) to form a single stranded molecule of the RNA. Three types of RNAs are formed from a single piece of the DNA including messenger RNA (mRNA), transfer RNA (tRNA) and ribosomal RNA (rRNA). The process of transcription occurs in the nucleus of a cell with the help of an enzyme called RNA polymerase. Three types of RNA polymerases namely RNA polymerase I, II and III are present in eukaryotes, which transcribes specific classes of genes. The transcription process is completed in three stages including initiation, elongation and termination. Before the transcription to start, the double stranded DNA molecule unwinds itself under certain conditions into two strands (single stranded) and these are termed as template strand and coding strand, respectively. A molecule of RNA polymerase uses template strand of the DNA to synthesise a complimentary copy of single stranded RNA, which is always in 5' to 3' direction. The newly formed RNA strand is almost identical to the coding strand of the DNA. The one major difference between the template DNA strand and newly formed RNA strand is that all the thymine (T) nucleotides are replaced with uracil (U) nucleotides in the sequencing of the RNA strand.

Initiation stage of the transcription starts when a molecule of RNA polymerase binds to the DNA template at a region called the promoter region. This promoter region contains a DNA sequence that helps RNA polymerase to bind with the DNA. Each gene has its own promoter region. After binding of RNA polymerase to the DNA, a bubble is formed called transcription bubble that is the sign of initiation of transcription. The second stage of transcription i.e. elongation is defined as the formation of an RNA strand by adding nucleotides in the complementary direction to the sequencing of template strand (in 3' to 5' direction). The newly formed RNA strand is similar to the coding strand of the DNA except the RNA strand have uracil (U) bases in place of thymine (T) in its sequencing. The last stage of transcription i.e. termination is the process that happens only when the RNA polymerase transcribes a specific sequence of DNA called the terminator. Transcription ends with the formation of an RNA transcript called pre messenger RNA (pre-mRNA). Thereafter, the Pre-mRNA is converted into fully mature mRNA post some modifications (RNA splicing etc.) and then this mature mRNA is further used to form new proteins in the process of translation (Figure 9-9).

Translation

The translation is the process of joining different amino acids to form proteins by utilizing the coding sequence of mRNA. It occurs in the cytoplasm of a cell unlike transcription that occurs in the nucleus of a cell. Translation requires two key types of molecules including transfer RNAs (tRNAs) and ribosomes (protein factories) to complete their process. Transfer RNAs are the building blocks of proteins that contain a sequence of three nucleotides called anticodon on the one side and a set of amino acids on the other side. Each codon of the mRNA strand connects with their respective anticodon present on the tRNA and encode for the amino acids to form new proteins. Ribosomes are the molecules where new proteins are built with the help of tRNAs and mRNA codons. They also catalyse the reaction of joining of amino acids together to make a functional protein.

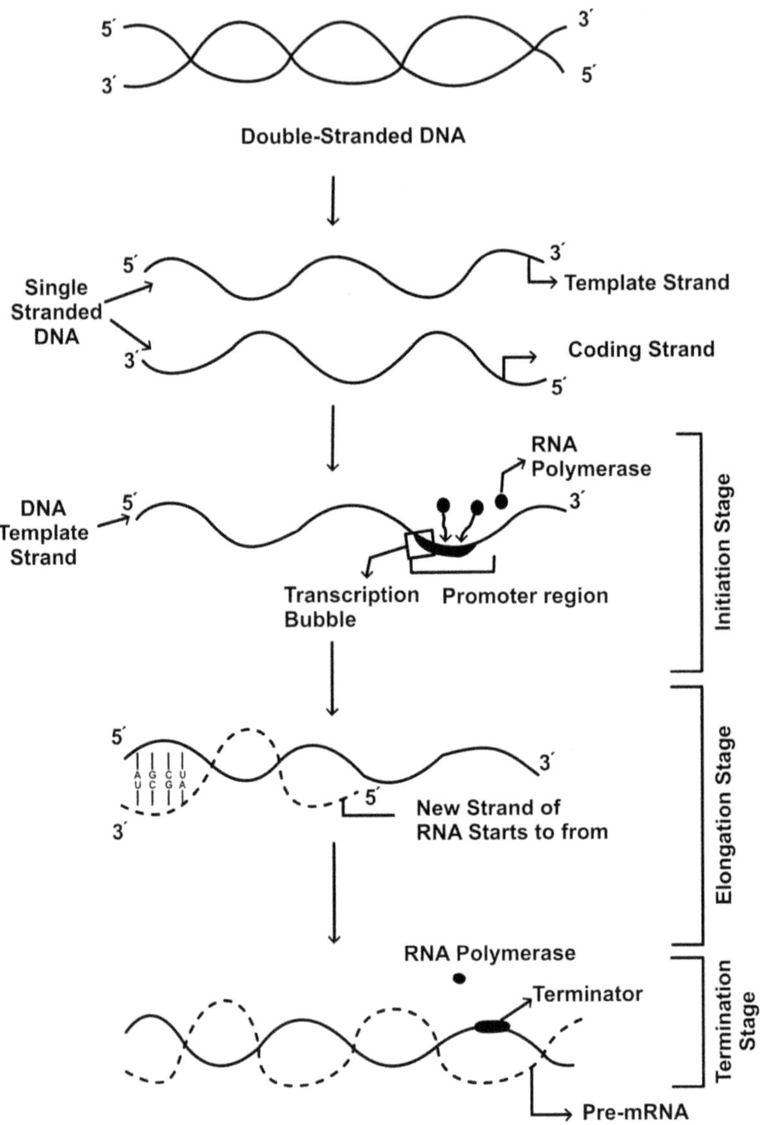

Figure 9-9 Flow chart of the process of transcription

Like transcription, the translation process is also divided into three stages including initiation, elongation and termination. The initiation stage starts when the ribosomes assemble around the mRNA strand, which read the first tRNA anticodon AUG (initiation codon) that carries methionine as an amino acid. After initiation, the chain of amino acids starts increasing in the form of polypeptides and this stage is known as the elongation stage. This stage comprises of many steps such as binding of tRNA to specific mRNA codon, linking of existing amino acid chain onto the amino acids of tRNA, exposing a new mRNA codon for reading an anticodon of tRNA etc. After the elongation of a polypeptide chain, when tRNA encodes for a stop codon (UAA, UAG or UGA), the translation reaction is terminated that leads to the release of a finished polypeptide chain. As a result, the new polypeptide chain is drifted out of the ribosome and get convert into a fully functional protein post translational modification.

Genetic Pattern of Inheritance

Genetic pattern of inheritance is defined as the pattern by which the basic characters or diseases are transmitted from one generation (parents) to the next generation (childs). Each cell of a body contains two copies of each chromosome (in case of autosomes but not in sex chromosomes) and consecutively two copies of each gene. The different forms of a gene present at a specific point (locus) on a chromosome are called alleles. There may be several alleles for a particular gene, and these can be similar or different across different individuals. The individuals with two copies of the same alleles are called homozygous for that allele and individuals with copies of different alleles are called heterozygous for that allele. Moreover, these alleles are responsible for the transmission of characters or diseases across different generations. The basic models of the genetic pattern of inheritance include

Autosomal dominant inheritance

Autosomal recessive inheritance

X-linked dominant inheritance

X-linked recessive inheritance

Mitochondrial inheritance

Autosomal dominant inheritance

The allele of a gene is said to be autosomal dominant when an individual has only one copy of that allele (i.e. heterozygous) and the characters (phenotype) associated with that allele are observed in the next generation. The disorders associated with the transmission of an autosomal dominant allele include0020Huntington's disease, neurofibromatosis, achondroplasia and familial hypercholesterolemia. In autosomal dominant inheritance pattern, there are 50% chances of transmission of disorders to the next generation.

Autosomal recessive inheritance

The allele of a gene is said to be autosomal recessive when an individual has two copies of the same allele (i.e. heterozygous) and the phenotype associated with that allele is observed in the next generation. The disorders associated with the transmission of an autosomal recessive allele include Tay-sachs disease, sickle cell anaemia, cystic fibrosis and phenylketonuria.

X-linked dominant inheritance

It is also called sex-linked inheritance. The pattern of X-linked dominant inheritance is observed when an abnormal allele of a gene present on the X chromosome is dominant over the normal allele of the same gene. The medical conditions associated with X-linked dominant inheritance include vitamin D-resistant rickets and ornithine transcarbamylase deficiency.

X-linked recessive inheritance

It is the more common form of X-linked inheritance. In this model, an abnormal allele of a gene located on the X chromosome is recessive over the normal allele of the same gene. The diseases transmitted by X-linked recessive inheritance include colour blindness, haemophilia A and Duchene muscular dystrophy.

Mitochondrial inheritance

Mitochondria are the cell bodies/organelles that are scattered throughout the cytoplasm of a cell. They contain their own DNA, which is replicated during the process of mitochondrial division. The replicated mitochondria are transmitted from the mother to the newly formed embryo. Therefore, mitochondrial inheritance is passed across the generations through females only. The diseases associated with this type of inheritance include Leber's hereditary optic neuropathy and Kearns-Sayre syndrome.

9.2 Chapter at a Glance

Term	Description
Chromosomes	Thread-like structures of DNA molecules
DNA	Deoxyribose nucleic acid
RNA	Ribose nucleic acid
Histone proteins	Positively charges basic proteins
Centromere	Constriction point present on the structure of chromosome
Isobrachial chromosomes	Chromosomes having two equal sized arms
Heterobrachial chromosomes	Chromosomes having two unequal sized arms
Homologous chromosomes	Chromosomes having similar size, shape and arrangement of genes

Contd...

Term	Description
Autosomes	First 22 pairs of chromosomes other than sex chromosomes
Allosomes/sex chromosomes	23rd pair of chromosomes (XX or XY)
Chromatin	Complex of DNA and histone proteins
Replication of DNA	Copying of DNA
Transcription	Conversion of DNA into mRNA
Translation	Formation of proteins from mRNA
Gene	A unit of inheritance made up of DNA sections
Genome	Total genetic information contained in a single cell
Cistron	A term used to denote a 'gene'
rRNA	Ribosomal RNA
tRNA	Transfer RNA
mRNA	Messenger RNA
Exons	Coding region of a gene
Introns	Non-coding region of a gene
A	Adenine
G	Guanine
C	Cytosine
T	Thymine
U	Uracil
Nucleosome	Structural and functional unit of chromatin
Linker DNA	DNA that links two nucleosomes
Euchromatin	Loosely packed DNA
Heterochromatin	Tightly packed DNA
Alleles	Different forms of a gene present at a specific point on chromosomes

Exercises

Multiple Choice Questions

1. The major component(s) of the chromosomes are
   (a) DNA (b) RNA
   (c) Histone proteins (d) Both a and b
   (e) Both a and c

2. The longer arm of the chromosome structure is called
   (a) S arm   (b) T arm
   (c) Q arm   (d) P arm

3. How many chromosomes are present in humans?
   (a) 23 chromosomes   (b) 46 chromosomes
   (c) 22 pairs of chromosomes (d) None of the above

4. Chromosomes are best visualized in which phase of the cell division
   (a) Interphase   (b) Prophase
   (c) Metaphase   (d) None of the above

5. Different types of non-constitutive genes
   (a) Housekeeping genes   (b) Repressible genes
   (c) Inducible genes   (d) Both b and c

6. The nitrogenous/chemical bases are the same in both the DNA and the RNA except
   (a) Adenine   (b) Cytosine
   (c) Thymine   (d) Guanine

7. A nucleotide contains
   (a) A sugar moiety   (b) Base pairs
   (c) A phosphate group   (d) All of the above

8. The two strands of a nucleotide run in a direction
   (a) Parallel direction   (b) Opposite direction
   (c) None of the above   (d) Straight direction

9. In a nucleosome, how much of the DNA is wrapped over protein octamer
   (a) 2 turn of DNA   (b) 1.6 turns of DNA
   (c) 1.7 turns of DNA   (d) 3 turns of DNA

10. The building blocks of proteins are
    (a) Transfer RNAs   (b) Messenger RNAs
    (c) Ribosomal RNAs   (d) All of the above

Short Answer Questions

1. What are chromosomes? Give their composition.

2. What is centromere? Classify chromosomes depending on the position of centromeres.

3. What are autosomes and allosomes?

4. Describe the functions of chromosomes?

5. What are genes? Describe their functions.

6. What are processed genes?

7. Write the names of different chemical/nitrogenous bases of DNA.

8. What is a nucleotide?

9. Write two differences between euchromatin and heterochromatin.
10. Give two differences between transcription and translation.

Long Answer Questions

1. Differentiate between the chromatin and the chromosomes.
2. Write a short note on constitutive, non-constitutive and split genes.
3. Write a note on DNA.
4. Write a short note on the packaging of DNA.
5. Write a note on transcription and translation.
6. What is the genetic pattern of inheritance? Brief about different methods of inheritance transmission.

Bibliography

Costanzo LS. Physiology. 4th Edition. Lippincott Williams & Wilkins.

Guyton AC, Hall JE. Textbook of Medical Physiology. 11th Edition. Elsevier Saunders. 2006.

Jaggi AS, Bali A, Singh N. Pathophysiology. 1st Edition. Vallabh Prakashan. 2019.

Jain AK. Human Anatomy and Physiology for Pharmacy. 3rd Edition. Arya publications. 2017.

Lodish H, Berk A, Kaiser CA. Molecular Cell Biology. 6th Edition. W. H. Freeman & Co Ltd. 2007.

Tortora GJ, Derrickson B. Principles of Anatomy and Physiology. 15th Edition. John Wiley and Sons, Inc. 2017.

Waugh A, Grant A. Ross and Wilson Anatomy and Physiology in Health and Illness. 12th Edition. Churchill Livingstone. 2014.

Answer Key MCQs

1. (e)	2. (c)	3. (b)	4. (c)	5. (d)
6. (c)	7. (d)	8. (b)	9. (c)	10. (a)

Index

T

U

V

W